CLINICAL HANDBOOK IN

ENDOCRINOLOGY, DIABETES AND METABOLISM

CASTLE CONNOLLY GRADUATE BOARD REVIEW SERIES

FOCUS: Diabetes - 4th Edition 2011

Editors-in-Chief:
David M. Kendall, MD
International Diabetes Center at Park Nicollet
Minneapolis, MN
Chief Scientific and Medical Officer
The American Diabetes Association

Richard M. Bergenstal, MD
Executive Director,
International Diabetes Center at Park Nicollet
Minneapolis, MN
Clinical Professor, Department of Medicine
University of Minnesota

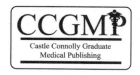

Castle Connolly Graduate Medical Publishing, Ltd.

17 Battery Place, Suite 643 • New York, NY 10004 • Tel: 212.644.9696 • Fax: 646.827.6443 • www.ccgmp.com • e-mail: info@ccgmp.com

Castle Connolly Graduate Medical Publishing, Ltd., publishes review manuals to assist residents and fellows in preparing for board certification exams, and practicing physicians in preparing for board recertification.

NOTICE

Our thanks to Copy Editor Sarah Herndon

ISBN: 978-0-9840551-8-0

Contents

Robert Cuddihy, MD
Adjunct Associate Professor,
University of Minnestoa Medical School
Medical Director,
International Diabetes Center at Park Nicollet
Minneapolis, MN

David M. Kendall, MD
International Diabetes Center at Park Nicollet
Minneapolis, MN
Chief Scientific and Medical Officer
The American Diabetes Association

John B. Buse, MD, PhD
Professor of Medicine
Chief, Division of Endocrinology
University of North Carolina School of Medicine
Chapel Hill, NC

David C. Goff Jr, MD, PhD
Professor,
Epidemology and Prevention, Social Sciences and
Health Policy, and Internal Medicine
Wake Forest University Health Services
Winston-Salem, NC

William C. Cushman, MD
Chief, Preventive Medicine
Memphis Veterans Affairs Medical Center
Professor, Preventive Medicine
University of Tennessee College of Medicine
Memphis, TN

Gissette Soffer, MD
Assistant Professor in Translational Research
Columbia University Medical Center
New York, NY

Henry N. Ginsberg, MD
Irving Professor of Medicine
Columbia University College of Medicine /
Irving Institute for Clinical and
Translational Research
New York, NY

A. Melissa Solum MD
Fellow, University of North Carolina, Chapel Hill
Durham, NC

John B Buse MD, PhD
Professor of Medicine
Chief, Division of Endocrinology
University of North Carolina School of Medicine
Chapel Hill, NC

Thomas O'Connell, MD
Assistant Clinical Professor of Medicine,
Div of Endocrinology
University of North Carolina School of Medicine
Durham, NC

Robert Cuddihy, MD
Adjunct Associate Professor,
University of Minnesota Medical School
Medical Director,
International Diabetes Center at Park Nicollet
Minneapolis, MN

Amy Criego, MD, MS
Pediatric Endocrinologist
International Diabetes Center at Park Nicollet
Minneapolis, MN

Betsy Schwartz, MD, MS
Pediatric Endocrinologist
Park Nicollet Clinic
St. Louis Park, MN

Gregg Simonson, PhD
Adjunct Assistant Professor of Medicine
University of Minnesota Medical School
International Diabetes Center at Park Nicollet
Minneapolis, MN

Pam Tompos, MS, RD, LD
Consultant
International Diabetes Center
Minneapolis, MN

Jan Pearson, BAN, RN, CDE
Senior Consultant
International Diabetes Center
Minneapolis, MN

Judy L. Shih, MD PhD
Clinical Fellow
Beth Israel Deaconess Medical Center/
Joslin Diabetes Center
Boston, MA

Howard Wolpert, MD
Senior Physician
Director, Insulin Pump Program
Joslin Diabetes Center
One Joslin Place
Boston, MA

Introduction

The enthusiastic response to the previous editions of the *Educational Review Manual in Endocrinology, Diabetes and Metabolism* prompted the editors and publisher to develop a separate volume focusing on diabetes mellitus. This current edition provides an update to the very valuable edition edited by Drs. Martin Abrahamson and Norman Ertel.

The reasons for a diabetes focus of the Endocrine Manual are obvious to anyone involved in diabetes care. Diabetes is increasingly common - now affecting nearly 25 million persons in the United States and more than 200 million individuals worldwide. Diabetes affects nearly 10% of the US adult population and it has been estimated that children born in 2000 have an approximately 33% lifetime risk of developing diabetes.

The increased prevalence of diabetes is associated with increasing numbers of individuals with both microvascular and macrovascular complications - resulting in significant diabetes related morbidity and mortality. The health care and indirect costs of type 2 diabetes in the United States in 2007 were estimated at more than $170 billion.[1] While estimates of the worldwide prevalence of diabetes vary, it is anticipated that by 2030, diabetes (predominantly type 2 diabetes) will affect approximately 365 million persons, or more than 5% of the population.[2] In addition, there are increasing numbers of individuals with pre-diabetes (including both impaired glucose tolerance and impaired fasting glucose)[1].

With the emerging diabetes epidemic in mind, additional training on diabetes management is essential. Our understanding of the basic pathophysiology of diabetes and obesity - along with the emergence of a broader array of therapies - necessitates careful attention to diabetes clinical care. The emerging role of the diabetes clinical care specialist and the endocrinologist will focus on a leadership role in both direct care and sharing responsibility with the primary care provider.[3]

In this edition of the Manual, we have expanded the clinical focus - while emphasizing the core components of pathophysiology of both type 1 and type 2 diabetes. Key elements of this edition include:

- Pathophysiology and management of type 1 diabetes in children and adults (Chapters 1 and 13)

- Pathophysiology and management of obesity, pre-diabetes and type 2 diabetes (Chapters 2, 5, 6, 7 and 11)

- Clinical management of diabetes microvascular complications (Chapters 3 and 4)

- A focus on cardiovascular disease - including management of glycemia, dyslipidemia and hypertension (Chapters 8, 9, 10)

- Hospital management of diabetes (Chapter 12)

- Unique features of diabetes in adolescents and children (Chapter 13)

- Pre-diabetes and diabetes prevention (Chapter 11)

- Diabetes care delivery (Chapter 14)

- Diabetes technology (Chapter 15)

Highlights of this edition include a detailed description of type 1 diabetes provided by Gilliam and Hirsch. The authors note that "while type 1 diabetes (T1D) comprises a relatively small fraction of the overall number of diabetes cases (5-10%), it is important that providers…understand the unique pathogenesis and treatment modalities for type 1 diabetes as compared to the much more common type 2 diabetes". They review pathogenesis, classification and principles of management. Schwartz and Criego add to this edition by focusing on the unique features of management in children and adolescents with diabetes.

Contributions from Steven Smith and colleagues focus on the emerging importance of obesity management, while John Buse and colleagues discuss the diagnosis, screening and treatment of pre-diabetes. A series of chapters on pathophysiology and pharmacologic and non-pharmacologic management of type 2 diabetes have been provided by clinicians and investigators at the International Diabetes Center. These chapters focus on the natural history of type 2 diabetes and the central role of insulin resistance and beta cell dysfunction, and discuss the management of type 2 diabetes as it relates our understanding of this natural history.

Carol Wysham, Agbor Ngip and Andrew Boulton provide an excellent summary of microvascular and peripheral neuropathic complications of diabetes, emphasizing the role of glycemic control on prevention of these disabling consequences of diabetes. Data from DCCT, UKPDS and other studies are reviewed, and the practical clinical management of diabetes microvascular complications is emphasized. A series of chapters discuss the management of cardiovascular risk in diabetes, including the role of glycemic control, hypertension management and the treatment of dyslipidemia. Unique to this volume of the Manual are chapters on hospital management, diabetes care delivery models and the use of newer technologies in diabetes care. We trust that all of these contributions will be helpful educationally and will provide support of your clinical practice.

The publication of the Manual was graciously supported by educational funding from Santarus, Inc. We thank them for their continued commitment to medical education and clinical excellence. Each of the contributors is an acknowledged expert and we thank them for their thoughtful presentation of material that was deemed to be most important for the endocrinologist entering practice, the diabetes clinician and anyone preparing for Board examinations.

We especially wish to thank Michael D. Wolf, PhD, Executive Vice President of Castle Connolly Graduate Medical Publishing, whose editorial expertise, perseverance and gentle prodding were critical in bringing this first edition to fruition. We welcome comments and suggestions for changes or additions. They will be carefully considered in the preparation of future editions.

David Kendall

Richard Bergenstal

References

1. http://www.cdc.gov/diabetes/pubs/pdf/ndfs _2007.pdf. American Diabetes Association, Inc., National Diabetes Fact Sheet, 2007.

2. http://www.who.int/diabetes/facts/world _figures/en/. Prevalence of Diabetes Worldwide: Country and Regional Data. World Health Organization.

3. Graber AL, et al. Improving glycemic control in adults with diabetes mellitus: Shared responsibility in primary care practices. South Med. 2002;J95(7):684-690.

Chapter 1: Type 1 Diabetes: Pathogenesis and Treatment

Lisa K. Gilliam, MD
Irl B. Hirsch, MD

Contents

Overview

A solid understanding of the disease process and management of diabetes is necessary for care providers in every medical specialty. While type 1 diabetes (T1D) comprises a relatively small fraction of the overall number of diabetes cases (5%-10%),[1] it is important that providers of adolescent and adult patients understand the unique pathogenesis and treatment modalities for T1D, as compared to the much more common type 2 diabetes (T2D).

1. Classification and Diagnosis of Type 1 Diabetes (T1D)

T1D, formerly called juvenile-onset diabetes and insulin-dependent diabetes mellitus (IDDM), is a disease of insulin deficiency. The lack of insulin is a consequence of the autoimmune destruction of the beta-cells in the pancreas. This type of diabetes is more precisely termed type 1a diabetes, to differentiate it from non-autoimmune etiologies of insulinopenic diabetes (discussed below). However, for the purposes of this review, we will refer to diabetes of autoimmune etiology as T1D, which is standard terminology in the literature and in clinical practice. T2D, in contrast, is a disease of insulin resistance, in the setting of a relative insulin deficiency due to a non-autoimmune beta-cell lesion. Although T1D and T2D are generally considered to be distinct disease processes (a distinction which is currently debated by some diabetologists),[2-4] differentiating them clinically can occasionally be difficult. Patients, particularly children with T1D, generally have abrupt onset of disease, symptomatic presentation with polyuria, polydipsia and weight loss, thin body habitus, high levels of glycosylated hemoglobin at presentation, ketoacidosis, and no or minimal family history (Table 1). On the other hand, patients with T2D tend to have a gradual disease onset, which is often asymptomatic or mild in presentation, with elevated BMI, clinical signs of insulin resistance (ie, acanthosis nigricans) and a significant family history of diabetes.

The limitation of a disease classification which is based on clinical symptoms, rather than on the etiology and pathogenesis of the disease, is that many patients present with mixed features of T1D and T2D, and none of the clinical features described above are specific for a particular diabetes type. For example, with the increasing prevalence of world-wide obesity, a growing number of patients with T1D are overweight at presentation. Likewise, a subset of African American patients with T2D present acutely, with very high glucose levels and ketoacidosis. The etiology of this form of diabetes, termed atypical diabetes, or "Flatbush diabetes",[5] is unknown, but after an initial period of insulin requirement, their beta-cell function recovers and these patients can be treated with oral agents, like other T2D patients. Another clinical feature that classically differentiates patients with T1D and T2D is age at onset. Until recently, T2D was extremely rare in children. However, with the greater occurrence of obesity in the pediatric population, 15% of teenagers with diabetes in the U.S. are now classified as having T2D, with even higher rates in minority populations.[6] Conversely, diabetes that presents in adulthood, particularly later adulthood, is almost always initially diagnosed as T2D. While T2D is certainly far more common in this population, T1D does present in adulthood; in fact, as many patients with T1D are diagnosed at >18 years of age as are diagnosed during childhood.[7] Because T1D and T2D are treated very differently at onset, it is important for care providers to take into account multiple patient characteristics before assigning a diagnosis of T1D vs. T2D. It is therefore not uncommon for patients to be misclassified, although the exact frequency of this is not known.

At the present time, no specific guidelines exist in the U.S. for the classification of T1D vs. T2D, beyond assessment of clinical features and insulin requirement at diagnosis. 1 tool that can assist the clinician in the differentiation between the 2 diabetes types is the measurement of diabetes autoantibodies (DAA), a marker of the autoimmune disease process, in the patient's serum. The specific antibodies that can be measured clinically and challenges with these measures are discussed later in this chapter. In practice, DAAs are often used to classify patients who present with mixed clinical features of T1D and T2D. The application of these measures in population-based research studies of diabetic patients has further muddied the waters in terms of classification of T1D and T2D, by identifying patients with clinically diagnosed T1D who are DAA-negative (termed type 1b, or idiopathic diabetes),[1] as well as patients with clinically diagnosed T2D who are DAA-positive. The pathophysiology of type 1b diabetes is not well understood. These patients, by definition, have absolute insulin deficiency resulting from beta-cell destruction. However, the lack of DAAs and T1D-associated risk HLA markers suggest that this diabetes type is non-autoimmune in etiology. On the other end of the spectrum, the finding of clinically defined T2D patients who are positive for DAAs is far more common and clinically relevant. DAA

positivity is found in approximately 10% of the adult T2D population, with reports of frequency ranging from 5%-30%, depending on the age and ethnicity of the study group.[8] This entity is most commonly termed *latent autoimmune diabetes in adults* (LADA), but has many other names in the literature (Table 2). The nomenclature is clearly confusing and in need of clarification, as other authors only refer to LADA as generally thin adults with T1D with positive DAA who maintain residual insulin secretion for many years. However, for this discussion, we will refer to LADA as the clinically defined T2D patient with DAA-positivity. DAA-positivity is even more common in children with clinically-defined T2D, with a frequency of 32% in the population-based SEARCH study for Diabetes in Youth.[9]

The finding of DAA-positivity in patients with clinically-defined T2D raises 2 important questions. First, are DAA measures necessary to identify these patients, or are there clinical clues that could have helped the practitioner to distinguish these patients from those with classical, non-autoimmune T2D? Second, is it clinically important to make this distinction? In answer to the first question, there do appear to be phenotypic differences between these DAA-positive T2D patients and classical non-autoimmune T2D patients. Comparisons between study groups, as a whole, have shown that LADA patients tend to have a decreased prevalence of metabolic syndrome characteristics, more severely impaired b-cell function, lower BMI, more common presentation with polyuria, polydipsia and weight loss, poorer glycemic control as assessed by HbA1C and a higher frequency of type 1 DM–associated risk human leukocyte antigen (HLA) genotypes.[10-12] These patients also have a shorter duration of insulin independence following their diagnosis, compared with classical T2D patients.[13] Unfortunately, while these differences can be demonstrated on a population basis, they are much less helpful in determining whether an individual has T2D vs. LADA, due to the large degree of overlap in clinical features between the 2 groups.[11,14] Thus, to correctly classify these patients for the majority of the time, DAAs would have to be measured in all clinically diagnosed T2D patients, a proposition which is not economically

Table 1

**Differing Clinical and Biochemical Features of Patients with T1D and T2D
(note that there are *many* exceptions)**

	T1D	T2D
Clinical onset	Acute	Non-acute
Age at onset	Childhood	Adulthood
Clinical features at onset	Polyuria, polydipsia, weight loss	Often asymptomatic
Features noted on clinical examination	Normal or low BMI	Elevated BMI, acanthosis nigricans
Laboratory evaluation	Low or absent fasting C-peptide, diabetes autoantibodies, ketoacidosis, very high HbA1C	Normal or high fasting C-peptide, no diabetes autoantibodies, no ketoacidosis, moderately elevated HbA1C
Family history	Usually no or sparse family history	Often strong family history

Table 2

Various Terminology for DAA-positive Clinically-defined T2D[25]

Adults	Children
• Latent autoimmune diabetes in adults (LADA)	• Latent autoimmune diabetes in the young (LADY)
• Type 1.5 diabetes	• Type 1.5 diabetes
• Slowly progressive type 1 diabetes	• Hybrid diabetes
• Slowly progressive insulin-dependent diabetes mellitus (SPIDDM)	• Double diabetes
	• Atypical diabetes
	• Indeterminate diabetes

feasible. Furthermore, the measurement and interpretation of autoantibody levels in the clinical setting is not always straightforward (see discussion below on the humoral immune response).

Regarding whether it is clinically important to identify LADA patients, several studies have demonstrated a more aggressive disease course for these patients, characterized by a shorter time to failure of oral hypoglycemic therapy[15-20] and progressive β-cell failure leading to insulin deficiency.[21-24] The majority of LADA patients will require insulin within the first few years after diagnosis, and many practitioners believe that insulin is the appropriate therapy for these patients from the outset. However, it has become clear that, compared to classical type 1A diabetes, those with LADA have extremely variable progression to complete insulin deficiency. Consequently, to predict clinical course and provide appropriate treatment, it is important to identify patients with apparent type 2 DM who fall into this category. Given the challenges of identifying these patients based on clinical features alone, but also given the unrealistic option of measuring DAAs in every patient with clinically diagnosed T2D, there is no perfect solution. The practitioner should just be aware of this population, whose pathophysiology and treatment is much more akin to that for T1D than T2D, and should have a low threshold for performing DAA measures based on clinical suspicion.

The average annual incidence rates of T1D vary from 0.1 per 100,000 children in parts of Asia and South America to 36.5 per 100,000 children in Finland, the nation with the highest incidence rates in the world.[26] These numbers are derived from a worldwide study reported nearly a decade ago; more recent estimates of incidence rates in Finland are now even higher, at 42.9 per 100,000.[27] Like T2D, an increase in the annual incidence of T1D has been observed over the past few decades. Studies in European and Scandinavian countries have suggested a 4%-6% annual increase in incidence rates,[26,28,29] and similar data are being collected in other countries, including the U.S.[6] The incidence rates vary by geographic region (with higher incidence in regions of more northern latitude, Figure 1), by age at diagnosis,[32] by gender (male predominance in regions with high incidence, with a 1.8:1 male:female ratio),[33,34] by increasing parental age at delivery[35-38] and by birth order (15% risk reduction per child born).[37-39] In addition, T1D is oftentimes a "disease of the wealthy," with higher rates in affluent countries compared with third world countries.[40] Rates are also higher in Caucasian populations, although it should be noted that a majority of the available data on incidence rates has been collected in Caucasian populations, with limited information for other racial and ethnic groups. Current studies, including the US-based SEARCH Study for Diabetes in Youth, are seeking to better define T1D incidence rates in minorities. The geographic and socioeconomic variations have prompted hypotheses about specific environmental factors that may trigger the onset of disease in genetically susceptible individuals, as described later in this chapter.

Association of T1D with Other Autoimmune Diseases

Several autoimmune diseases occur at higher frequency in patients with T1D compared with individuals from the general population. These include: thyroid autoimmunity (Hashimoto's thyroiditis and Graves' disease), adrenal autoimmunity (Addison's disease) and celiac disease. Less common diseases, including vitiligo, chronic atrophic body gastritis, pernicious anemia, chronic hypoparathyroidism, premature ovarian failure, alopecia, autoimmune hepatitis and Stiff-person syndrome may be seen in T1D patients.[41] The

Figure 1

Geographic variation in T1D incidence (1990-1994)

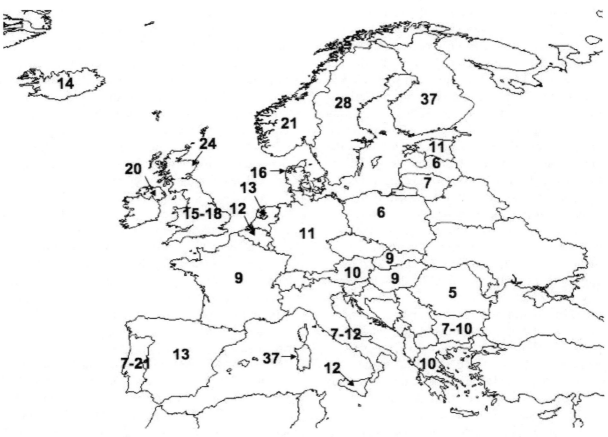

The age-adjusted incidence of T1D (per 100,000 per year) from 1990 to 1994 was determined in children 14 years of age from 100 centers in 50 countries as a part of the Diabetes Mondiale (DiaMond) Project Group.[26] Incidence data from Europe is depicted on this map, with data from some countries having multiple clinic sites shown as ranges. Note the general trend towards an increase in incidence with increasing latitude, with some exceptions (eg: Finland and Iceland, Sardinia and continental Italy). Incidence rates in Europe are high compared with rates in some other parts of the world (eg: Pakistan 0.7, Venezuela 0.1).

grouping of Addison's disease in addition to autoimmune thyroid disease and/or T1D carries a clinical designation, autoimmune polyendocrine syndrome type 2 (APS-2), with the triad historically termed Carpenter's syndrome.[42] APS-2 differs from APS-1 (described below), in that APS-1 is a monogenic disorder of which T1D may be a component, whereas APS-2 is a clustering of diseases of different etiologies, which have shared genetic factors. Frequency in patients with T1D of some of the more common T1D-associated autoimmune disorders and screening recommendations for adults with T1D, are described later in this chapter (Table 17).

The understanding that T1D is an autoimmune disease dates back to observations in the early 20th century, that in diabetic patients who died shortly after clinical onset, their pancreatic islets were altered by fibrosis, hyalinosis, atrophy and infiltration of inflammatory cells.[43] This inflammatory lesion was termed insulitis (Figure 2),[44] and it was later shown that the insulin-producing beta-cells in the islets of Langerhans are specifically targeted for destruction, with preservation of the other cell types in the islet.[45, 46] 2 animal models established in the 1970s have been used to study the pathogenesis of spontaneously-occurring T1D: the nonobese diabetic (NOD) mouse and the BioBreeding (BB) rat. These animal models made it possible to directly observe the selective destruction of the beta-cells in the islets, and to study the process by which that occurs. We have learned a tremendous amount about the pathogenesis of human T1D by studying these animal models, with the caveat that not everything learned in these models is translatable to human disease.

In humans, T1D usually develops gradually over a long prodromal period, with DAAs appearing in the sera of patients up to a decade prior to the clinical onset of disease.[47,48] The stages of development of T1D (Figure 3) are hypothesized to take place as follows: in susceptible individuals with genetic risk, an inciting (likely environmental) event triggers the initial destruction of pancreatic b-cells, exposing b-cell antigens to the immune system. As a consequence, the autoimmune process is initiated, and silent, progressive b-cell loss begins to occur. Clinical manifestations of diabetes do not appear until an individual has lost >90% of his or her b-cell function,[49] therefore, the silent b-cell loss can continue for a long period of time. Research studies in which pre-diabetic individuals have been followed prior to the development of their disease have shown that the first preclinical defect observed is impaired glucose tolerance.[50] This is followed by the development of impaired fasting glucose and, eventually, frank diabetes. At the time of diagnosis, most patients have some residual insulin secretion, manifested by detectable fasting C-peptide. Over the next few years, continued destruction of the b-cells results in the decline and eventual disappearance of C-peptide, and the end result is unstable diabetes,

Figure 2

Insulitis

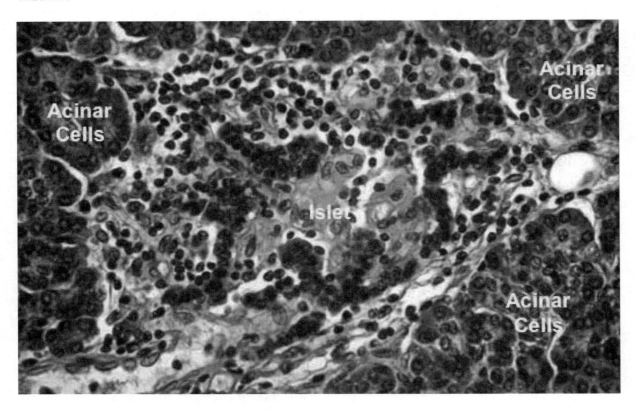

Inflammatory infiltrate of mononuclear cells in the islet of a patient with recent-onset T1D. The photomicrograph comes from the collection of W. Gepts and was provided with permission by Danny Pipeleers.

with the potential for large variability in blood glucose values.

Immunological Aspects of T1D

The autoimmune process of T1D involves both the cellular and humoral branches of the immune system, with the generation of islet-specific T-cell reactivity, as well as autoantibodies directed against islet cell antigens. The cellular immune response is thought to play the primary role in disease pathogenesis, with contributions from both CD4+ and CD8+ cells in the process of destroying the pancreatic beta-cells; hence, T1D is termed a "T-cell dependent" organ-specific autoimmune disease. On the other hand, the humoral response (generation of autoantibodies by B cells) was traditionally thought to be a byproduct of the beta-cell destruction, with anti-islet autoantibodies developing during the prodromal stage of the disease process, in response to and as a marker of, the ongoing T-cell destructive process. Recent studies have suggested that B cells and anti-islet autoantibodies may also play a role in disease pathogenesis.[51,52]

Many theories exist to explain the etiology of the pathogenic immunological response in T1D, as outlined in Table 3. In addition, some important lessons about the breakdown of immunological tolerance have been learned from the identification of genes causing 2 monogenic T1D-associated disorders, APS-1 (Autoimmune Polyendocrine Syndrome type 1) and IPEX (immune dysregulation, polyendocrinopathy, enteropathy, X-linked), as outlined in Table 4. For example, the molecular defect in APS-1 involves mutation of a gene that

Figure 3

The stages of development of T1D

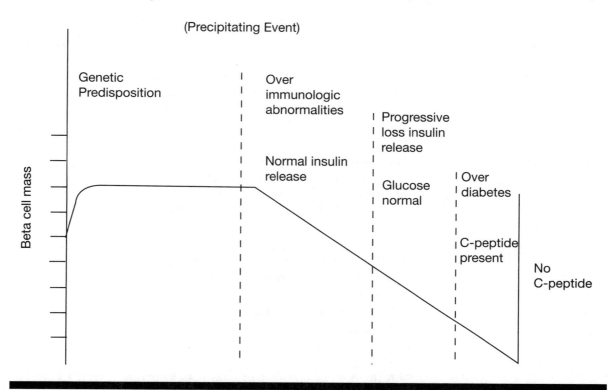

(Provided and used with permission from George Eisenbarth)

controls the process whereby autoreactive T-cells are deleted within the thymus, via transcriptional regulation of tissue-restricted antigens. This results in widespread, multi-organ autoimmunity. Similarly, polymorphisms in the insulin gene promoter have been associated with an increased risk for developing T1D (see Section 4). The monogenic human APS-1 example, which has been further illuminated by studies in knock-out animals, provides an attractive mechanism by which the insulin VNTR polymorphisms may contribute to T1D risk (see Figure 4).[53,54]

Cellular immune response
The cellular immune response plays a major role in the pathogenesis of T1D. Studies in the 1970s using tests for leukocyte migration inhibition and blast formation indicated that T1D patients are sensitized to pancreatic antigens.[72-75] In addition, immunosuppressive drugs with anti-T-cell activity, such as cyclosporine[76] or humanized monoclonal antibodies against CD3,[77] have been shown to

delay the development of disease. Unfortunately, reproducible tests of blood T-cell reactivity to specific antigens have been difficult to establish, and those that are in use are limited to the research setting.

Figure 5 depicts the hypothesized mechanism by which an aberrant immune response leads to the development of T1D. Pancreatic autoantigens (green triangles) are taken up by local APCs and presented as small fragments on the surface of these cells in the context of HLA class II molecules. CD4+ T-helper (Th) cells with the appropriate self-reactive specificity recognize this complex, become activated, and stimulate both B lymphocytes and cytotoxic T lymphocytes (CTLs). Activated B-cells begin to generate diabetes autoantibodies and activated CTLs, which recognize endogenous pancreatic autoantigens in the context of HLA class I molecules and target the beta cells for destruction. Natural killer (NK) cells also play a role, via recognition of HLA class I by

Table 3

Mechanisms for the Pathogenic Immunological Response in T1D

Mechanism	Explanation	Reference
Molecular mimicry	Common epitopes shared between islet antigens and foreign (eg, viral) antigens lead to loss of T-cell tolerance to these epitopes when the immune system is exposed to that virus	55, 56
Bystander damage	Local viral infections in the pancreas lead to inflammation, tissue damage and the release of sequestered islet antigen, resulting in the re-stimulation of resting autoreactive T-cells	57
Pathogenic cytokine milieu	Evidence from animal studies: • Animal studies in which T1D is accelerated by Th1 cytokines and prevented with Th2 cytokines in animal models • Disease transfer in animal models is mediated by Th1 cells Evidence in humans: • A Th1 polarization of autoreactive T-cell response has been observed in patients with T1D	58-62
Aberrant beta-cell expression of co-stimulatory molecules, adhesion molecules and MHC	• Biopsy specimens from new-onset T1D patients demonstrated hyperexpression of HLA class I and II, ICAM-1 and LFA-3	63, 64

Abbreviations: T helper 1 (Th1), T helper 2 (Th2), Human leukocyte antigen (HLA), intercellular adhesion molecule 1 (ICAM-1), lymphocyte function-associated antigen 3 (LFA-3)

killer immunoglobulin-like receptors (KIR) on these cells.

This pathogenic autoimmune response does not occur in healthy individuals. The reason for the aberrant immune response may be due to failure to induce central tolerance to these autoantigens (ie, lack of deletion of self-reactive T-cells in the thymus; see previous discussion of APS-1 and the T1D correlate insVNTR), failure to achieve peripheral tolerance or both. A subset of T-cells, CD4+ and CD25+ regulatory T-cells (Treg), play an important role in the induction of peripheral tolerance by suppressing autoreactive Th function.[78] The importance of Tregs in maintaining immune tolerance has become apparent in recent years. For example, their absence in patients with IPEX (see Table 4) results in severe, multi-organ autoimmune disease. Studies in animals have shown that transfer of Tregs into diabetes-susceptible animals can prevent and even reverse disease.[79] And finally, it has been hypothesized that the mechanism by which recent prevention studies in humans have achieved success, including the anti-CD3 and GAD-ALUM trials, is by

Table 4

Monogenic T1D-associated Diseases

Disorder	Clinical presentation	Genetic defect	Normal function of mutated gene
APS-1 (Autoimmune polyendocrine syndrome type 1)	• Tissue-specific multi-organ autoimmunity resulting in a variety of clinical diseases, including T1D in 20% of cases[65] • Most commonly characterized by the following triad: autoimmune hypoparathyroidism, autoimmune adrenal disease and mucocutaneous candidiasis[66]	AIRE (autoimmune regulator gene)[66, 67]	• Controls the process whereby autoreactive T-cells are deleted within the thymus, via transcriptional regulation of tissue-restricted antigens[53] • Mutations have been linked to defects in both **central** and **peripheral** tolerance
IPEX (immune dysregulation, polyendocrinopathy, enteropathy, X-linked)	• Autoimmune endocrinopathies, most commonly T1D mellitus and autoimmune thyroid disease[68] • Enteropathy that manifests as chronic, watery diarrhea • Dermatitis, most commonly eczematous	FoxP3[69,70]	• Encodes a protein that is required for the development and suppressive function of CD4+ and CD25+ regulatory T-cells, which suppress effector T-cell responses, including those directed at self antigens[71] • Mutations thus lead to a defect in **peripheral** tolerance

Figure 4

Mechanism by which AIRE and insVNTR may contribute to immunological tolerance

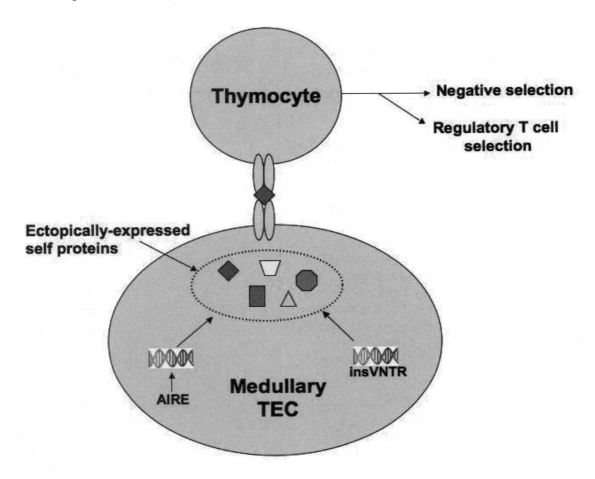

AIRE controls the expression of certain organ-specific genes in the medullary thymic epithelial cells (TEC). These ectopically expressed organ-specific proteins are presented to developing T-cells in the context of MHC, resulting in negative selection of these self-reactive T cells. It has also been hypothesized that some thymocytes which recognize the MHC/self-antigen complex may become regulatory T-cells. The same mechanism of tolerance has been suggested for insulin, in which the insulin protein is ectopically expressed in the thymus and presented to developing thymocytes to induce negative selection. The insVNTR class I allele may confer disease susceptibility due to the fact that it is a weaker promoter, resulting in reduced expression of the insulin protein in the thymus and thus decreased induction of central tolerance (Adapted from Su MA. *Current Opin Immunol.* 2004;16:746)[223]

Reprinted from Su MA, Anderson MS. Aire: an update. Current Opinion in Immunology. *2004; 16(6):746-752., with special permission from Elsevier.*

Table 5

Characteristics and Clinical Utility of DAAs

Autoantibody	Characteristics/Clinical utility
ICA (islet cell antibody)	• Found in 80% of T1D patients at diagnosis • Disappear after diagnosis, not useful to measure in patients with long-standing disease • Not currently used in clinical practice
IAA (insulin autoantibody)	• Found in 50%-90% of T1D patients at diagnosis • Prevalence is inversely correlated with age at diagnosis, so IAA are more useful to measure in children <12 years of age at onset • Commonly the first DAA to develop • Can only be assessed at or before diagnosis, prior to insulin treatment which induces insulin antibodies that cannot be easily discriminated from insulin autoantibodies
GAD65Ab (glutamic acid decarboxylase autoantibody	• Found in 70% of T1D patients at diagnosis • Persist in the sera of many patients with T1D for years following diagnosis, despite the progressive decline in β-cell function → thus, a good retrospective marker of autoimmunity • More prevalent in women, in patients with other types of autoimmunity and in LADA patients • High titers predict rapid β-cell failure, whereas low titers predict a slowly progressive β-cell insufficiency
IA-2Ab (islet antigen 2 autoantibody)	• Found in 32%-75% of T1D patients at diagnosis • Prevalence is higher in males and inversely correlated with age at diagnosis
ZnT8Ab (Zinc transporter 8 autoantibody)	• Found in 60%-80% of T1D patients at diagnosis • Found in 25% of T1D patients who are negative for GAD65Ab, IA-2Ab, IAA and ICA • Adding this measure to GAD65Ab, IA-2Ab and IAA increases detection rate for T1D to 98% at disease onset • Newly described, not currently used in clinical practice

Figure 5

Mechanism by which an aberrant immune response may lead to the development of T1D[78]

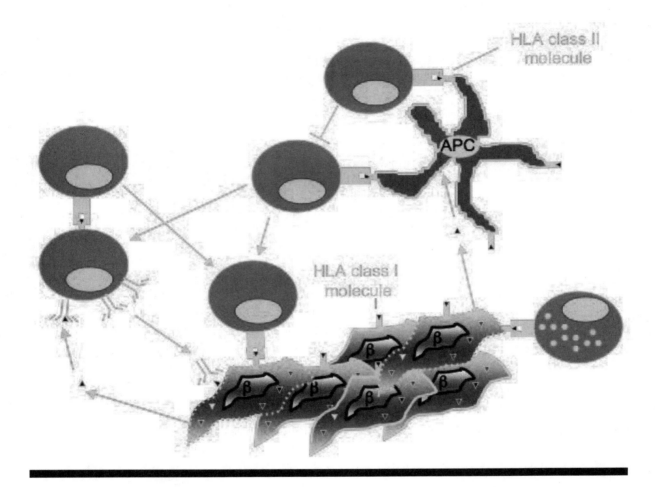

enhancing the immunoregulatory effects of endogenous Tregs.[80] It is possible that the future of T1D prevention will lie in the use of *in vitro*, expanded, antigen-specific Tregs to harness the unrestrained anti-islet immune response.[80]

Another important mechanism of immunotolerance is based on the balance between the "type 1" and "type 2" adaptive cellular immune response in an individual. Type 1 responses, directed by T helper type 1 (Th1) cells, normally function to protect against infections via intracellular pathogens, by activating CTLs and macrophages. Type 2 responses, directed by Th2 cells, normally function to protect against infections via parasites, by activating B cells. Each response is character-

ized by particular cytokine profile, with the Th1-mediated immune response identified by the cytokines interferon gamma (IFN-g), interleukin 2 (IL-2), interleukin 12 (IL-12) and tumor necrosis factor alpha (TNF-a). The Th2 response is identified by the cytokines interleukin 4 (IL-4), interleukin 5 (IL-5), interleukin 10 (IL-10) and transforming growth factor beta (TGF-b). The development of T1D has been ascribed to a shift in the Th1/Th2 balance towards a Th1 response (see Table 3 and Figure 6).

Humoral immune response/Diabetes autoantibodies (DAAs)

The idea that the humoral branch of the immune system plays a role in T1D pathogenesis, rather

Figure 6

A shift in the Th1/Th2 balance towards a Th1 response is a permissive factor for the development of T1D

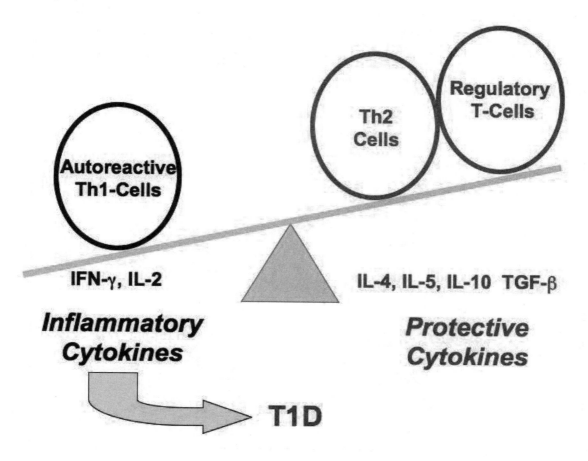

Maintaining tolerance requires that autoreactive Th1 cells be held in check by Th2 and regulatory CD4+/CD25+ T cells. When the balance is tipped in the direction of the autoreactive Th1 cells, either by forces that enhance the inflammatory response or those that diminish the protective, regulatory response, the consequence may be the development of an autoimmune disease, such as T1D.

than simply serving as a useful marker of the autoimmune process, is a recent concept. Studies in the NOD mouse model of disease have shown that B cells act as important antigen-presenting cells (APCs) in the process of stimulating the pathogenic CD4+ T-cells.[52] Furthermore, autoantibodies themselves might be responsible for influencing the autoimmune process. A potential important role played by autoantibodies is their effect on autoantigen processing and presentation. Antigen-specific Fc receptors on APCs increase the efficiency of antigen capture, and thus lower the threshold for a T-cell response.[81] It has been suggested that DAA-mediated antigen internalization may shift transport and processing events in the APCs. This could result in the presentation of different T-cell epitopes and potentially unmask "cryptic" self-determinants, thus altering the focus of the T-cell response and resulting in the breakdown of immunological tolerance (Figure 7).[51]

Figure 7

Autoantibody-mediated effects on antigen presentation

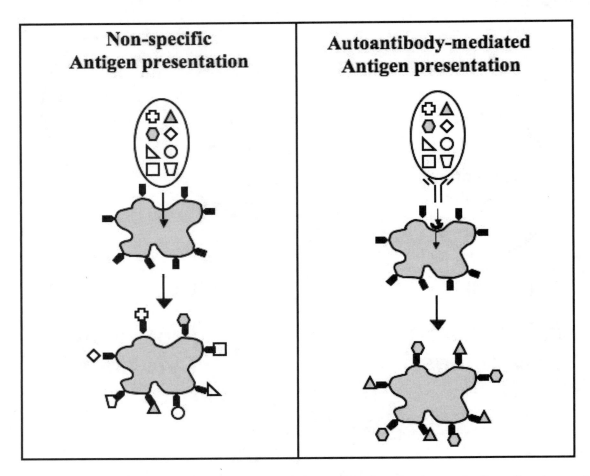

A.) In the classical pathway for antigen presentation (left panel), antigen is taken up by the antigen presenting cell (APC) via a non-specific mechanism, either endocytosis or pinocytosis. Once in the cell, the antigen is processed in specialized lysosomes and certain epitopes bound to class II MHC molecules are presented on the surface of the APC to T-helper cells.

B.) In the presence of an antibody specific to the antigen of interest (right panel), antigen is taken up by the APC via a more efficient and specific Fc-receptor mechanism, which targets the antibody/antigen complex for processing through a different set of intracellular compartments and, consequently, a different set of epitopes are expressed in the context of MHC on the surface of the APC.

DAAs are measured in humans for 2 primary reasons: to classify diabetes type in cases which are not clear based on clinical grounds alone, and for risk assessment, to predict the future development of T1D. The use of DAAs to establish a diagnosis of T1D (or similar disease processes, like LADA) is imperfect, but it remains the best tool we currently have for this purpose. Many clinicians lack an understanding of which autoantibodies to measure for which clinical scenario, how to interpret results (particularly in borderline cases) and how to evaluate the validity of results from a particular clinical laboratory. Regarding risk assessment, this is currently practiced only in research settings. Prospective studies performed in pre-diabetic individuals have shown that diabetes autoantibodies begin to appear between 9 months and 3 years of age, with insulin autoantibodies (IAA) often being the first to appear, followed by glutamic acid decarboxylase 65 autoantibodies (GAD65Ab) and islet antigen 2 autoantibodies (IA-2Ab), formerly called ICA-512.[82,83] Patients may be positive for GAD65Ab, IA-2Ab or insulin antibodies for many years without developing T1D. However, the presence of 2 or more of these autoantibodies strongly predicts T1D, with 3 antibodies predicting the development of T1D within 5 years in nearly 100% of patients (Figure 8).[84]

Islet cell antibodies (ICA) were the first disease-specific autoantibodies to be described in patients with T1D.[85] These DAAs are important to discuss for historical reasons, but for practical purposes they are not currently used in clinical practice. ICA are measured immunohistochemically, by incubating patients' serum with post-mortem

Figure 8

Effect of multiple autoantibodies (GAD65, IA-2, or insulin) on the risk of developing type 1 diabetes[88]

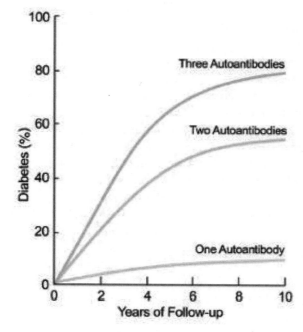

Reprinted from Notkins AL, Lernmark Å. Autoimmune type 1 diabetes: resolved and unresolved issues. J Clin Invest. 2001; 108(9):1247-1252., with permission.

human blood group O pancreas, followed by a fluorescently-labeled anti-human immunoglobulin secondary antibody.[85] On average, ICA are found in 80% of newly diagnosed T1D patients, and they gradually disappear after diagnosis.[86] ICA have been used in many of the important T1D studies (eg, as inclusion criteria in the Diabetes Prevention Trial for Type 1 Diabetes [DPT-1]). As a result, much of the information we currently have, defining the ability of DAAs to predict the development of disease, includes the measurement of ICA. However, the ICA assay has proven difficult to standardize,[87] so clinically, this method has largely been replaced by assays measuring specific autoantigens.

The 3 principal autoantigens measured in T1D patients include insulin, glutamic acid decarboxylase (GAD65) and islet antigen 2 (IA-2). 80%-90% of subjects newly diagnosed with T1D have antibodies to 1 or more of these 3 antigens.[88] The absence of any of these 3 autoantibodies does not preclude T1D, as other antigenic targets (either discovered or undiscovered) may predominate in a particular patient. The characteristics and the clinical utility of each of these autoantibodies differ, depending on the specific clinical scenario (Table 5). In addition, it is important to keep in mind that assays run by clinical laboratories can vary in their sensitivity and specificity, depending on the method employed. A harmonization effort, funded by the Centers for Disease Control, called the Diabetes Antibody Standardization Program (DASP), has been evaluating the relative performance of assays from reference laboratories around the world over the past several years. The most recent report found a median sensitivity for the GAD65Ab assay of 88% and specificity of 98% for all the participating labs, and a median sensitivity for the IA-2Ab assay of 74% and specificity of 98%.[89] The workshop concluded that there was good concordance among labs in categorization of samples, in spite of the use of different assay formats, including some commercial assay kits. The important lesson for practitioners is that GAD65Ab and IA-2Ab tests can be performed by commercial labs, but that it is important to evaluate the performance of a lab's assay in the DASP workshop. The IAA assay has proven much more difficult to perform, with wide variation in the sensitivity of IAA assays between laboratories participating in the DASP workshop. It appears that measuring IAA affinity significantly improves the sensitivity, specificity and concordance of the assays.[90] While these findings are promising for the future use of this test in clinical practice, the measurement of IAA is not currently a viable option outside the research setting.

While autoantibodies directed against these 3 autoantigens are found in the vast majority of newly diagnosed T1D patients, 10%-20% of patients do not have measurable antibody responses again GAD65, IA-2 or insulin. Another major autoantigen was recently identified, the cation efflux transporter ZnT8 (Slc30A8), with autoantibodies against this molecule seen in 60%-80% of recent-onset T1D patients.[91] Of importance, ZnT8 antibodies were found in 25% of T1D subjects who were negative for all other measured antibodies (ie, GAD65Ab, IA-2Ab, IAA and ICA). Combining the measurement of ZnT8 autoantibodies with the other 3 biochemical autoantibodies increased detection rates for T1D to 98% at disease onset.[91] The population of individuals with diabetes identified by ZnT8 autoantibodies alone may therefore explain some cases of type 1b diabetes, the etiology of which has been previously unexplained. While the measurement of ZnT8 autoantibodies is not currently available outside the research setting, it seems likely that these autoantibodies will be used for clinical screening and classification purposes in the future.

T1D is a complex genetic disease, meaning that it results from the effects of multiple genes in combination with lifestyle and environmental factors. Twin studies suggest that genes and environment each explain approximately 50% of the causality of T1D, since for identical twins who are discordant for disease, the non-diabetic twin has a 50%-65% likelihood of developing T1D over his or her lifetime.[92,93] While a family history of diabetes is far less common in T1D compared with T2D, the overall lifetime risk for first-degree relatives has been estimated at about 8% for siblings and 5% for children of parents with type 1 diabetes.[94] Interestingly, the offspring of affected fathers have an increased risk for developing T1D (6%-8%) compared with the offspring of affected mothers (2%-4%).[39,95,96] The reason for this is not understood.

The most important genetic contributor to the development of T1D, termed IDDM1, is based in the class II region of the human leukocyte antigen (HLA) system located on chromosome 6. The class II HLA complex comprises a group of genes that encode cell-surface antigen-presenting proteins which, in combination with fragments of foreign antigens, stimulate T-helper cells to proliferate and modulate immune responses (Figure 9). Studies mapping genetic susceptibility loci have confirmed that the HLA locus accounts for 40% of the genetic risk seen in families.[97] The identification of particular alleles that confer risk has proven difficult, because of the strong linkage disequilibrium in this region of the genome, meaning that HLA haplotypes tend to be inherited in complete sets, making it very difficult to establish which of the alleles in that set is the actual diabetogenic factor. The highest genetic risk is conferred by the DQB1*0302-A1*0301/DQB1*0201-A1*0501 genotype.[98,99] More than 40% of children with T1D have this genotype, and 95% of patients diagnosed as children or young adults carry at least 1 of these risk alleles. These genotype and allele frequencies compare with 3% and 45% of the background population, respectively.[88] While the risk for T1D is highest when an individual inherits the complete genotype, each allele also confers individual risk. Other alleles have been shown to have a negative association with risk for diabetes (a protective effect), most notably HLA

DQB1*0602-A1*0102 (DQ6). This allele is present in 15% of the general population, but only 3% of adult-onset T1D patients. A summary of the genotypes associated with risk and protection is shown in Table 6, and a comparison of genotype frequencies in patients with T1D vs. DAA-negative controls is shown in Figure 10.

The mechanism by which HLA haplotypes exert their risk for T1D is under investigation. The underlying defect in T1D is thought to be a disorder in antigen presentation which generates self-reactive T-helper cells specific for islet cell antigens. The "risk" HLA molecules could theoretically be involved in 1 of 2 ways: either they are ineffective at presenting relevant peptides to immature T cells in the thymus, failing to induce tolerance to these antigens, or they are better able than "non-risk" alleles to present relevant peptides to these self-reactive T cells in the periphery.

Table 6

HLA Genotypes Positively or Negatively Associated with T1D Risk

Genotype		Risk
Allele #1	Allele #2	
DR 4/DQB1 *0302	DR3/DQB1 *0201	High
DR 4/DQB1 *0302	DR 4/DQB1 *0302	Moderate
DR3/DQB1 *0201	DR3/DQB1 *0201	Moderate
DR 4/DQB1 *0302	X	Moderate
X	X	Neutral
DR 2/DQ *0602	X	Protective

Figure 9

Structure of human and mouse MHC complexes

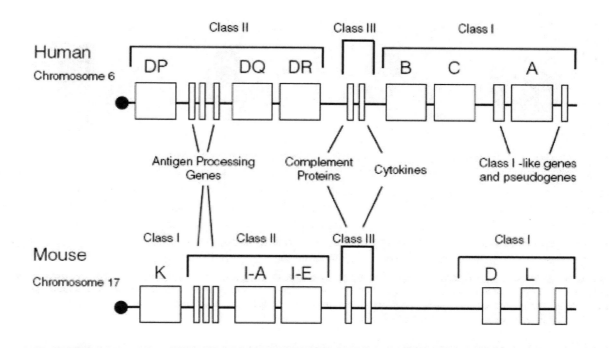

(Provided and used with permission from George Eisenbarth)

The non-HLA genetic factors involved in T1D include many types of inherited defects in immunomodulation. No single non-HLA locus contributes more than 10% towards disease risk. Much of our understanding of the genetics of this disease derives from the recent efforts of the T1D Genetics Consortium, an international, multicenter program organized to identify novel T1D genes. Other important lessons have been learned by studying the shared genetic susceptibility factors for T1D and other diseases that occur at greater frequency in these patients, such as autoimmune thyroiditis.100 The defined and putative T1D non-HLA loci are shown in Table 7.

Figure 10

Frequency of T1D-associated HLA genotypes in T1D patients compared with non-diabetic patients

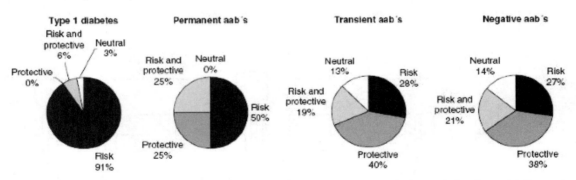

Subjects in the All Babies In Southeast Sweden (ABIS) study, a prospective population-based follow-up study, were divided into 4 categories: those who developed diabetes during the follow-up period, those who developed permanent autoantibodies, those who developed transient autoantibodies and those who remained autoantibody-negative. The figure depicts the percentage of individuals with the risk, protective, combination of risk + protective and neutral HLA genotypes in each of these 4 categories. The frequency of high-risk genotypes in the group of children who developed T1D was significantly higher, and the frequency of protective genotypes significantly lower, compared with the non-diabetic cohorts.[224]

Gullstrand C, Wahlberg J, Ilonen J, Vaarala O, Ludvigsson J. Progression to type 1 diabetes and autoantibody positivity in relation to HLA-risk genotypes in children participating in the ABIS study. Pediatric Diabetes. 2008; 9(3pt1):182-190. Reprinted with permission of Blackwell Publishing, Ltd.

Table 7

Non-HLA Genetic Susceptibility Genes for T1D

Gene/marker	Locus (Chromosome)	Description	References

insVNTR (insulin variable number of tandem repeats)	IDDM2 (11p15.5)	• Polymorphism in the insulin gene promoter
		
		• Estimated to contribute ~10% towards disease risk
		
		• Class I – III (depending on number of repeats)
		
		  * Increased risk – homozygosity for Class I
		
		  * Protection – homozygosity for Class III
		
		• Size of VNTR influences the expression of insulin in the thymus, increased expression with increased number of repeats
			101

CTLA-4	IDDM12 (2q33)	• CTLA4 protein is expressed on T helper cells and limits the proliferative response of activated T cells. • This susceptibility factor is shared by other autoimmune diseases, such as autoimmune thyroid disease and vitiligo • Significant ethnic heterogeneity, with stronger effects in Italian, Spanish and French, as well as Mexican American and Korean populations; almost no effect in Danish, British, Sardinian and Chinese populations	100, 102
LYP/PTPN22	(1p13)	• LYP (lymphoid-specific phosphatase) is encoded by PTPN22 and serves as a suppressor of T-cell activation • LYP variant associated with T1D does not bind the negative regulatory kinase Csk, resulting in hyper-reactive T cells • Also associated with Graves' disease, rheumatoid arthritis and systemic lupus erythematosus	103, 104

5. Environmental Factors in T1D

Teasing out the genetic vs. environmental contributions to complex genetic diseases can be very difficult. As noted above, twin concordance studies have suggested a major role for environmental contributors to the development of T1D. In addition, many T1D experts have argued that changes in environmental factors must be the primary basis for the recent increase in T1D incidence, since population genetics do not change on such a short time scale.[105] In 1 UK study, HLA genotypes in a modern cohort of T1D patients was compared with those of a cohort diagnosed >50 years ago. These investigators found a decline in the proportion of high-risk HLA genotypes in the modern cohort, with a relatively greater proportion of "moderate risk" genotypes.[106] These findings have been replicated in other populations[107,108] and suggest that the rising incidence of T1D in children is a consequence of exposure of a genetically susceptible subgroup of the population to an increasingly diabetogenic environment.

Environmental factors that have been hypothesized to play a role in the development of T1D are listed in Table 8. One risk determinant that has received a great deal of attention is early infant diet (cow's milk vs. breast milk). Several epidemiological and *in vitro studies indicated that intact cow's milk, if given* before 3 months of age, may induce an immune response towards beta-cells (Table 8).[109] However, trials in the U.S. and Germany did not support these findings,[110,111] and this point remains controversial. A multicenter trial attempting to answer this question is currently underway (see Section 7). Another environmental factor that may have an effect on T1D incidence is body weight, or factors associated with obesity. If obesity is associated with the development of T1D, then in light of the current obesity epidemic, there will likely be significant changes in the epidemiology of the disease. Other putative environmental factors include: early exposure to gluten, environmental toxins, lack of exposure to vitamin D, sanitation, season and psychological stress.

The concept that viral infections might play a role in triggering T1D is based on numerous case-control studies in which infectious outbreaks are temporally associated with a higher incidence of diabetes as well as studies showing seasonality of

T1D onset. Furthermore, congenital infections with rubella and enterovirus have been strongly implicated in the subsequent development of diabetes by infants exposed in utero. Candidate viruses involved in the pathogenesis of T1D are listed in Table 9.

More prospective studies are needed to better define environmental triggers for T1D, as these have been very difficult to characterize. The NIH-funded TEDDY study (The Environmental Determinants of Diabetes in the Young) is an international effort currently underway to identify these determinants, including the study of gestational infection or other gestational events, as well as the study of childhood infections or other environmental factors after birth.

Table 8

Environmental Factors That Play a Role in the Development of T1D

Environmental factor	Evidence	Reference
Obesity/Weight Gain	• The **"accelerator hypothesis"** suggests that obesity (insulin resistance) results in a decrease in age at onset of T1D in genetically "at risk" individuals • Several studies have suggested that a child's BMI may play an important role in determining disease risk, with an increased risk for developing T1DM in individuals who were heavier as young children or experienced rapid early growth	2,112-122
Early Infant Diet: Cow's Milk vs. Breast Milk	• Observational studies (1980s) suggested that breastfeeding was associated with lower rates of T1D • T-cells from T1D children are sensitized to bovine serum albumin • Cow's milk proteins cause diabetes in animals • Decreased rates of T1D in animals weaned to hydrolyzed proteins instead of intact foreign proteins • TRIGR study – results pending	109-111
Early Infant Diet: Exposure to Gluten	• Increased association between type 1 DM and celiac disease • Reduced prevalence of T1D autoimmunity after gluten deprivation in patients with celiac disease • **BABYDIAB study:** Ingestion of gluten-containing foods before age 3 months was associated with significantly increased islet autoantibody risk, while this risk was abrogated if gluten-containing foods were started after age 6 months • **DAISY study:** Children initially exposed to cereals (both gluten and non-gluten containing) between ages 0 and 3 months and those who were exposed at >7 months had increased islet autoantibody risk compared with those who were exposed during the 4th through 6th month	110,123-125

---

continued

Table 8 (continued)

Environmental Factors That Play a Role in the Development of T1D

Environmental factor	Evidence	Reference
Vitamin D	• T1D incidence demonstrates a "north-south gradient" (countries in which children get little exposure to sunlight have higher rates of T1D) *Children from Finland are 400x more likely to develop T1D than are children from Venezuela • Epidemiological data: T1D patients have lower levels of vitamin D at diagnosis, compared to matched individuals without diabetes • Meta-analysis of 1 cohort and 4 case-control studies: infants who received vitamin D supplementation were significantly less likely to have developed T1D by age 15-30, with an OR of 0.71	126-129
Environmental Toxins	Toxins that may cause T1D in humans: • Dietary N-nitroso compounds – found in cured meat, and may be found in drinking water • Vacor – rodenticide • Cycasin – from cycad seeds found in the islands of Micronesia Toxins shown to cause T1D in other animals (may cause T1D in humans, but no direct evidence): • Streptozotocin – agent that preferentially kills islet β-cells, commonly used to induce experimental diabetes in rodents • Alloxan – oxidized product of uric acid, commonly used to induce experimental diabetes in rodents • Bafilomycin – antibiotic that can infest tuberous vegetables, including potatoes and sugar beet	130

continued

Table 8 (continued)

Environmental Factors That Play a Role in the Development of T1D

Environmental factor	Evidence	Reference
Sanitation/Hygiene	• Hygiene hypothesis: improved sanitation and living conditions, combined with vaccination strategies, our exposure to infectious agents and development of disease has been markedly diminished • Some infectious agents may have immunomodulatory properties that protect against the development of immune-mediated disorders • Positive associations have been found between T1D incidence and average male and female life expectancy, gross domestic product, and accessibility of the water supply and sewage systems • While evidence also exists in animal models to support this hypothesis, there is no evidence in human T1D to date, beyond correlative studies	131-133
Vaccinations	• **No evidence for a role of vaccines in diabetes**	134
Season	• Several studies have documented higher rates of T1D onset in late autumn, winter and early spring, with lower rates in summer • This suggests a role of environmental exposure, such as virus infections, variation of sunshine hours, or temperature	34, 135-138
Psychological Stress	• Psychological stress, measured as psychosocial strain in families, is associated with diabetes-related autoimmunity during infancy	139

Table 9

Viruses Implicated in the Development of T1D

Virus	Evidence in humans for a relationship between viral infection and triggering of T1D	Reference
Rubella	• T1D develops in 12%-20% of cases of congenital rubella	140, 141
Coxsackie B (enterovirus)	• Coxsackie B4 virus isolated from the pancreas of a child who died at presentation with T1D was propagated in *in vitro* cultures of endocrine pancreatic cells, and then shown to have diabetic activity in certain mouse strains • A sequence in GAD65 is identical to that in a Coxsackie virus antigen • Prospective epidemiological studies have supported a role for enteroviral infection in the pathogenesis of T1D • Anti-enteroviral T-cell response, enteroviral RNA and anti-viral IgM have been demonstrated in patients with T1D	142-151
Cytomegalovirus	• Correlation between the presence of CMV genome in the blood of patient with recent onset T1D and DAAs • High titres of anti-CMV IgG antibodies positively correlate with the presence of DAAs in healthy siblings of diabetic children • However, several studies did NOT find a correlation between CMV infection and T1D onset, suggesting that if CMV has a role in the pathogenesis of T1D, it is limited to a subset of children	152-154
Mumps	• A high frequency of children with mumps have islet cell antibodies and some go on to develop overt diabetes • Mumps outbreaks have been associated with an increase in the incidence of T1D 2-4 years later	155, 156
Rotavirus	• Increased levels of rotavirus-specific IgG and IgA antibodies are correlated with the appearance or increase in autoantibodies against islets in children at risk for T1D • This finding has *not* been replicated by all groups • The rotavirus protein VP7 shows sequence homology with the autoantigens tyrosine phosphatase IA-2 and GAD	157-159

6. Treatment of T1D

The effective treatment of a patient with type 1 diabetes requires that the practitioner understand the unique pathogenesis of T1D, compared with T2D. T1D is primarily a disease of insulin deficiency, rather than a combination of insulin deficiency and insulin resistance. While insulin resistance may play a prominent role in some patients with T1D (and should be taken into consideration when designing a treatment regimen), the cornerstone of T1D therapy is physiological insulin replacement. Beyond that, the practitioner needs to keep in mind the association between T1D and other autoimmune diseases, and do appropriate monitoring for those other conditions. Finally, the long-term complications of diabetes always need to be kept in mind, and multimodal therapies targeting glycemia, blood pressure, cholesterol control and other cardiovascular disease prevention strategies should be part of routine care for patients with T1D.

Treatment Recommendations

In the early 1990s, the Diabetes Control and Complications trial (DCCT) established the standard of care for the treatment of patients with T1D, by clearly demonstrating that intensive glucose control could delay, and even possibly prevent, the development of renal, retinal and neurological complications in patients with T1D.[160] Patients who received intensive therapy compared with conventional therapy experienced a 39% risk reduction for the development of microalbuminuria, a 54% reduction for albuminuria and a 60% reduction for clinical neuropathy (Figure 11).[160] In a follow-up observational study of the same population, the Epidemiology of Diabetes Interventions and Complications (EDIC), the investigators found that this beneficial effect of intensive glycemic control started soon after diagnosis and lasting for a mean of 6.5 years was long-lasting, even if a patient's control deteriorated after completion of the intervention trial. Nearly a decade after the end of the DCCT trial, patients who had been randomized to the intensive control arm continued to have a reduced risk of progression of microvascular complications, even though their HbA1C levels were, at that time, no different from that of the former control group: at about 8%.[161] Furthermore,

Figure 11

Reduction in the incidence of microvascular complications in the DCCT

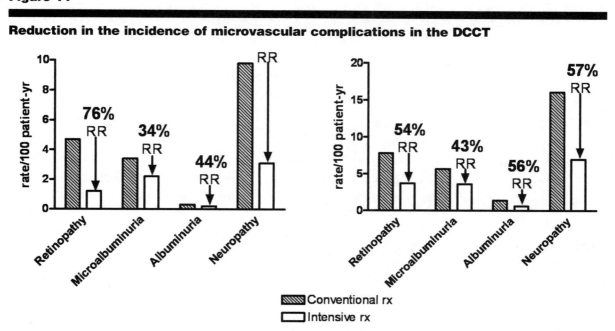

Incidence rates per 100 patient-years are shown for conventional therapy vs. intensive therapy arms in the DCCT. In both the primary prevention cohort (no pre-existing complications) and the secondary prevention cohort (pre-existing complications), there were significant risk reductions (RR) in retinopathy, microalbuminuria and neuropathy, ranging from 34%-76%.[160]

after even a longer follow-up period, the former intensive control group demonstrated a 57% risk reduction for nonfatal myocardial infarction, stroke or death, compared to the former control group.[162] This finding has been termed "metabolic memory" and has important implications for the treatment of patients with T1D, namely that blood glucose control needs to be managed aggressively early in the course of the disease, in order to have long-lasting effects on lowering complication rates. The exact mechanism of metabolic memory is not known, but is under active study. Since the original DCCT did not include prepubertal children, there still is controversy about the impact of metabolic memory in this population, and thus less agreement about glycemic targets for these patients.

The American Diabetes Association currently recommends a general glycemic target of <7% for adults with T1D.[163] For an individual patient, the goal is to obtain an HbA1C as close to normal as possible, without inducing significant hypoglycemia. This may mean a goal of closer to 6% or lower in patients with no significant comorbidities, some residual insulin production and/or an insulin regimen that is well-matched with the patient's insulin requirements. In other patients, the goal may be higher (eg, in patients with a history of hypoglycemia unawareness, in children and in patients with pre-existing cardiovascular disease, in whom the risk of detrimental consequences of hypoglycemia outweighs the benefit of very tight glucose control). Other glycemic and non-glycemic targets put forth by the ADA are listed in Table 10.

Insulins

Insulins can be broadly divided into 2 categories. "Basal insulin," sometimes called the "background insulin," provides a steady, low level of insulin in the circulation that mimics the basal insulin secret-

Table 10

Glycemic and Non-glycemic Treatment Goals for Patients with T1D (ADA Guidelines)[163]

Glycemic control	1. HbA1C <7.0%[a] for patients in general
	2. HbA1C <6.0% (as close to normal as possible without significant hypoglycemia) for the individual patient
	3. Preprandial capillary plasma glucose 90-130 mg/dl (during pregnancy: <105 mg/dl)
	4. Peak postprandial capillary plasma glucose (1-2 hours after starting a meal) <180 mg/dl (during pregnancy: either <155 mg/dl 1 hour post-meal or <130 2 hours post-meal)
Blood pressure	<130/80 mmHg
Lipids	1. LDL <100 mg/dl (ideally <70 mg/dl in high-risk patients with cardiovascular disease)
	2. Triglycerides <150 mg/dl
	3. HDL >40 mg/dl in men, >5 mg/dl in women

[a]Referenced to a nondiabetic range of 4.0%-6.0% using a DCCT-based assay.

Table 11

Factors That Affect Insulin Pharmacokinetics

	Factor	Comment/Tips for Patients

Absorption	Injection site	• Absorption differs at different sites[a]
		  * Abdominal injection (especially upper abdomen) → quickest absorption
		  *Arm injection intermediate absorption
		  *Thigh/hip injection → slowest absorption
		• Differences are primarily related to blood flow differences at various sites
		• Patients: be consistent with injection sites
		• Exercise caution when injecting into scar tissue/areas of lipohypertrophy

	Injection depth	• IM injections absorbed more rapidly than SQ injections
	Exercise of injected area	• Strenuous exercise of a limb within 1 hour of injection results in more rapid absorption
	Local massage	• Vigorous rubbing or massage following an injection can result in more rapid absorption
	Temperature	• Heat can increase absorption rate (eg, sauna, shower, hot bath), cold can decrease absorption rate
	Insulin dose	• Non-linear relationship between dose and effect on blood glucose • Large doses of injected insulin may form a depot that delays the onset action and prolongs the duration of action

Distribution	Insulin antibodies (rare in patients who have only received insulin analogues)	• The presence of insulin antibodies may have the following effects:
		  *Delay the onset of insulin activity
		  *Reduce the peak concentration of free insulin
		  *Prolong the biologic half-life of insulin

Elimination	Renal insufficiency (severe)	• Reduces the clearance of insulin • Prolongs the effect of insulin

[a]Note that data on variability in absorption at different sites mostly refers to studies using human insulins. These differences are not as pronounced with insulin analogues.

Table 12

Currently Available Insulin Preparations

Category/ Generic name	Brand name	Comparison with human insulin	Onset of acton (h)	Peak action (h)	Effective duration of action (h)	Maximum duration (h)
Rapid-acting analogs						
Insulin aspart	Novolog	Substitution of aspartic acid for proline at position 28 of the insulin B-chain	¼ - ½	½ - 1 ¼	3-4	4-6
Insulin lispro	Humalog	Inversion of amino acids lysine and proline at positions 28 and 29 of the insulin B-chain	¼ - ½	½ - 1 ¼	3-4	4-6
Insulin glulisine	Apidra	Substitution of lysine for asparagine at position 3 and substitution of glutamic acid for lysine at position 29 of the insulin B-chain	¼ - ½	½ - 1 ¼	3-4	4-6
Short-acting						
Regular human insulin	Novolin R Humulin R		½ - 1	2-3	3-6	6-8
Intermediate-acting						
Neutral protamine hagedorn (NPH)	Humulin N Novolin N	Addition of protamine to regular insulin	2-4	6-10	10-16	14-18
Long-acting analogs						
Insulin glargine	Lantus	Substitution of glycine for alanine at position 21 of the insulin A-chain; addition of 2 extra AAs (arginines) at the end of the insulin B-chain	3-4	8-16	18-20	20-24
Insulin detemir	Levemir	Removal of threonine from terminal position 30 of insulin B-chain; acylation of lysine at position 29 with 14-C myristic acid	3-4	6-8	14	~20

Figure 12

Approximate pharmacokinetic profiles of human insulin and insulin analogues[225]

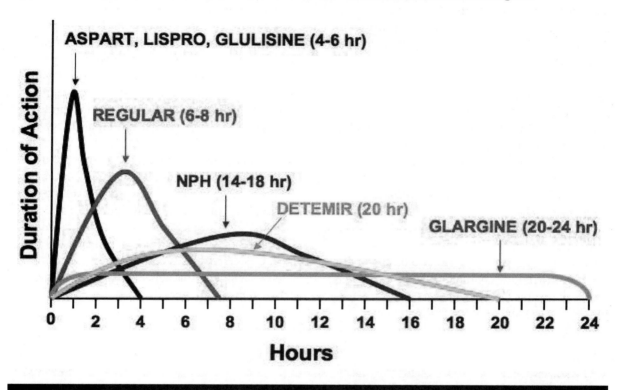

ed in healthy subjects between meals and during fasting, which serves to modulate basal hepatic glucose production. "Prandial insulin" (also called "bolus" or "meal-time") mimics the burst of insulin secreted during a meal, that serves to dispose of ingested glucose and other nutrients. The ideal insulin regimen for a patient with T1D simulates the non-diabetic insulin delivery pattern as closely as possible, using what is termed "physiological insulin replacement," consisting of a basal insulin component and a prandial insulin component. Many traditional insulin regimens, such as twice daily NPH alone, do not replace insulin in a physiological manner, making it very difficult to achieve meticulous control using these regimens, unless the patient has some residual endogenous insulin production.

The design of a regimen using physiological insulin replacement requires an understanding of insulin pharmacokinetics and the pharmacodynamics of the different insulins available.[164]

Pharmacokinetics refers to the rate at which insulin is absorbed, distributed and eliminated from the body. The absorption of insulin is the rate-limiting step of insulin activity, and this can vary tremendously within an individual from one injection to another,[165] and even more significantly between individuals. Factors that influence the absorption are listed in Table 11.[166] A general principle is that when local blood flow in the subcutaneous tissue is altered, the absorption rate of insulin will also be affected. Thus, something that increases subcutaneous blood flow will increase the absorption rate, and vice versa. The rate of insulin distribution is not as variable as absorption, although some factors, such as the presence of insulin antibodies (not to be confused with DAAs),[167] can influence this step. Elimination occurs via degradation in the kidneys and liver. Under normal physiological circumstances, the liver degrades the majority of endogenous insulin, which first reaches the liver via the portal vein before entering the non-portal circulation. In contrast, in T1D patients, the kidney degrades the majority of exogenously injected insulin. Consequently, renal insufficiency can influence the pharmacokinetic profile of insulin by reducing the clearance and prolonging its effect. However, this is generally not a clinically significant effect unless the renal insufficiency is severe.[168]

Pharmacodynamics describes the metabolic effect of specific insulin formulations, ie, onset, peak and duration. Insulins are categorized as rapid-acting, short-acting, intermediate-acting and long-acting, as summarized in Table 12 and Figure 12.

Twice-daily insulin regimens vs. multiple daily injections (MDI)
In the DCCT, patients in the intensive therapy arm were randomized to a physiological insulin replacement regimen, with either multiple daily injections (MDI) or continuous subcutaneous insulin infusions (CSII). This was a sharp departure from the standard treatment regimen at the

time (and the treatment regimen still used today in many non-specialty clinics), which consisted of either basal insulin injections (ie, NPH) given BID, or pre-mixed (or free-mix) short- and intermediate-acting insulins (ie, 70/30 NPH/Regular) given BID. The theory behind the BID split mix popularized in the 1960s is that regular insulin serves as the prandial insulin for breakfast, and NPH serves as both basal insulin for the late morning and afternoon and prandial insulin for lunch. In reality, the regular insulin also serves as basal insulin for the late morning and early afternoon because of its long effective duration of action (6-8 hours). Thus, there is no clear separation between the basal and prandial insulin components, and this overlapping action of the 2 insulins (insulin stacking) means that the patient is forced to be extremely rigid with injection times, meal times, meal sizes and snack times, to avoid hypoglycemia or unacceptable hyperglycemia between meals (Figure 13).

Figure 13

Combined prandial and basal effects of both regular and NPH insulin

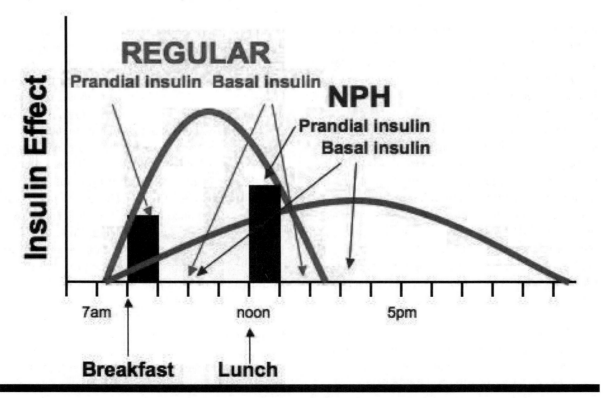

MDI regimens, in contrast, are a much more effective way to obtain good diabetes control, while maintaining some flexibility as to meal times and meal sizes. MDI, also called "basal-bolus" therapy, is based on the concept of physiological insulin replacement described above, in which separate insulins are used for basal and prandial requirements (Figure 14). This requires more injections per day, since patients must take 1 (sometimes 2) injections of basal insulin and 3+ injections of prandial insulin, depending on the number of meals and large snacks consumed. In the DCCT, the patients in the intensive control arm on MDI regimens used NPH or *ultralente* insulin for basal components, and *regular* insulin for prandial requirements. Ultralente insulin is no longer available. Aside from CSII, this was the best physiological replacement regimen possible with the insulin preparations available on the market at that time. Achieving targets established by

the DCCT and set out by the ADA has become much more feasible with the use of newer insulins, including longer-acting and smaller-peaked basal insulins and shorter-acting analogues (see Table 12). While these insulin preparations are far from perfect in mimicking normal insulin secretion, in general they do reduce the risk of hypoglycemia, particularly in patients with lower HbA1C levels.

It should also be emphasized with all of our physiologic insulin regimens, that even though we classify the insulins as "basal" or "prandial" due to the pharmacodynamics of the insulin, there still is significant overlap. For example, with a high-carbohydrate meal the food might be absorbed in 2-3 hours, whereas the insulin action is present for at least 5 hours. The same insulin dose for a high-fat meal may generally do a better job of actually mimicking a prandial dose. Even more common are patients unintentionally on high doses of basal

Figure 14

Idealized diagrammatic representation of a multiple daily injection insulin regimen, using insulin analogues

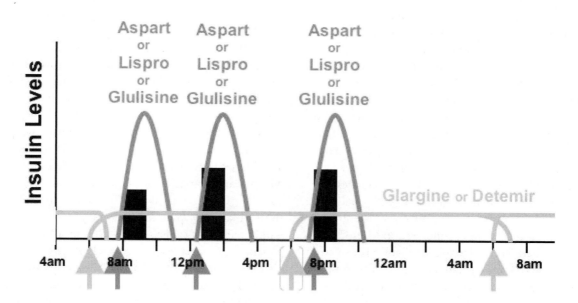

Red arrows show injections with rapid-acting analogs, and purple arrows show injections with long-acting analogues. Meals are depicted as black rectangles. As illustrated, MDI regimens require at least 4-5 injections per day, but provide a much better match of insulin action with insulin requirements, compared to a BID NPH and regular insulin regimen.

insulin, which in essence are managing prandial needs. While part of the problem is that current insulin preparations are still not ideal in replicating normal insulin secretion, the advent of continuous glucose monitoring has allowed us to use our insulins more effectively. Furthermore, there is active research to develop longer and "flatter" basal insulins and quicker prandial insulins to better match physiological needs.

Continuous subcutaneous insulin infusion (CSII)

Insulin pump therapy (or CSII as noted above), is the optimal means of achieving physiological insulin replacement because of the precision with which normal basal insulin secretion can be mimicked by programming basal rates, usually in 1-hour segments over a 24-hour period. Thus, rather than giving a single injection of long-acting insulin that theoretically reaches a stable plateau over the 24-hour period, the patient can program precise doses to match differing insulin demands at different times of the day. (In reality, none of the basal insulins are perfectly peakless, and none last for precisely 24 hours.) For example, many patients have lower requirements at night (from ~11 pm to ~4 am) but then have higher requirements in the morning (from ~4 am to ~9 am), due to the "dawn phenomenon" caused by an early morning surge in growth hormone.[169] In addition to these regularly scheduled dose adjustments, patients can easily make changes in the basal rates on a day-to-day basis to accommodate physiological changes, such as illness, exercise, food, menstrual periods or varying schedules. A meta-analysis evaluating 12 randomized controlled trials comparing CSII vs. intensive therapy with MDI found that better control was achieved by patients on CSII, with lowered mean glucose concentrations and HbA1C levels, compared to MDI.[170] In addition, there is good evidence that CSII use reduces the risk for hypoglycemia.[171] Thus, for a patient who is interested in wearing one of these devices and is willing to be actively involved with their diabetes care, CSII is the best possible means of providing insulin therapy.

Perhaps the most critical point about CSII, also important for MDI, is that this therapy is best performed with a multi-disciplinary diabetes team,

ideally with access to 1 or more certified diabetes educators (CDEs). Successful insulin therapy in general, and CSII in particular, is difficult without assistance from trained nursing and nutritional experts in insulin therapy. The CDEs could be based at the local hospital, and in the case of CSII, each pump company has trainers (who are usually CDEs) to assist patients. CSII is covered in greater detail in another chapter in this educational review.

Physiological insulin replacement regimens and key concepts

Determining the Appropriate Basal Dose

The approach to determining insulin doses is similar for both MDI and CSII. Most T1D patients with little or no residual beta-cell function will require 0.4-0.8 units of insulin/kg/day for both basal and prandial insulin combined. Patients who are in their pubertal years, are obese, have a family history of T2D or are sedentary will likely need a dose on the higher end of that range, and patients who are thinner, active and female will require less. The basal insulin dose should be ≤50% of the total. 1 mistake often made by practitioners is to provide the majority of insulin as basal insulin. This situation may come about when post-prandial spikes are not being adequately treated, resulting in a misdirected increase in the basal insulin dose, rather than addressing the prandial issue. As a result of using basal insulin to treat prandial spikes, patients may find that they become hypoglycemic if they skip a meal, and they may even have to snack in between meals to avoid hypoglycemia. The best way to determine whether an appropriate basal dose has been selected is to perform a basal test. To do this, the patient starts on a night when the bedtime glucose falls within the target range (ie, 90-130 mg/dl). The patient then measures 1, preferably 2, glucose levels through the night. In the morning after awakening, the patient skips breakfast and continues to measure the glucose on an hourly basis until early afternoon. We generally stop then, as it is quite unusual for basal requirements to change the rest of the day (the most common exception is regular afternoon or evening exercise). In the event that the patient becomes hypoglycemic during the basal test, the patient consumes food and the basal dose is subsequently lowered. If the glucose levels climb over the test period, the basal dose is raised. Obviously, this type of testing is best suited for CSII therapy, as there is minimal ability to change basal doses for different time periods with MDI. On the other hand, some practitioners take advantage of the imperfect basal pharmacodynamic profiles and split the doses to twice daily, to obtain better basal insulinemia for a particular situation. For example, for the patient with a significant dawn phenomenon not wishing to use CSII, we will commonly use the shorter-acting insulin detemir (instead of insulin glargine, see below) in a higher dose at bedtime with a lower dose in the morning. While this is totally anecdotal, the subtle differences in these basal insulins make dealing with these situations possible.

Differences Between Different Basal Insulins

The options currently available for basal insulins in patients on MDI therapy include intermediate-acting insulin (NPH) and long-acting analogues (glargine and detemir). The ideal basal insulin is thought to be peakless and has a very consistent duration of action. However, we have quickly learned with real-time continuous glucose monitoring that it is difficult to truly replicate an "ideal basal insulin," since these insulin requirements can be quite variable in some patients. None of the available insulins are ideal, although glargine and detemir come much closer to mimicking normal basal insulin secretion than NPH, which has a peak activity occurring within 6-10 hours after subcutaneous injection. This peak is associated with an increased risk of hypoglycemia, particularly when the NPH is given at bedtime to lower fasting glucose. NPH also has a high degree of variability in its absorption profile.[166] "Patient factors" further contribute to this variability, due to the need to resuspend NPH insulin prior to injection in a very consistent manner. Glargine, in the other hand, has a nearly peakless profile and reduced absorption variability compared to NPH.[164,172] While glargine does not appear to improve overall glycemic control compared to NPH, as measured by HbA1C reduction, it has been shown to reduce nocturnal hypoglycemia.[173] Similarly detemir, as compared to NPH, demonstrates no significant reduction in glycemia, but a significant lowering of hypoglycemia.[174]

Although often considered interchangeable by many practitioners, detemir and glargine have some important differences. Detemir does not achieve the same peakless action seen with glargine.[174] Secondly, the duration of action is not as long, meaning that most T1D patients require twice-daily dosing.[175] Thirdly, detemir has a relatively lower affinity for the insulin receptor as compared to human insulin. It has been formulated in its own units to match the biological potency of NPH, however, its potency is 30% lower than that of glargine,[175] which means that a higher dose of detemir is often required to achieve an equivalent hypoglycemic response. On the other hand, some studies have suggested that detemir is associated with less weight gain compared to NPH, and possibly compared to glargine.[174] The finding of reduced weight gain is currently under investigation. In addition, 1 randomized, double-blind study comparing detemir with glargine and NPH insulin in T1D patients demonstrated decreased within-subject variability using insulin detemir.[176] Nevertheless, we feel that glargine should be the first-line basal insulin for most adult patients with T1D, with detemir being a second choice, followed by NPH. The main exception to this recommendation are those patients (as noted above) with a significant dawn phenomenon not wishing to pursue CSII. What is clearly needed is a "head-to-head, treat-to-target" study comparing detemir to glargine in T1D. Ideally, to reduce any bias, both insulins would be given BID and the study would be double-blinded. Until that happens, by necessity we need to base our recommendations on insulin clamp data. Finally, as opposed to T2D, where hypoglycemia risk is extremely low with high A1C levels (especially over 9%) and it is difficult to rationalize the cost-effectiveness of either insulin analog compared to NPH insulin, the much higher risk for hypoglycemia, particularly nocturnal hypoglycemia in T1D, suggests that NPH should have minimal, if any, use in most patients with T1D.

Determining the Appropriate Prandial Dose – Insulin to Carbohydrate Ratios

Once an appropriate basal insulin and dose have been selected, the remainder of the daily insulin should be given as prandial insulin: boluses in the case of CSII and meal-time injections (either with an insulin pen device or traditional syringe) in the case of MDI. Ideally, prandial insulin doses are determined based on calculations made by the patient of how many carbohydrates they are ingesting for a particular meal, and then applying a pre-established carbohydrate to insulin ratio to calculate the required insulin dosage. If the patient is not able or motivated to count carbohydrates, other methods need to be employed to best match the insulin dose with the calorie content of each meal. 1 option is to take a diet history and assign insulin doses based on "typical" meals. The typical dose of rapid-acting analogue in patients with T1D is 1 unit of insulin for every 10-15 grams of carbohydrates. Obese patients may require higher insulin doses (ie, lower ratios down to 1:5), and insulin-sensitive patients may require lower doses (ratios up to 1:20). The insulin to carbohydrate ratios are best fine-tuned after an appropriate basal insulin dose has been determined, and in conjunction with a good diet history. Some patients may even require different insulin to carbohydrate ratios at different times of the day, due to varying levels of insulin sensitivity.

Timing of Prandial Injections: "Lag Time"
1 important key to success with prandial insulin injections is the correct determination of an appropriate time interval (lag time) between the insulin injection and eating, taking into consideration insulin bioavailability with respect to the glycemic excursion after a meal. Assuming the blood glucose levels are normal and not trending up or down, the rapid-acting analogues should ideally be given within 10 minutes before eating, due to their rapid onset of action. These insulin may even be given immediately prior to eating, or just after eating if the planned amount of food ingestion is uncertain, such as in children. Regular insulin, on the other hand, should be given 20-30 minutes prior to eating, in order to allow the slower onset of action to better match the glycemic excursion.

Factors that should prompt changes in the planned lag time include: hyper- or hypoglycemia prior to eating, the relative content in the meal of pure carbohydrate and the quality of the carbohydrate ingested. For prandial boluses given when a patient is hypoglycemic, regular insulin should be administered immediately prior to eating, and rapid-acting analogues should be delayed until after some carbohydrate has been consumed. On the other hand, for prandial boluses given when a patient is hyperglycemic, the lag time between insulin administration and eating should be increased, to: at least 20 minutes for blood glucose levels in the 200s, a minimum of 30 minutes for blood glucose levels in the 300s for analogues and at least 30-60 minutes for this degree of hyperglycemia for regular insulin. The higher the blood glucose level, the longer the lag time.

Determining a Hyperglycemia Correction Dose (Insulin Sensitivity Factor)
In addition to changing the timing of insulin injections for pre-meal hyperglycemia, the patient should add a pre-determined "correction dose" to the prandial dose, to effectively bring the blood glucose level down into the normal range. A typical hyperglycemia correction dose would be 1 unit of insulin (rapid-acting analogue) for every 30-50 mg/dl the glucose needs to be lowered to get down to the target range. The target might be 100 mg/dl during the day and higher (120-130 mg/dl) at night. This is also called the *insulin sensitivity factor*. The correction dose can also be used to treat between-meal hyperglycemia, with the caveat mentioned below regarding the need to take into account the amount of active insulin on board. The ADA recommends a 1- to 2-hour postprandial target of <180 mg/dl[163] and the American Association of Clinical Endocrinologists (AACE) recommends a lower target of 140 mg/dl.[177]

Insulin on Board/Stacking
In order to safely give between-meal correction doses, it is important that the patient be taught the concept of *insulin on board* (IOB). This concept takes into account insulin action times, or the pharmacodynamics of insulin after injection (Figure 15). Insulin activity of a rapid-acting analogue is typically 4-6 hours in adults, with the activity of regular insulin being even longer, 6-8 hours (see Table 12). Thus, a planned dose of between-meal insulin injected during this time frame needs to be reduced, based on a calculation of how much IOB is still available. In our clinic, we distribute handouts to MDI patients with the graph shown in Figure 15, in order for them to calculate the dose for between-meal hyper-

Figure 15

The timing of action for insulin aspart

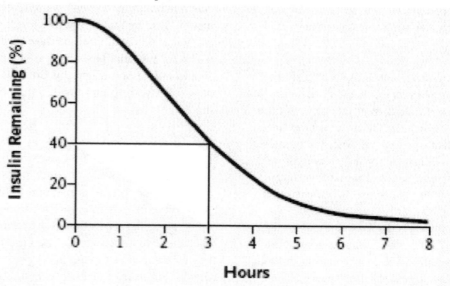

The use of this graph helps patients avoid "insulin stacking." For example, 3 hours after the administration of 10 units of insulin aspart, one can estimate that there is still 40% x 10 units, or 4 units of insulin remaining.[225,226] Adapted from Mudaliar S, et al. *Diabetes Care.* 1999;22:1501-1506.[226]

Mudaliar S, Lindberg F, Joyce M, Beerdsen P, Strange P, Lin A, et al. Insulin aspart (B28 asp-insulin): a fast-acting analog of human insulin: absorption kinetics and action profile compared with regular human insulin in healthy nondiabetic subjects. Diabetes Care. 1999; 22(9):1501-1506. Copyright ©1999 Massachusettes Medical Society. All rights reserved.

glycemia using the following formula:

Total correction dose – IOB = suggested correction dose

CSII users have a simpler task when giving between-meal correction doses, because modern-day insulin pumps take this concept into account with the bolus calculator. However, for those CSII patients who don't use the bolus calculator and MDI patients who don't take the IOB concept into account, the administration of between-meal correction can lead to insulin "stacking." This can result in hypoglycemia, due to the combined effects of IOB and unadjusted between-meal correction dose insulin. This topic of insulin stacking is also why we generally don't ask nurses to measure between-meal blood glucose levels during hospitalization, as we have found keeping track of IOB is too complex for many care providers uninitiated to insulin principles for T1D.

Non-insulin therapies

Pramlintide
Pramlintide (trade name Symlin) is a recent addition to the T1D therapy armamentarium. Patients with T1D are deficient for a hormone called amylin, which is normally co-secreted with insulin. Amylin functions to reduce postprandial hyperglycemia by reducing mealtime glucagon secretion, delaying gastric emptying and reducing satiety.[178] Pramlintide has been shown to have a modest effect on reducing HbA1C, with mean reductions of 0.5%-0.7% in clinical trials.[179-181]

Pramlintide is very effective at reducing post-prandial spikes, and might be considered for T1D patients who struggle with HbA1C lowering with physiological insulin replacement regimens alone. Often, these are patients who have difficulty limiting the amount of carbohydrates eaten at a sitting. In addition, this drug might be considered for T1D patients with imperfect glycemic control who are overweight, as 1-2 kg of weight loss over 6 months is seen on average due to the satiety effects mentioned above, and some patients experience much greater weight losses of up to 5-10 kg.

Pramlintide is given pre-prandially at a starting dose of 15 mcg per meal, and the dose is increased as tolerated every 3 days to a final dose of 60 mcg per meal. Unlike insulin, the dose of pramlintide remains constant once a final dose has been established, without adjusting for the carbohydrate content of a meal, with the caveat that this drug is only given prior to "major meals" consisting of 250 calories or 30 grams of carbohydrate. The company recommends decreasing the prandial insulin dose by 50% when starting pramlintide to avoid hypoglycemia, due to a reduction in food intake and delayed gastric emptying.[182] This reduction may be too aggressive initially for patients who are on appropriate basal insulin doses, so we generally start with a 25% reduction upon pramlintide initiation. Other changes that may need to be made to the insulin regimen include reducing the lag time of a prandial dose, and even potentially switching to regular insulin for the prandial insulin, which some patients find provides a smoother postprandial glycemic profile. In this situation, we still tend to have patients use the rapid-acting analogues for their correction doses. For this situation, it is usually easier to use syringe therapy and we want to ensure the brand of regular insulin matches the brand of analogue insulin. (Novo Regular is mixed with insulin aspart and Lilly Regular is mixed with insulin lispro.)

Limiting effects on the use of pramlintide include nausea and hypoglycemia. Nausea, or abdominal fullness, is very common upon initiation of this drug, seen in 1/3 to 1/2 of patients,[181] but it generally remits with time. If a patient is experiencing nausea, the practitioner is advised to hold off on upward titration of the dose until the nausea subsides. Some patients are more sensitive to this drug than others, and may require a very slow dose titration. Hypoglycemia is another adverse effect of this drug, with severe hypoglycemia occurring in 2.3% of patients in the first 3 months

of the open-label clinical trials.[181] In order to avoid this, it is important to ensure an appropriate basal dose prior to initiation of pramlintide, and to check the appropriateness of the reduced prandial insulin dose by measuring post-meal glucose levels. Patients who do not measure blood glucose levels on a regular basis (at least 4 times a day) should not be prescribed this drug, due to the risk of severe hypoglycemia with infrequent monitoring.

Diet and Exercise

Diet and exercise are 2 lifestyle factors that play a very prominent role in the treatment of T2D, but should not be forgotten in patients with T1D. The ADA recommends monitoring carbohydrate intake, whether by carbohydrate counting, exchanges or experienced-based estimation, as a key element of achieving good glycemic control. In addition, it may be beneficial to consider the glycemic index and glycemic load of a meal, rather than simply total carbohydrate content. Detailed nutrition-related recommendations are reviewed in the ADA position statement,[162] and every T1D patient should meet with a registered dietician who has expertise in the management of diabetes in order to implement these recommendations. The importance of medical nutritional therapy (MNT) in patients with T1D is illustrated by clinical trials demonstrating a ~1% decrease in HbA1C with MNT (REF),[182] as well as reductions in other risk factors, such as dyslipidemia and hypertension.[183]

Similarly, regular exercise in patients with diabetes can improve glycemic control, reduce cardiovascular risk factors, contribute to weight loss and improve well-being. The ADA position statement recommends 150 minutes per week of moderate-intensity aerobic physical activity (50%-70% of maximal heart rate) for patients with diabetes.[162] However, the physician should assess patients for comorbidities that might contraindicate certain forms of exercise, as outlined in Table 13. For older patients and those in poor physical condition, the exercise regime should be started at low intensity, with a gradual increase in intensity and duration over time. 2 special considerations for patients with T1D include the effects of exercise on ketosis (Table 13) and on blood glucose levels.

Table 13

Contraindications to Exercise in T1D Patients

Contraindication	Justification/Recommendation
Uncontrolled hypertension	• Exercise may exacerbate uncontrolled hypertension • Get hypertension under control before initiating an exercise regime
Severe autonomic neuropathy	• Decreased cardiac responsiveness to exercise, postural hypotension, impaired thermoregulation, impaired night vision and unpredictable carbohydrate delivery from gastroparesis may predispose patients to adverse exercise-related events, including hypoglycemia
	• Because of a strong association of autonomic neuropathy (AN) with CVD, patients with severe AN should undergo cardiac evaluation before increasing physical activity levels
Severe peripheral neuropathy or history of foot lesions	• Decreased pain sensation in the extremities puts patients at risk for skin breakdown and infection or Charcot joint destruction
	• Encourage non-weight bearing activities, such as swimming, bicycling or arm exercises
Advanced retinopathy	• In the case of PDR or severe non-PDR, vigorous aerobic or resistance exercise may be contraindicated because of the risk of triggering vitreous hemorrhage or retinal detachment • Recommend lower-intensity or non-resistance forms of exercise
Ketoacidosis	• Avoid vigorous activity in the presence of ketosis, as exercise can worsen the problem • This does not preclude exercising during hyper glycemia, as long as the patient is not ketotic

Table 14

Clinical Situations in Which HbA1C Monitoring is Not Useful

Short-term changes in glycemic control	HbA1C should not be measured more frequently than every 2-3 months, as changes in glycemic control are not reflected in a shorter time frame. Short-term changes in glycemic control may occur in the following clinical scenarios: • Rapid changes in diabetes treatment • Acute illness that may change glucose levels and insulin requirements over a short period of time
Diabetes in pregnancy	The insulin requirements in a pregnant woman change rapidly and significantly, and meticulous control throughout the pregnancy is essential for fetal wellbeing.
Increased red blood cell (RBC) turnover or RBC loss	Conditions in which the average life of RBCs is decreased will falsely lower the HbA1C measure, due to the decrease in exposure time of circulating RBCs to elevated levels of blood glucose. This occurs in the following clinical scenarios: • Hemolytic anemias and hemoglobinopathies, such as sickle cell disease • Iron-deficiency anemias following initiation of treatment[a] • Renal insufficiency treated with erythropoietin • Blood transfusion (HbA1C measured soon after transfusion reflects the donor's glycemic control)

[a]*Iron deficiency anemia may artificially lower or raise HbA1C, depending on the clinical scenario. In untreated iron-deficiency anemia, when RBC turnover is low, HbA1C levels are falsely elevated, but they decline significantly and may become falsely low after imitating treatment, as the rate of reticulocytosis increases.[186] Similarly, HbA1C levels may be falsely elevated during late pregnancy in the setting of iron-deficiency anemia caused by increased demands.[187]*

Hypoglycemia can be a problem during or after exercise in patients with T1D. To avoid this, it is recommended that patients ingest some carbohydrates prior to starting exercise if glucose levels are low (<100 mg/dl). In addition, many T1D patients find that they need to alter their insulin doses during, before and/or after exercise, whether by activating a lower temporary basal rate in CSII users or by adjusting their prandial doses before or after exercise. The individual glycemic response to exercise can be variable, so patients and their providers may need to experiment with the best strategies for preventing exercise-induced hypoglycemia.

Monitoring tools

Hemoglobin A1C (HbA1C) and Fructosamine
Hemoglobin A1C (HbA1C, or glycated hemoglobin) is 1 of the cornerstones of monitoring glycemic control. The HbA1C value represents the integration of fasting and postprandial glucose levels over the preceding 3 months and measures the amount of glucose nonenzymatically bound to hemoglobin in circulating erythrocytes in a concentration-dependent fashion. Thus, it provides an overall measure of long-term diabetes control. There are several methods for measuring HbA1C, and results using 1 method cannot be directly

compared with those using another method. The National Glycohemoglobin Standardization Program (NGSP, http://www.ngsp.org/) is seeking to standardize these test results, so that clinical laboratory results are comparable to those reported in DCCT trial, where relationships to mean blood glucose and risk for microvascular complications have been established. It should be noted that HbA1C does not provide any information on the degree of glucose excursions or glycemic variability, valuable information which can only be obtained by using other monitoring tools. The ADA recommends measuring HbA1C at least every 6 months in patients who have achieved good glycemic control, and every 3 months in patients who are not at goal or whose therapy has changed.[163]

The HbA1C measure is not useful in some clinical settings, as outlined in Table 14. In these cases, fructosamine levels (which measure glycemic control over a shorter time frame, 2-3 weeks) are more useful.[185] Fructosamine measures the amount of glucose bound to serum albumin. This measure is not often used clinically outside the scenarios listed in Table 14, because there is little standardization between test methods and laboratories, and normal values are dependent on several factors, including age and gender. Furthermore, practitioners should be aware that high levels of vitamin C (ascorbic acid), lipemia, hemolysis and hyperthyroidism can interfere with fructosamine test results.

Self-monitoring of Blood Glucose (SMBG)

The process of monitoring one's own blood glucose using a glucose meter is termed self-monitoring of blood glucose (SMBG). SMBG is an important component of modern T1D therapy, with the goal of collecting detailed information about blood

Table 15

SMBG Recommendations for Patients with T1D[191]

Clinical scenario	Recommended SMBG frequency
T1D on any insulin regimen	At *least* 3 times daily
T1D on physiological insulin replacement (MDI or CSII)	3-4 times daily
Clinical situations requiring increased SMBG frequency:	>3-4 times daily

- Presence of hypo- or hyperglycemic symptoms
- Hypoglycemic unawareness
- Illness
- Gastroparesis
- Use of medications that can affect glucose levels (ie, steroids)
- Pregnancy and preconception planning
- Periods of insulin dosage adjustments
- Strenuous physical activity
- A change in living environment resulting in differences in food, exercise and sleeping amounts (common with adolescents and business travelers)

glucose levels at many times points throughout the day to establish glycemic patterns, prevent hypoglycemia and enable improvements in the insulin regimen. In addition to a mean blood glucose level over a particular period of monitoring, SMBG also provides an estimate of glycemic variability, or blood glucose fluctuations, by enabling the calculation of a standard deviation. The mean blood glucose and standard deviation measure was shown to predict severe hypoglycemia independently from HbA1C in the DCCT trial.[188] In addition, some recent studies have indicated that acute blood glucose fluctuations and the consequent oxidative stress and superoxide formation may have important implications for the development of diabetes complications, independent of HbA1C.[189] Thus, the measure of standard deviation, provided by most glucose meter software programs, is important for the assessment of risk for clinically significant hypo- or hyperglycemia, as well as potentially the risk for developing complications. A target that may be easily employed in the clinical setting is SD x 2 < mean glucose (ideally SD x 3 < mean glucose, although this can be a very difficult goal for T1D patients to achieve), with the caveat that the SD measurement requires at least 5 (preferably 10) blood glucose measures to be meaningful.

A recent consensus statement written by a group of diabetes experts has put forth recommended SMGB frequency, as outlined in Table 15. It is important to note that these are minimum frequency recommendations. Increased SMBG frequency has been shown to correlate directly with better metabolic control in T1D patients in a large, standardized, prospective database documenting diabetes care and outcome.[190] In this study, each additional daily BG measurement improved the HbA1C level by 0.26%. These guidelines do not delineate when SMBG should take place. For patients doing minimal self-monitoring, testing before meals and at bedtime is the usual recommendation, in order to determine the amount of prandial insulin required for each meal and to minimize nocturnal hypoglycemia. For patients doing more frequent monitoring, postprandial testing can be very useful in order to assess the prandial insulin doses, and to achieve postprandial blood glucose target levels by treating between-

meal hyperglycemia. More frequent testing also provides important information about glucose trend (ie, whether the blood glucose level is going up or down). This information can be very helpful when deciding whether or not to give supplemental correction dose insulin, or to determine whether an increased or decreased lag time is needed between the administration of a prandial insulin dose and eating a meal.

Real-time Continuous Glucose Monitoring (rt-CGM)

Real-time continuous glucose monitoring (rt-CGM) has been a recent revolutionary advance in diabetes care. This technology involves the insertion of a small sensor under the skin, which is worn for 3-7 days and allows patients to view an approximation of their blood glucose levels every 5 minutes. Thus, rt-CGM permits fine-tuning of a patient's glycemic control that is not possible with SMBG. The more times per day that a patient performs SMBG, the better their understanding of their glycemic "pattern"; however, a single BG measurement remains a snapshot in time, with no information about where the BG has recently been, or where it is going. rt-CGM adds that critical piece of information about glycemic trend that is not available from SMGB alone (ie, direction *and* rate of BG change). The end result is that patients can make much more effective diabetes management decisions, based not only on the glucose value, but also on whether the glucose level is rising or falling, and how quickly. Other benefits of rt-CGM over SMBG include safety alarms for high and low blood glucose thresholds, as well as the rigorous measures of glycemic variability made possible by a vastly greater amount of data. While there are challenges with the use of the currently available devices, both on the part of the physician and the patient[192], this technology may become the standard of care for management for T1D patients in the future. Rt-CGM is discussed in greater detail elsewhere in this educational review.

Monitoring for diabetes complications
Diabetes complications, including retinopathy, nephropathy, neuropathy (microvascular complications) and cardiovascular disease (macrovascular complications), confer significant contributions to

Table 16

Recommended Screening Modalities, Frequency and Treatment for T1D Complications in Adults[163]

Complication	Screening Recommendations	Treatment
	Microvascular complications	
Diabetic retinopathy	• Undergo comprehensive dilated eye examination by an ophthalmologist within 5 years after the onset of T1D and annually thereafter • Less frequent exams (every 2-3 years) can be considered following one or more normal eye exams • More frequent exams are required if retinopathy is progressing • Women with T1D who are planning pregnancy should undergo a comprehensive eye examination in the first trimester with close follow-up throughout pregnancy and for 1 year postpartum	If any macular edema, severe NPDR, or any PDR: • Prompt referral to an ophthalmologist with experience in treating diabetic retinopathy If high-risk PDR, clinically significant macular edema and, occasionally, severe NPDR: • Laser photocoagulation thearpy
Diabetic nephropathy	• Measure urine albumin excretion (spot urine microalbumin to creatinine ratio) annually in all patients with diabetes duration of ≥5 years • Measure serum creatinine at lease annually	If micro- or macroalbuminuria: • ACE inhibitors or ARBs If early stages of chronic kidney disease: • Reduce protein intake to 0.8-1.0 g/kg body weight
Neuropathy	• Screen for DPN at diagnosis and at least annually thereafter using clinical tests • Screen for signs and symptoms of autonomic neuropathy 5 years after the diagnosis of TID	If DPN: • Educate about self-care of the feet • Refer for special footwear If DPN or autonomic neuropathy: • Offer medications for the relief of specific symptoms related to the neuropathy

continued

Table 16 (continued)

Recommended Screening Modalities, Frequency and Treatment for T1D Complications in Adults[163]

Complication	Screening Recommendations	Treatment
	Microvascular complications	
CVD	• In asymptomatic patients, evaluate risk factors to stratify patients by 10-year risk and treat risk factors accordingly	<u>If any macular edema, CVD or patients >40 years of age with another CVD risk factor</u>[a]: • Begin ACE-inhibitor, ASA and statin therapy (if not contraindicated) <u>In patients with prior MI:</u> • Add beta-blockers (if not contraindicated)

Abbreviations: Non-proliferative diabetic retinopathy (NPDR); proliferative diabetic retinopathy (PDR); distal symmetric polyneuropathy (DPN); cardiovascular disease (CVD); myocardial infarction (MI)

[a]*CVD risk factors include hypertension, family history, dyslipidemia, microalbuminuria, cardiac autonomic neuropathy or smoking.*

the morbidity and mortality associated with T1D. The major risk in T1D is for microvascular complications, although macrovascular complications are also increased later in the course of disease. The primary early risk factor is hyperglycemia, although other risk factors, including hypertension and dyslipidemia, may occur as a result of uncontrolled hyperglycemia or renal disease. Thus, in contrast to T2D, complications in T1D are usually acquired after diagnosis. The key to reducing the impact of diabetic complications is to optimize blood glucose and blood pressure control, institute appropriate screening and commence treatment when indicated (see Table 16). Diabetes complications are discussed in greater detail elsewhere in this education review, but T1D-specific screening and treatment guidelines for adults are shown in Table 16.

Monitoring for other autoimmune diseases

Several autoimmune disorders occur with increased frequency in patients with T1D. For example, patients with T1D are at high risk for the development of autoimmune thyroid disease, with 15%-30% of patients manifesting clinical disease

and 25% manifesting thyroid autoantibody positivity.[193] For this reason, the practitioner needs to be aware of the signs and symptoms of the associated autoimmune diseases, and be knowledgeable about screening recommendations in asymptomatic patients. Autoimmune disorders that are associated with T1D include, in order of frequency: thyroid disease (autoimmune hypo- and hyperthyroidism), celiac disease, pernicious anemia (vitamin B12 deficiency) and Addison's disease (autoimmune adrenal insufficiency). A summary of these disorders and screening recommendations for adults with T1D are shown in Table 17.

Transplantation

Transplantation is a treatment option that may be considered for certain patients with T1D. 2 types of transplantation can be performed: islet transplantation and whole organ (pancreas alone, simultaneous pancreas-kidney or pancreas after kidney) transplantation. The decision to refer a patient for transplantation should be made based on knowledge of the patient criteria, and the risks and benefits of each procedure.

Table 17

T1D-associated Autoimmune Disorders and Screening Recommendations for Adults with T1D

Disease	Autoantibody	Disease frequency in the general population	Disease frequency in T1D	Recommendation for screening	References
Autoimmune thyroid disease	TPO, Tg	<1% overt, 5% subclinical	15%-30%	<u>Diagnosis:</u> • In patients who become symptomatic measure TSH and free thyroxine <u>Screening:</u> • Measure TPO and Tg Abs at diagnosis • Meausre THS after metabolic control has been established and repeat every 3 years (or sooner if suspicious symptoms develop)	163, 194
Celiac disease	TTg, EMA	0.3%-1%	1%-16%	<u>Diagnosis:</u> • In patients who become symptomatic, measure TTg Abs or EMA + IgA levels • Consider small bowel biopsy when clinical suspicion is high and Abs are negative • Considser evaluation for difficult to manage hypothyroidism, early unexplained fracture and iron deficiency anemia (especially in males) <u>Screening:</u> • In children, measure Abs at diagnosis and consider periodic subsequent measures	65, 163

(continued)

Table 17 (continued)

T1D-associated Autoimmune Disorders and Screening Recommendations for Adults with T1D

Disease	Autoantibody	Disease frequency in the general population	Disease frequency in T1D	Recommendation for screening	References
Autoimmune gastritis/ Pernicious anemia	PCA	2%/0.1%-2%	6%/2.5%-4%	Diagnosis: • In patients who become symptomatic: measure iron, vitamin B12 levels, a complete blood count and gastrin levels • Consider evaluation in patients with early onset or unexplained neuropathy Screening: • Some authors recommend measurement of PCA at diagnosis and periodically thereafter, but there is no consensus on this practice	195, 196
Addison's Disease	21-OH	0.005%	<0.5%	Diagnosis (ACTH stimulation test): • Evaluate in patients who become symptomatic • Consider evaluation in the case of unexplained hypoglycemia Screening (21-OH Abs): • When other autoimmune diseases are present consider screening 1x (ie, at diagnosis)	65, 197

Abbreviations: Thyroid peroxidase (TPO), thyroglobulin (Tg), autoantibodies (Abs) thyroid stimulating hormone (TSH), tissue transglutaminase (TTg), Endomysial antibodies (EMA), parietal cell antibodies (PCA), 21-hydroxylase (21-OH)

Islet transplantation involves the transfer of insulin-secreting beta-cells from cadaveric donor pancreases into the recipient's portal vein, for the purpose of restoring endogenous insulin secretion. Candidates for islet transplantation include: patients with frequent episodes of severe hypoglycemia in the setting of hypoglycemia unawareness, those with severe glycemic variability and those with progressive diabetic complications, in spite of optimized insulin and other non-insulin therapies. A great advance in this field was made in the late 1990s, with the publication of the *Edmonton protocol*, in which islet transplantation using a steroid-free immunosuppressive regimen led to insulin independence in 100% (n=7) of subjects enrolled in the study.[198] This report generated a great deal of excitement among the T1D community; unfortunately, the excellent outcome of the patients in that trial proved very difficult to replicate in other, less experienced transplantation centers. In addition, in a follow-up, international, multicenter trial following the Edmonton protocol, only 58% of patients achieved insulin independence and this was not sustainable in the majority of patients.[199] The reasons for the decline or loss of islet function are under investigation, and may include immunosuppressive toxicity, allo- or recurrent autoimmune rejection or islet cell apoptosis.[200] The good news is that, even with a decline in rates of insulin independence, most patients (80%) maintain production of C-peptide, which has important implications for glycemic variability and risk for hypoglycemia.[201] Thus, at this time, it is unclear whether the successes of islet transplantation in a few specialized centers are generalizable, and there are several challenges that need to be overcome in order for this therapy to transition from an investigational therapy to a common clinical procedure (see Table 18).

Whole organ pancreas transplantation alone (PTA), simultaneous pancreas-kidney (SPK) and pancreas after kidney (PAK) transplantation are other options for T1D patients with complications from their disease, in particular end-stage renal disease. Eligibility criteria for SPK includes T1D with end-stage renal disease on dialysis, or expected to require dialysis in the next 12 months. Eligibility criteria for solitary pancreas transplant includes T1D with (PAK) or without (PTA) a prior kidney transplantation, with debilitating, frequent severe hypoglycemia. The majority (78%) of pancreas transplantations are performed in combination with a kidney transplantation, with 16% PAK and 7% solitary PTA.[202] While the first SPK and PTA procedures were performed in the 1960s, the history of pancreas transplantation has been fraught with technical challenges, including the management of pancreas exocrine drainage, duct management, venous failure and toxic effects of immunosuppressive regimens.[203] Recent advances in immunosuppression and surgical techniques have improved the overall outcomes of these procedures, with 1-year pancreas graft survival rates of >80%-85%.[202] Compared with islet transplantation, whole organ transplantations are much more invasive and thus confer higher mortality rates (~5% survival at 1 year).[202] The population for whom solid organ pancreas transplantation is optimal is those individuals with end-stage renal disease, in whom renal transplantation is the preferred treatment over dialysis. Importantly, the combination of SPK compared to renal transplantation alone has been shown to increase the chances of long-term renal allograft and patient survival.[204] In addition, long-term studies have shown that pancreas transplantation decreases progression of, or improves, most diabetic end-organ complications.[205] Thus, when determining whether transplantation is the best option for a particular patient, many factors must be taken into consideration.

Table 18

Benefits and Challenges of Islet Transplantation

Benefits	Challenges
• Initial insulin independence is achieved in a majority of patients (1-year insulin independence rates currently ~75% [REF])	• Usually at least 2 donor pancreases are required for each islet transplant recipient
• Even with a decline in graft function over time, most patients (80%) remain C-peptide positive	• The procedure can only be performed at transplant centers with specific experience
• Long-term benefits of physiologic insulin secretion in those who maintain graft function, including reduction in complications (theoretical benefit: not proven)	• Requires toxic immunosuppressive therapy
	• Gradual decline in insulin independence rates over time (5-year insulin independence rates ~10%)
• Immediate and long-term benefits of decreased glycemic variability	
	• Procedure-associated adverse events include: abdominal pain/nausea (>50%), intraperitoneal hemorrhage (10%) and mucosal ulceration (96%)
• Less invasive than whole pancreas transplantation; thus generally safer	

7. Prevention of T1D

The prevention of T1D is not yet possible, but this is the thrust of many research projects at the current time. The goals of prevention are 3-fold: first, to prevent T1D in genetically at-risk individuals who have no evidence of autoimmunity at the start of the trial (primary prevention); second, to prevent T1D onset in genetically at-risk individuals who already have evidence of ongoing autoimmunity (ie, the presence of DAAs) but do not yet have diabetes; and third, to halt or reverse the autoimmune process in individuals with recent-onset diabetes, with the goal to preserve beta-cell function.

The prevention of the initial development of autoimmunity in genetically at-risk individuals would be the ideal means of preventing T1D. However, this is a very difficult task, because it requires an intervention in a large population of individuals, of whom a very small number would normally progress to develop T1D. One proposed prevention strategy is the use of vitamin D supplementation in infancy and early childhood, a strategy that has received recent attention in the literature (see Table 8). No prospective studies have evaluated the influence of vitamin D on the underlying genetic propensity for T1D, but the evidence to date is compelling, and the American Academy

Table 19

Completed Secondary Prevention Trials in T1D

Prevention	Trial	Did the Strategy Prevent T1D?	References
Completed trials			
Parenteral insulin	Diabetes prevention trial type 1 (DPT-1)-completed	• No. Low-dose insulin injections do not prevent T1D in people with completed impaired insulin secretion who have a high (≥50%) risk of developing diabetes in 5 years	208
Oral insulin	Diabetes prevention trial type 1 (DPT-1)-completed	• No. Oral insulin does not delay or prevent T1D in individuals at moderaterisk (26%-50%) of developing diabetes in 5 years • In a subgroup with high insulin autoantibody levelss, there wa the	209
Nasal insulin	Type 1 Diabetes Prediction and Prevention study (DIPP)- completed	• No. Administration of nasal insulin, started soon after the detection of autoantibodies, did not prevent or delay T1D in children at moderate-to-high risk of developing diabetes	210
Nicotinamide	European Nicotinamide Diabetes Intervention Trial (ENDIT)	• No. Nicotinamide did not prevent or delay the development of T1D in moderate risk (40%) of developing diabetes in 5 years	211

of Pediatrics has recommended that infants who are exclusively breast-fed (unlike formula, breast milk contains very little vitamin D) should receive daily vitamin D supplementation.[206] Another topic of primary prevention for T1D that has long been debated in the literature is the issue of early infant diet; in particular, early exposure to cow's milk proteins. (See Section 5 and Table 8). An international, multicenter, randomized, controlled trial, the Trial to Reduce Insulin-dependent diabetes mellitus in the Genetically at Risk (TRIGR), is currently underway to test the hypothesis that hydrolyzed infant formula, compared to cow's milk-based formula, decreases risk of developing T1D in children with increased genetic susceptibility. Recruitment for this trial ended in 2006, and children are being followed until they reach 10 years of age.

A third primary prevention strategy that is currently being tested is the use of docosahexaenoic acid, or DHA, an omega-3 fatty acid found in some foods, such as pumpkin seeds, coldwater fish, soybeans, walnuts and eggs. It is hypothesized that DHA may have anti-inflammatory benefits which prevents development of the autoimmunity that leads to type 1 diabetes. A recent study found that dietary intake of omega-3 fatty acids was associated with reduced risk of DAAs in children who were at increased genetic risk for T1D.[207] A pilot study (the Nutritional Intervention to Prevent Diabetes [NIP] Study) is currently underway to test this hypothesis.

As far as preventing the progression to T1D in genetically at-risk individuals who already manifest evidence of an ongoing autoimmune process, no interventions have been successful to date. These studies are summarized in Table 19, and studies that are underway or in planning stages are summarized in Table 20.

A final prevention strategy is the treatment of new onset patients with an agent that is intended to halt or reverse the autoimmune process, with the result of preserving the remaining beta-cells (Table 21). Early studies examining the effect of agents such as cyclosporine and azathioprine on new-onset T1D found that these agents did increase remission rates and preserve beta-cell function. However, this occurred at the expense of serious side effects (nephrotoxicity, in the case of cyclosporine), and the beneficial effect did not last after discontinuing the immunomodulatory agent.

Table 20

Trials Underway and in Planning Stages for Secondary Prevention of T1D

Intervention	Objective
Oral insulin in individuals with high IAA Levels	Determine whether oral insulin will prevent or delay the development of clinical T1D in IAA-positive non-diabetic relatives of patients with T1D who do not have a metabolic defect
GAD-Alum	Determine whether GAD-Alum vaccine will prevent or delay the development of clinical T1D in non-diabetic GAD65Ab-positive relatives of patients with T1D
anti-CD3	Determine whether anti-CD3 will prevent or delay the development of clinical T1D in non-diabetic relatives of patients with T1D who have dysglycemia, and are thus at very high risk for developing T1D

Table 21

Trials in Newly Diagnosed T1D to Prevent Further Loss of C-peptide

Agent	Did the strategy halt or reverse the autoimmune process?	References
Cyclosporine	• Yes, increased rate of remission, enhanced insulin secretion • Caveats: effects not sustained when immunotherapy was discontinued; side effects were intolerable (nephrotoxicity)	212-214
Azathioprine ± glucocorticoids	• Yes, increased rate of remission, enhanced insulin secretion • C–aveat: effects not sustained when immunotherapy was discontinued	215-217
Anti-CD3	• Y–es, preserves residual beta-cell function in patients with recent-onset T1D	77, 218
GAD-Alum	• Y–es, preserves residual insulin secretion in patients with recent-onset T1D • Larger study in planning stages	219
DiaPep277	• Y–es, preserves beta-cell function in patients with recent onset T1D	220
Anti-CD20 (Rituximab)	• Unknown, study underway	
CTLA-4 Ig (Abatacept)	• Unknown, study underway	
Early intensive glucose control	• Insulin treatment in T1D at the time of disease onset can preserve β-cell function • Patients in the DCCT trial who were randomized to intensive insulin therapy maintained higher stimulated C-peptide levels compared with those individuals assigned to conventional therapy • Larger, definitive study in planning stages	221 222
MMF/DZB	• Unknown, study underway	

8. Conclusions

Some recent studies, including those testing anti-CD3 and GAD-Alum have shown promising results with regards to the preservation of beta-cell function, but these studies have been small and require further proof that the benefits outweigh the risks. Several studies testing other prevention strategies in newly diagnosed patients are currently underway, under the direction of the NIH-funded TrialNet consortium.

No prevention strategies are yet ready for general clinical application. However, every trial teaches us more about the pathogenesis of T1D and paves the way for studying better, more directed prevention strategies. Hopefully, some successful strategies will emerge over the next decade, so that T1D will become a preventable disease, or at least 1 that can be stabilized early to prevent the progression to complications.

Type 1 diabetes is a T-cell dependent autoimmune disease, characterized by the autoimmune destruction of the insulin-producing beta-cells in the pancreas. Both genetics and environmental factors contribute to the development of T1D, although environmental factors are currently playing a more prominent role, as evidenced by the widespread "epidemic" that has occurred over the past several decades. Treatment recommendations are based on the findings from the DCCT trial, which showed that achieving near-normal glycemic levels with the use of intensive insulin therapy was associated with a significant reduction in the long-term complications of diabetes. Importantly, the DCCT trial was performed with a multi-disciplinary team, which is still the model we use for the treatment of T1D today. Thus, patients with T1D should be treated with physiological insulin regimens (MDI or CSII) in order to reach this goal of near-normal blood glucose levels. In addition to managing glycemic control, the diabetes practitioner must monitor for diabetes complications, as well as for other associated autoimmune diseases. In patients with severe hypoglycemia or end-stage renal disease, islet or pancreas-kidney transplants may be considered. Finally, the ideal treatment for T1D would be prevention, and several trials are underway with the goals of preventing the development of autoimmunity, preventing progression of autoimmunity or preserving beta-cell function in patients with new-onset T1D.

9. References

1. American Diabetes Association. Diagnosis and Classification of Diabetes Mellitus. *Diabetes Care*. 2009;32(Supplement 1):S62-S67.

2. Kibirige M, Metcalf B, Renuka R, Wilkin TJ. Testing the accelerator hypothesis: The relationship between body mass and age at diagnosis of type 1 diabetes. *Diabetes Care*. 2003;26(10):2865-2870.

3. Wilkin TJ. Diabetes mellitus: Type 1 or type 2? The accelerator hypothesis. *J Pediatr*. 2002;141(3):449-450.

4. Becker D, Libman I, Pietropaolo M, Dosch M, Arslanian S, LaPorte R. Changing phenotype of IDDM. Is it type 1 or type 2? *Pediatric Research*. 2001;49:93A.

5. Banerji MA, Chaiken RL, Huey H, et al. GAD antibody negative NIDDM in adult black subjects with diabetic ketoacidosis and increased frequency of human leukocyte antigen DR3 and DR4: Flatbush diabetes. *Diabetes*. 1994;43(6):741-745.

6. Dabelea D, Bell RA, D'Agostino RB, Jr, et al. Incidence of diabetes in youth in the United States. *JAMA*. 2007;297(24):2716-2724.

7. Molbak AG, Christau B, Marner B, Borch-Johnsen K, Nerup J. Incidence of insulin-dependent diabetes mellitus in age groups over 30 years in Denmark. *Diabet Med*. 1994;11(7):650-655.

8. Stenstrom G, Gottsater A, Bakhtadze E, Berger B, Sundkvist G. Latent Autoimmune Diabetes in Adults: Definition, Prevalence, {beta}-Cell Function, and Treatment. *Diabetes*. 2005;54(suppl 2):S68-S72.

9. Pihoker C LJ, Dolan L, Williams D, et al for the SEARCH for Diabetes in Youth Study Group. Biochemical vs provider-assigned diabetes type in youth: a population-based assessment. *Diabetes*. 2005; 54(supple 1):A458.

10. Monge L, Bruno G, Pinach S, et al. A clinically orientated approach increases the efficiency of screening for latent autoimmune diabetes in adults (LADA) in a large clinic-based cohort of patients with diabetes onset over 50 years. *Diabetic Medicine*. 2004;21(5):456-459.

11. Juneja R, Hirsch IB, Naik RG, Brooks-Worrell BM, Greenbaum CJ, Palmer JP. Islet cell antibodies and glutamic acid decarboxylase antibodies, but not the clinical phenotype, help to identify type 1[frac12] diabetes in patients presenting with type 2 diabetes*1. Metabolism. 2001;50(9):1008-1013.

12. Genovese S, Bazzigaluppi E, Goncalves D, et al. Clinical phenotype and {beta}-cell autoimmunity in Italian patients with adult-onset diabetes. *Eur J Endocrinol*. 2006;154(3):441-447.

13. Gilliam LK, Palmer JP, Lernmark Å. Autoantibodies and the disease process of type 1 diabetes mellitus. In: LeRoith D, Taylor SI, Olefsky JM, eds. Diabetes Mellitus: A fundamental and clinical text. Philadelphia, PA: Lippincott Williams & Wilkins; 2004: 499-518.

14. Gilliam LK, Palmer JP. How useful is autoantibody screening in adult-onset diabetes? *Nat Clin Pract Endocrinol Metab*. 2006;2(9):490-491.

15. Irvine WJ, McCallum CJ, Gray RS, Duncan LJ. Clinical and pathogenic significance of pancreatic-islet-cell antibodies in diabetics treated with oral hypoglycaemic agents. *Lancet*. 1977;1(8020):1025-1027.

16. Di Mario U, Irvine WJ, Borsey DQ, Kyner JL, Weston J, Galfo C. Immune abnormalities in diabetic patients not requiring insulin at diagnosis. *Diabetologia*. 1983;25:392-395.

17. Groop LC, Bottazzo GF, Doniach D. Islet cell antibodies identify latent type I diabetes in patients aged 35-75 years at diagnosis. *Diabetes*. 1986;35(2):237-241.

18. Hagopian WA, Karlsen AE, Gottsater A, et al. Quantitative assay using recombinant human islet glutamic acid decarboxylase (GAD65) shows that 64K autoantibody positivity at onset predicts diabetes type. *J Clin Invest*. 1993;91(1):368-374.

19. Turner R, Stratton I, Horton V, et al. UKPDS 25: Autoantibodies to islet-cell cytoplasm and glutamic acid decarboxylase for prediction of insulin requirement in type 2 diabetes. UK Prospective Diabetes Study Group. *Lancet*. 1997;350(9087):1288-1293.

20. Littorin B, Sundkvist G, Hagopian W, et al. Islet cell and glutamic acid decarboxylase antibodies present at diagnosis of diabetes predict the need for insulin treatment. A cohort study in young adults whose disease was initially labeled as type 2 or unclassifiable diabetes. *Diabetes Care*. 1999;22(3):409-412.

21. Gottsater A, Landin-Olsson M, Fernlund P, Lernmark A, Sundkvist G. Beta-cell function in relation to islet cell antibodies during the first 3 yr after clinical diagnosis of diabetes in type 2 diabetic patients. *Diabetes Care*. 1993;16(6):902-910.

22. Niskanen LK, Tuomi T, Karjalainen J, Groop LC, Uusitupa MI. GAD antibodies in NIDDM. Ten-year follow-up from the diagnosis. *Diabetes Care*. 1995;18(12):1557-1565.

23. Borg H, Gottsater A, Landin-Olsson M, Fernlund P, Sundkvist G. High levels of antigen-specific islet antibodies predict future beta-cell failure in patients with onset of diabetes in adult age. *J Clin Endocrinol Metab*. 2001;86(7):3032-3038.

24. Borg H, Gottsater A, Fernlund P, Sundkvist G. A 12-year prospective study of the relationship between islet antibodies and beta-cell function at and after the diagnosis in patients with adult-onset diabetes. *Diabetes*. 2002;51(6):1754-1762.

25. Gilliam LK, Palmer JP. Latent autoimmune diabetes in adults. *Insulin*. 2006;1(3):122-127.

26. Karvonen M, Viik-Kajander M, Moltchanova E, Libman I, LaPorte R, Tuomilehjto J. Incidence of childhood type 1 diabetes worldwide. Diabetes Mondiale (DiaMond) Project Group. *Diabetes Care*. 2000;23:1516-1526.

27. Harjutsalo V, Sjöberg L, Tuomilehto J. Time trends in the incidence of type 1 diabetes in Finnish children: a cohort study. *Lancet*. 2008; 371(9626):1777-1782.

28. EURODIAB ASG. Variation and trends in incidence of childhood diabetes in Europe. *Lancet*. 2000;355(9207):873-876.

29. Green A, Patterson CC. Trends in the incidence of childhood-onset diabetes in Europe 1989-1998. *Diabetologia*. 2001;44(suppl 3):B3-B8.

30. Diabetes Epidemiology Research International Group. Geographic patterns of childhood insulin-dependent diabetes mellitus. *Diabetes*. 1988; 37(8):1113-1119.

31. Green A, Gale EA, Patterson CC. Incidence of childhood-onset insulin-dependent diabetes mellitus: the EURODIAB ACE Study. *Lancet*. 1992;339(8798):905-909.

32. Karvonen M, Pitkaniemi M, Pitkaniemi J, Kohtamaki K, Tajima N, Tuomilehto J. Sex difference in the incidence of insulin-dependent diabetes mellitus: an analysis of the recent epidemiological data. World Health Organization DIAMOND Project Group. *Diabetes Metab Rev*. 1997; 13(4):275-291.

33. Gale EA, Gillespie KM. Diabetes and gender. *Diabetologia*. 2001;44(1):3-15.

34. Östman J, Lönnberg G, Arnqvist HJ, et al. Gender differences and temporal variation in the incidence of type 1 diabetes: results of 8012 cases in the nationwide Diabetes Incidence Study in Sweden. *Journal of Internal Medicine*. 2008;263(4):386-394.

35. Blom L, Dahlquist G, Nyström L, Sandstrom A, Wall S. The Swedish childhood diabetes study--social and perinatal determinants for diabetes in childhood. *Diabetologia*. 1989;32(1):7-13.

36. Harjutsalo V, Reunanen A, Tuomilehto J. Differential transmission of type 1 diabetes from diabetic fathers and mothers to their offspring. *Diabetes*. 2006;55(5):1517-1524.

37. Bingley PJ, Douek IF, Rogers CA, Gale EA. Influence of maternal age at delivery and birth order on risk of type 1 diabetes in childhood: prospective population based family study. Bart's-Oxford Family Study Group. *BMJ*. 2000;321(7258):420-424.

38. Bottini N, Meloni GF, Lucarelli P, et al. Risk of type 1 diabetes in childhood and maternal age at delivery, interaction with ACPI and sex. *Diabetes Metab Res Rev*. 2005; 21(4):353-358.

39. Tuomilehto J, Podar T, Tuomilehto-Wolf E, Virtala E. Evidence for importance of gender and birth cohort for risk of IDDM in off-spring of IDDM parents. *Diabetologia*. 1995;38(8):975-982.

40. Tedeschi A, Airaghi L. Is affluence a risk factor for bronchial asthma and type 1 diabetes? Pediatric *Allergy and Immunology*. 2006;17(7):533-537.

41. Betterle C, Lazzarotto F, Presotto F. Autoimmune polyglandular syndrome Type 2: the tip of an iceberg? *Clin Exper Immunol*. 2004;137(2):225-233.

42. Carpenter C, Solomon N, Silverberg S, et al. Schmidt's syndrome (thyroid and adrenal insufficiency): a review of the literature and a report of fifteen new cases including ten instances of coexistent diabetes mellitus. *Medicine*. 1964;43:153-180.

43. Weichselbaum A. Über die Veränderungen des Pankreas bei Diabetes Mellitus. Sitzungsber. Akad. Wiss. Wien, Math. Naturw. Klasse. 1910; 119:73-281.

44. von Meyenburg H. Über "Insulitis" bei Diabetes. Schweitz Med Wochenschr. 1940;21:554-561.

45. Gepts W. Pathologic anatomy of the pancreas in juvenile diabetes mellitus. *Diabetes*. 1965;14:619-633.

46. Gepts W, De Mey J. Islet cell survival determined by morphology. *Diabetes*. 1978;27:251-261.

47. Gorsuch AN, Spencer KM, Lister J, et al. Evidence for a long prediabetic period in Type 1 (insulin-dependent) diabetes mellitus. *Lancet*. 1981;ii:1363-1365.

48. Landin-Olsson M, Karlsson A, Dahlquist G, Blom L, Lernmark Å, Sundkvist G. Islet cell and other organ-specific autoantibodies in all children developing type 1 (insulin-dependent) diabetes mellitus in Sweden during one year and in matched controls. *Diabetologia*. 1989; 32:387-395.

49. Bekris LM, Kavanagh TJ, Lernmark A. Targeting type 1 diabetes before and at the clinical onset of disease. Endocr Metab Immune *Disord Drug Targets*. 2006;6(1):103-124.

50. Sosenko JM, Palmer JP, Greenbaum CJ, Mahon J, Cowie C, Krischer JP, et al. Patterns of metabolic progression to type 1 diabetes in the diabetes prevention trial-type 1. *Diabetes Care*. 2006;29(3):643-649.

51. Pihoker C, Gilliam LK, Hampe CS, Lernmark A. Autoantibodies in diabetes. *Diabetes*. 2005;54(suppl 2):S52-S61.

52. Silveira PA, Grey ST. B cells in the spotlight: innocent bystanders or major players in the pathogenesis of type 1 diabetes. *Trends Endocrin Metab*. 2006;17(4):128-135.

53. Anderson MS. Update in Endocrine Autoimmunity. *J Clin Endocrinol Metab*. 2008;93(10):3663-3670.

54. Vafiadis P, Bennett S, Todd J, et al. Insulin expression in human thymus is modulated by INS VNTR alleles at the IDDM2 locus. *Nature Genetics*. 1997;15:289-292.

55. Maclaren NK, Alkinson MA. Insulin-dependent diabetes mellitus: the hypothesis of molecular mimicry between islet cell antigens and microorganisms. *Mol Med Today*. 1997;3(2):76-83.

56. Roep BO, Hiemstra HS, Schloot NC, et al. Molecular mimicry in type 1 diabetes: immune cross-reactivity between islet autoantigen and human cytomegalovirus but not coxsackie virus. *Ann NY Acad Sci*. 2002;958(1):163-165.

57. Horwitz MS, Bradley LM, Harbertson J, Krahl T, Lee J, Sarvetnick N. Diabetes induced by Coxsackie virus: initiation by bystander damage and not molecular mimicry. *Nat Med*. 1998;4(7):781-785.

58. Debray-Sachs M, Carnaud C, Boitard C, et al. Prevention of diabetes in NOD mice treated with antibody to murine IFN[gamma]. *J Autoimmun*. 1991;4(2):237-248.

59. Healey D, Ozegbe P, Arden S, Chandler P, Hutton J, Cooke A. In vivo activity and in vitro specificity of CD4+ Th1 and Th2 cells derived from the spleens of diabetic NOD mice. *J Clin Invest*. 1995;95(6):2979-2985.

60. Katz J, Benoist C, Mathis D. T helper cell subsets in insulin-dependent diabetes. *Science*. 1995;268(5214):1185-1188.

61. Trembleau S, Penna G, Gregori S, Giarratana N, Adorini L. IL-12 administration accelerates autoimmune diabetes in both wild-type and IFN-{gamma}-deficient nonobese diabetic mice, revealing pathogenic and protective effects of IL-12-induced IFN-{gamma}. *J Immunol*. 2003;170(11):5491-5501.

62. Arif S, Tree TI, Astill TP, et al. Autoreactive T cell responses show proinflammatory polarization in diabetes but a regulatory phenotype in health. *J Clin Invest*. 2004;113(3):451-463.

63. Itoh N, Hanafusa T, Miyazaki A, et al. Mononuclear cell infiltration and its relation to the expression of major histocompatibility complex antigens and adhesion molecules in pancreas biopsy specimens from newly diagnosed insulin-dependent diabetes mellitus patients. *J Clin Invest*. 1993;92:2313-2322.

64. You S, Alyanakian M-A, Segovia B, et al. Immunoregulatory Pathways Controlling Progression of Autoimmunity in NOD Mice. *Annals of the New York Academy of Sciences*. 2008;1150(Immunology of Diabetes V From Bench to Bedside):300-310.

65. Barker JM. Type 1 diabetes-associated autoimmunity: natural history, genetic associations, and screening. *J Clin Endocrinol Metab*. 2006;91(4):1210-1217.

66. Perheentupa J. Autoimmune Polyendocrinopathy-Candidiasis-Ectodermal Dystrophy. *J Clin Endocrinol Metab*. 2006;91(8):2843-2850.

67. Nagamine K, Peterson P, Scott HS, et al. Positional cloning of the APECED gene. *Nat Genet*. 1997; 17(4):393-398.

68. Ochs HD, Gambineri E, Torgerson TR. IPEX, FOXP3 and regulatory T-cells: a model for autoimmunity. *Immunol Res*. 2007;38(1-3):112-121.

69. Hori S, Nomura T, Sakaguchi S. Control of regulatory T cell development by the transcription factor Foxp3. *Science*. 2003;299(5609):1057-1061.

70. Fontenot JD, Gavin MA, Rudensky AY. Foxp3 programs the development and function of CD4+CD25+ regulatory T cells. *Nat Immunol*. 2003;4(4):330-336.

71. Sakaguchi S, Yamaguchi T, Nomura T, Ono M. Regulatory T cells and immune tolerance. *Cell*. 2008;133(5):775-787.

72. Nerup J, Binder C. Thyroid, gastric and adrenal autoimmunity in diabetes mellitus. *Acta Endocrinol*. 1973;72:279-286.

73. MacCuish AC, Irvine WJ. Autoimmunological aspects of diabetes mellitus. *Clin Endocrinol Metab*. 1975;4:435-471.

74. Nerup J, Andersen OO, Bendixen G, Egeberg J, Poulsen JE. Antipancreatic cellular hypersensitivity in diabetes mellitus. *Diabetes*. 1971; 20:424-427.

75. Nerup J, Andersen OO, Bendixen G. Antipancreatic cellular hypersensitivity in diabetes mellitus. Experimental induction of an antipancreatic, cellular hypersensitivity and associated morphological β-cell changes in the rat. *Acta Endocrinol (Copenh)*. 1973;28:231-249.

76. Bougneres PF, Carel JC, Castano L, et al. Factors associated with early remission of type 1 diabetes in children treated with cyclosporine. *N Engl J Med*. 1988;318:663-667.

77. Herold KC, Hagopian W, Auger JA, et al. Anti-CD3 monoclonal antibody in new-onset type 1 diabetes mellitus. *N Engl J Med*. 2002;346(22):1692-1698.

78. Roep BO. Diabetes: Missing links. *Nature*. 2007;450(7171):799-800.

79. Bluestone JA, Tang Q. Therapeutic vaccination using CD4+CD25+ antigen-specific regulatory T cells. Proceedings of the National Academy of Sciences of the United States of America. 2004;101(suppl 2):14622-14626.

80. Putnam AL, Brusko TM, Lee MR, et al. Expansion of human regulatory T-cells from patients with type 1 diabetes. *Diabetes*. 2009;58(3):652-662.

81. Lanzavecchia A. Receptor-mediated antigen uptake and its effect on antigen presentation to class 11-restricted T lymphocytes. *Annu Rev Immunol*. 1990;8:773-793.

82. Rewers M, Norris JM, Eisenbarth GS, et al. Beta-cell autoantibodies in infants and toddlers without IDDM relatives: diabetes autoimmunity study in the young (DAISY). *J Autoimmun*. 1996;9(3):405-410.

83. Kimpimaki T, Kulmala P, Savola K, et al. Natural history of {beta}-cell autoimmunity in young children with increased genetic susceptibility to type 1 diabetes recruited from the general population. *J Clin Endocrinol Metab*. 2002;87(10):4572-4579.

84. Verge CF, Gianani R, Kawasaki E, et al. Prediction of type I diabetes in first-degree relatives using a combination of insulin, GAD, and ICA512bdc/IA-2 autoantibodies. *Diabetes*. 1996;45(7):926-933.

85. Bottazzo GF, Florin-Christensen A, Doniach D. Islet cell antibodies in diabetes mellitus with autoimmune polyendocrine deficiencies. *Lancet*. 1974;2:1279-1283.

119. Knerr I, Wolf J, Reinehr T, et al. The 'accelerator hypothesis': relationship between weight, height, body mass index and age at diagnosis in a large cohort of 9248 German and Austrian children with type 1 diabetes mellitus. *Diabetologia*. 2005; 48(12):2501-2504.

120. Kordonouri O, Hartmann R. Higher body weight is associated with earlier onset of Type 1 diabetes in children: confirming the 'Accelerator Hypothesis'. *Diabetic Medicine*. 2005;22(12):1783-1784.

121. Dabelea D, D'Agostino RB Jr, Mayer-Davis EJ, et al. Testing the accelerator hypothesis: body size, {beta}-cell function, and age at onset of type 1 (autoimmune) diabetes. *Diabetes Care*. 2006; 29(2):290-294.

122. Wilkin TJ. Diabetes: 1 and 2, or one and the same? Progress with the accelerator hypothesis. *Pediatric Diabetes*. 2008; 9(3:2):23-32.

123. Cronin CC, Shanahan F. Insulin-dependent diabetes mellitus and coeliac disease. *Lancet*. 1997;349(9058):1096-1097.

124. Ventura A, Neri E, Ughi C, Leopaldi A, Città A, Not T. Gluten-dependent diabetes-related and thyroid-related autoantibodies in patients with celiac disease. *Pediatrics*. 2000;137(2):263-265.

125. Norris JM, Barriga K, Klingensmith G, et al. Timing of initial cereal exposure in infancy and risk of islet autoimmunity. *JAMA*. 2003;290(13):1713-1720.

126. Gillespie KM. Type 1 diabetes: pathogenesis and prevention. *CMAJ*. 2006;175(2):165-170.

127. Littorin B, Blom P, Schölin A, et al. Lower levels of plasma 25-hydroxyvitamin D among young adults at diagnosis of autoimmune type 1 diabetes compared with control subjects: results from the nationwide Diabetes Incidence Study in Sweden (DISS). *Diabetologia*. 2006;49(12):2847-2852.

128. Pozzilli P, Manfrini S, Crino A, et al. Low levels of 25-hydroxyvitamin D3 and 1,25-dihydroxyvitamin D3 in patients with newly diagnosed type 1 diabetes. *Horm Metab Res*. 2005;37(11):680-683.

129. Zipitis CS, Akobeng AK. Vitamin D supplementation in early childhood and risk of type 1 diabetes: a systematic review and meta-analysis. *Arch Dis Child*. 2008;93(6):512-517.

130. Myers MA, Mackay IR, Zimmet PZ. Toxic Type 1 Diabetes. *Rev Endo Metab Dis*. 2003;4(3):225-231.

131. Gale E. A missing link in the hygiene hypothesis? *Diabetologia*. 2002;45(4):588-594.

132. Cooke A. Review series on helminths, immune modulation and the hygiene hypothesis: How might infection modulate the onset of type 1 diabetes? *Immunology*. 2009;126(1):12-17.

133. Jarosz-Chobot P, Polanska J, Polanski A. Does social and economical transformation influence the incidence of type 1 diabetes mellitus? A Polish example. *Pediatric Diabetes*. 2008;9(3:1):202-207.

134. Hviid A, Stellfeld M, Wohlfahrt J, Melbye M. Childhood vaccination and type 1 diabetes. *N Engl J Med*. 2004; 350(14):1398-1404.

135. Padaiga Z, Tuomilehto J, Karvonen M, et al. Seasonal variation in the incidence of Type 1 diabetes mellitus during 1983 to 1992 in the countries around the Baltic Sea. *Diabetic Medicine*. 1999;16(9):736-743.

136. Christau B, Kromann H, Christy M. Incidence of insulin-dependent diabetes mellitus (0-29 years at onset) in Denmark. *Acta Med Scand*. 1979; 624:54-60.

137. Nyström L, Dahlquist G, Rewers M, Wall S. The Swedish childhood diabetes study: an analysis of the temporal variation in diabetes incidence 1978-1987. *Int J Epidemiol*. 1990;19:141-146.

138. Joner G, Sovik O. The incidence of type 1 (insulin-dependent) diabetes mellitus 15-29 years in Norway 1978-1982. *Diabetologia*. 1991; 34(4):271-274.

139. Sepa A, Wahlberg J, Vaarala O, Frodi A, Ludvigsson J. Psychological stress may induce diabetes-related autoimmunity in infancy. *Diabetes Care*. 2005;28(2):290-295.

140. Menser MA, Forrest JM, Bransby RD. Rubella infection and diabetes mellitus. *Lancet*. 1978;1:57-60.

141. Ginsberg-Fellner F, Witt ME, Yagihashi S, et al. Congenital rubella syndrome as a model for type 1 (insulin-dependent) diabetes mellitus: increased prevalence of islet cell surface antibodies. *Diabetologia*. 1984;27(suppl):87-89.

142. Yoon JW, Austin M, Onodera T, Notkins AL. Virus-induced diabetes mellitus. Isolation of a virus from the pancreas of a child with diabetic ketoacidosis. *N Engl J Med*. 1979;300:1173-1179.

143. Atkinson MA, Bowman MA, Campbell L, Darrow BL, Kaufman DL, Maclaren NK. Cellular immunity to a determinant common to glutamate decarboxylase and coxsackie virus in insulin-dependent diabetes. *J Clin Invest*. 1994;94(5):2125-2129.

144. Lonnrot M, Korpela K, Knip M, et al. Enterovirus infection as a risk factor for beta-cell autoimmunity in a prospectively observed birth cohort: the Finnish Diabetes Prediction and Prevention Study. *Diabetes*. 2000;49(8):1314-1318.

145. Juhela S, Hyoty H, Hinkkanen A, et al. T cell responses to enterovirus antigens and to beta-cell autoantigens in unaffected children positive for IDDM-associated autoantibodies. *J Autoimmun*. 1999;12(4):269-278.

146. Yin H, Berg A-K, Tuvemo T, Frisk G. Enterovirus RNA Is Found in Peripheral Blood Mononuclear Cells in a Majority of Type 1 Diabetic Children at Onset. *Diabetes*. 2002;51(6):1964-1971.

147. Elfaitouri A, Berg A-K, Frisk G, Yin H, Tuvemo T, Blomberg J. Recent enterovirus infection in type 1 diabetes: Evidence with a novel IgM method. *Journal of Medical Virology*. 2007;79(12):1861-1867.

148. Hyöty H, Hiltunen M, Knip M, et al. A prospective study of the role of coxsackie B and other enterovirus infections in the pathogenesis of IDDM. Childhood Diabetes in Finland (DiMe) Study. *Diabetes*. 1995;44:652-657.

149. Kimpimaki T, Kupila A, Hamalainen AM, et al. The first signs of beta-cell autoimmunity appear in infancy in genetically susceptible children from the general population: the Finnish Type 1 Diabetes Prediction and Prevention Study. *J Clin Endocrinol Metab*. 2001;86(10):4782-4788.

150. Lonnrot M, Korpela K, Knip M, et al. Enterovirus infection as a risk factor for beta-cell autoimmunity in a prospectively observed birth cohort: the Finnish Diabetes Prediction and Prevention Study. *Diabetes*. 2000;49(8):1314-1318.

151. Salminen K, Sadeharju K, Lönnrot M, et al. Enterovirus infections are associated with the induction of beta-cell autoimmunity in a prospective birth cohort study. *Journal of Medical Virology*. 2003;69(1):91-98.

152. Ward KP, Galloway WH, Auchterlonie IA. Congenital cytomegalovirus infection and diabetes. *Lancet*. 1979;313(8114):497-497.

153. Pak C, McArthur RG, Eun H-M, Yoon J-W. Association of cytomegalovirus infection with autoimmune type I diabetes. *Lancet*. 1988;i:1-4.

154. Nicoletti F, Scalia G, Lunetta M, et al. Correlation between islet cell antibodies and anti-cytomegalovirus IgM and IgG antibodies in healthy first-degree relatives of type 1 (insulin-dependent) diabetic patients. *Clin Immunol Immunopathol*. 1990;55(1):139-147.

155. Helmke K, Otten A, Willems W. Islet cell antibodies in children with mumps infection. *Lancet*. 1980;ii:211-212.

156. Hyoty H, Leinikki P, Reunanen A, et al. Mumps infections in the etiology of type 1 (insulin-dependent) diabetes. *Diabetes Res*. 1988;9(3):111-116.

157. Honeyman MC, Coulson BS, Stone NL, et al. Association between rotavirus infection and pancreatic islet autoimmunity in children at risk of developing type 1 diabetes. *Diabetes*. 2000;49:1319-1324.

158. Blomqvist M, Juhela S, Erkkila S, et al. Rotavirus infections and development of diabetes-associated autoantibodies during the first 2 years of life. *Clin Exper Immunol*. 2002;128(3):511-515.

159. Honeyman MC, Stone NL, Harrison LC. T-cell epitopes in type 1 diabetes autoantigen tyrosine phosphatase IA-2: potential for mimicry with rotavirus and other environmental agents. *Mol Med*. 1998;4(4):231-239.

160. The Diabetes Control and Complications Trial Research Group. The effect of intensive treatment of diabetes on the development and progression of long-term complications in insulin-dependent diabetes mellitus. *N Engl J Med*. 1993;329(14):977-986.

161. The Writing Team for the Diabetes Control Complications Trial/Epidemiology of Diabetes Interventions Complications Research Group. Effect of intensive therapy on the microvascular complications of type 1 diabetes mellitus. *JAMA*. 2002;287(19):2563-2569.

162. The Diabetes Control Complications Trial/Epidemiology of Diabetes Interventions Complications Study Research Group. Intensive diabetes treatment and cardiovascular disease in patients with type 1 diabetes. *N Engl J Med*. 2005;353(25):2643-2653.

163. American Diabetes Association. Standards of medical care in diabetes--2009. *Diabetes Care*. 2009; 32(supple 1):S13-S61.

164. Lepore M, Pampanelli S, Fanelli C, et al. Pharmacokinetics and pharmacodynamics of subcutaneous injection of long-acting human insulin analog glargine, NPH insulin, and ultralente human insulin and continuous subcutaneous infusion of insulin lispro. *Diabetes*. 2000;49(12):2142-2148.

165. ter Braak EW, Woodworth JR, Bianchi R, et al. Injection site effects on the pharmacokinetics and glucodynamics of insulin lispro and regular insulin. *Diabetes Care*. 1996;19(12):1437-1440.

166. Binder C, Lauritzen T, Faber O, Pramming S. Insulin pharmacokinetics. *Diabetes Care*. 1984;7(2):188-199.

167. Francis AJ, Hanning I, Alberti KG. The influence of insulin antibody levels on the plasma profiles and action of subcutaneously injected human and bovine short acting insulins. *Diabetologia*. 1985;28(6):330-334.

168. Rabkin R, Ryan MP, Duckworth WC. The renal metabolism of insulin. *Diabetologia*. 1984;27(3):351-357.

169. Campbell PJ, Bolli GB, Cryer PE, Gerich JE. Pathogenesis of the dawn phenomenon in patients with insulin-dependent diabetes mellitus. Accelerated glucose production and impaired glucose utilization due to nocturnal surges in growth hormone secretion. *N Engl J Med*. 1985; 312(23):1473-1479.

170. Pickup J, Mattock M, Kerry S. Glycaemic control with continuous subcutaneous insulin infusion compared with intensive insulin injections in patients with type 1 diabetes: meta-analysis of randomised controlled trials. *BMJ*. 2002;324(7339):705.

171. Pickup JC, Sutton AJ. Severe hypoglycaemia and glycaemic control in Type 1 diabetes: meta-analysis of multiple daily insulin injections compared with continuous subcutaneous insulin infusion. *Diabetic Medicine*. 2008;25(7):765-774.

172. Heinemann L, Linkeschova R, Rave K, Hompesch B, Sedlak M, Heise T. Time-action profile of the long-acting insulin analog insulin glargine (HOE901) in comparison with those of NPH insulin and placebo. *Diabetes Care*. 2000;23(5):644-649.

173. Ratner R, Hirsch I, Neifing J, Garg S, Mecca T, Wilson C. Less hypoglycemia with insulin glargine in intensive insulin therapy for type 1 diabetes. U.S. Study Group of Insulin Glargine in Type 1 Diabetes. *Diabetes Care*. 2000;23(5):639-643.

174. Owens DR, Bolli GB. Beyond the era of NPH insulin — long-acting insulin analogs: chemistry, comparative pharmacology, and clinical application. *Diabetes Tech Therap*. 2008;10(5):333-349.

175. Porcellati F, Rossetti P, Busciantella NR, et al. Comparison of pharmacokinetics and dynamics of the long-acting insulin analogs glargine and detemir at steady state in type 1 diabetes: A double-blind, randomized, crossover study. *Diabetes Care*. 2007;30(10):2447-2452.

176. Heise T, Nosek L, Ronn BB, et al. Lower within-subject variability of insulin detemir in comparison to NPH insulin and insulin glargine in people with type 1 diabetes. *Diabetes*. 2004;53(6):1614-1620.

177. Rodbard HW, Blonde L, Braithwaite SS, et al. American Association of Clinical Endocrinologists medical guidelines for clinical practice for the management of diabetes mellitus. *Endocr Pract*. 2007;13(suppl 1):1-68.

178. Scherbaum WA. The role of amylin in the physiology of glycemic control. *Exp Clin Endocrinol Diabete*s. 1998;106(2):97-102.

179. Whitehouse F, Kruger DF, Fineman M, et al. A randomized study and open-label extension evaluating the long-term efficacy of pramlintide as an adjunct to insulin therapy in type 1 diabetes. *Diabetes Care*. 2002;25(4):724-730.

180. Hollander PA, Levy P, Fineman MS, et al. Pramlintide as an adjunct to insulin therapy improves long-term glycemic and weight control in patients with type 2 diabetes: A 1-year randomized controlled trial. *Diabetes Care*. 2003;26(3):784-790.

181. Ratner RE, Dickey R, Fineman M, et al. Amylin replacement with pramlintide as an adjunct to insulin therapy improves long-term glycaemic and weight control in Type 1 diabetes mellitus: a 1-year, randomized controlled trial. *Diabetic Med*. 2004;21(11):1204-1212.

182. Symlin® package insert. July 2008. Amylin Pharmaceuticals.

183. Pastors JG, Warshaw H, Daly A, Franz M, Kulkarni K. The evidence for the effectiveness of medical nutrition therapy in diabetes management. *Diabetes Care*. 2002;25(3):608-613.

184. Yu-Poth S, Zhao G, Etherton T, Naglak M, Jonnalagadda S, Kris-Etherton PM. Effects of the National Cholesterol Education Program's Step I and Step II dietary intervention programs on cardiovascular disease risk factors: a meta-analysis. *Am J Clin Nutr.* 1999;69(4):632-646.

185. Negoro H, Morley JE, Rosenthal MJ. Utility of serum fructosamine as a measure of glycemia in young and old diabetic and non-diabetic subjects. *Am J Med.* 1988;85(3):360-364.

186. Tarim Ö, Küçükerdogan A, Günay Ü, Eralp Ö, Ercan İ. Effects of iron deficiency anemia on hemoglobin A$_{1c}$ in type 1 diabetes mellitus. *Pediatrics International.* 1999;41(4):357-362.

187. Hashimoto K, Noguchi S, Morimoto Y, et al. A1C but Not Serum Glycated Albumin Is Elevated in Late Pregnancy Owing to Iron Deficiency. *Diabetes Care.* 2008;31(10):1945-1948.

188. Kilpatrick E, Rigby A, Goode K, Atkin S. Relating mean blood glucose and glucose variability to the risk of multiple episodes of hypoglycaemia in type 1 diabetes. *Diabetologia.* 2007;50(12):2553-2561.

189. Brownlee M, Hirsch IB. Glycemic Variability: a hemoglobin A1c-independent risk factor for diabetic complications. *JAMA.* 2006;295(14):1707-1708.

190. Schutt M, Kern W, Krause U, et al. Is the frequency of self-monitoring of blood glucose related to long-term metabolic control? Multicenter analysis including 24,500 patients from 191 centers in Germany and Austria. *Exp Clin Endocrinol Diabetes.* 2006;114(7):384-388.

191. Hirsch IB, Bode BW, Childs BP, et al. Self-monitoring of blood glucose (SMBG) in insulin- and non-insulin-ising adults with diabetes: consensus recommendations for improving SMBG accuracy, utilization, and aesearch. *Diabetes Tech & Therap.* 2008;10(6):419-439.

192. Hirsch I. Practical aspects of real-time continuous glucose monitoring. *Diabetes Technol Ther.* 2009;11(suppl 1).

193. Barker JM, Yu J, Yu L, et al. Autoantibody "subspecificity" in type 1 diabetes: risk for organ-specific autoimmunity clusters in distinct groups. *Diabetes Care.* 2005;28(4):850-855.

194. Roldan MB, Alonso M, Barrio R. Thyroid autoimmunity in children and adolescents with Type 1 diabetes mellitus. *Diabetes Nutr Metab.* 1999;12(1):27-31.

195. Tzellos TG, Tahmatzidis DK, Lallas A, Apostolidou K, Goulis DG. Pernicious anemia in a patient with Type 1 diabetes mellitus and alopecia areata universalis. *J Diabetes Complications.* 2008; epub.

196. De Block CEM, De Leeuw IH, Van Gaal LF. Autoimmune gastritis in type 1 diabetes: a clinically oriented review. *J Clin Endocrinol Metab.* 2008;93(2):363-371.

197. de Graaff LC, Smit JW, Radder JK. Prevalence and clinical significance of organ-specific autoantibodies in type 1 diabetes mellitus. *Neth J Med.* 2007;65(7):235-247.

198. Shapiro AM, Lakey JR, Ryan EA, et al. Islet transplantation in seven patients with type 1 diabetes mellitus using a glucocorticoid-free immunosuppressive regimen. *N Engl J Med.* 2000;343(4):230-238.

199. Shapiro AMJ, Ricordi C, Hering BJ, et al. International Trial of the Edmonton protocol for islet transplantation. *N Engl J Med.* 2006;355(13):1318-1330.

200. Drachenberg CB, Klassen DK, Weir MR, et al. Islet cell damage associated with tacrolimus and cyclosporine: morphological features in pancreas allograft biopsies and clinical correlation. *Transplantation*. 1999;68(3):396-402.

201. Ryan EA, Paty BW, Senior PA, et al. Five-rear follow-up after clinical islet transplantation. *Diabetes*. 2005;54(7):2060-2069.

202. Gruessner AC, Sutherland DE. Pancreas transplant outcomes for United States (US) and non-US cases as reported to the United Network for Organ Sharing (UNOS) and the International Pancreas Transplant Registry (IPTR) as of June 2004. *Clin Transplant*. 2005;19(4):433-455.

203. Ming C-S, Chen Z-HK. Progress in pancreas transplantation and combined pancreas-kidney transplantation. *Hepatobiliary Pancreat Dis Int*. 2007;6:17-23.

204. Morath C, Zeier M, Dohler B, Schmidt J, Nawroth PP, Opelz G. Metabolic control improves long-term renal allograft and patient survival in type 1 diabetes. *J Am Soc Nephrol*. 2008;19(8):1557-1563.

205. Lipshutz GS, Wilkinson AH. Pancreas-kidney and pancreas transplantation for the treatment of diabetes mellitus. *Endocrinol Metab Clin North Am*. 2007;36(4):1015-1038.

206. Gartner LM, Greer FR, Section on Breastfeeding, Committee on Nutrition. Prevention of rickets and vitamin D deficiency: new guidelines for vitamin D intake. *Pediatrics*. 2003;111(4):908-910.

207. Norris JM, Yin X, Lamb MM, et al. Omega-3 polyunsaturated fatty acid intake and islet autoimmunity in children at increased risk for type 1 diabetes. *JAMA*. 2007;298(12):1420-1428.

208. The DPT-1 Study Group. Effects of insulin in relatives of patients with type 1 diabetes mellitus. *N Engl J Med*. 2002;346(22):1685-1691.

209. The Diabetes Prevention Trial-Type 1 Study Group. Effects of oral insulin in relatives of patients with type 1 diabetes: the diabetes prevention trial-type 1. *Diabetes Care*. 2005;28(5):1068-1076.

210. Näntö-Salonen K, Kupila A, Simell S, et al. Nasal insulin to prevent type 1 diabetes in children with HLA genotypes and autoantibodies conferring increased risk of disease: a double-blind, randomised controlled trial. *Lancet*. 372(9651):1746-1755.

211. Gale EAM. European Nicotinamide Diabetes Intervention Trial (ENDIT): a randomised controlled trial of intervention before the onset of type 1 diabetes. *Lancet*. 2004;363(9413):925-931.

212. Feutren G, Papoz L, Assan R, et al. Cyclosporin increases the rate and length of remission in insulin-dependent diabetes of recent onset. Results of a multicenter double-blind trial. *Lancet*. 1986;ii:119-123.

213. Canadian-European Randomized Control Trial Group. Cyclosporin-induced remission of IDDM after early intervention : Association of 1 year of cyclosporin treatment with enhanced insulin secretion. *Diabetes*. 1988;37:1574.

214. Skyler J, Rabinovitch A, Miami Cyclosporin Study Group. Cyclosporine in recent onset type 1 diabetes mellitus: Effects on beta cell function. *Journal Diabetes Complications*. 1992;6:77.

215. Harrison LC, Colman PG, Dean B, Baxter R, Martin FIR. Increase in remission rate in newly diagnosed type 1 diabetic subjects treated with azathioprine. *Diabetes*. 1985;34:1306-1308.

216. Silverstein J, MacLaren N, Riley W, Spillar R, Radjenovic D, Johnson S. Immunosuppression with azathioprine and prednisone in recent-onset insulin-dependent diabetes mellitus. *N Engl J Med*. 1988;319:599-604.

217. Cook JJ, Hudson I, Harrison LC. A double-blind controlled trial of azathioprine in children with newly-diagnosed type 1 (insulin-dependent) diabetes. *Diabetologia*. 1987;30:509A.

218. Keymeulen B, Vandemeulebroucke E, Ziegler AG, et al. Insulin needs after CD3-antibody therapy in new-onset type 1 diabetes. *N Engl J Med*. 2005;352(25):2598-2608.

219. Ludvigsson J, Faresjo M, Hjorth M, et al. GAD treatment and insulin secretion in recent-onset type 1 diabetes. *N Engl J Med*. 2008;359(18):1909-1920.

220. Huurman VAL, Meide PE, Duinkerken G, et al. Immunological efficacy of heat shock protein 60 peptide DiaPep277TM therapy in clinical type I diabetes. *Clin Experiment Immunol*. 2008;152(3):488-497.

221. Shah SC, Malone JI, Simpson NE. A randomized trial of intensive insulin therapy in newly diagnosed insulin-dependent diabetes mellitus. *N Engl J Med*. 1989;320:550-554.

222. Diabetes Control and Complications Trial Study Group. Effect of intensive therapy on residual beta-cell function in patients with type 1 diabetes in the diabetes control and complications trial. A randomized, controlled trial. *Ann Intern Med*. 1998;128(7):517-523.

223. Su MA, Anderson MS. Aire: an update. *Current Opin Immunol*. 2004;16(6):746-752.

224. Gullstrand C, Wahlberg J, Ilonen J, Vaarala O, Ludvigsson J. Progression to type 1 diabetes and autoantibody positivity in relation to HLA-risk genotypes in children participating in the ABIS study. *Pediatric Diabetes*. 2008;9(3:1):182-190.

225. Hirsch IB. Insulin Analogues. *N Engl J Med*. 2005;352(2):174-183.

226. Mudaliar S, Lindberg F, Joyce M, et al. Insulin aspart (B28 asp-insulin): a fast-acting analog of human insulin: absorption kinetics and action profile compared with regular human insulin in healthy nondiabetic subjects. *Diabetes Care*. 1999;22(9):1501-1506.

Chapter 2: The Pathophysiology and Natural History of Type 2 Diabetes: A Clinical Perspective

David M. Kendall, MD

Acknowledgements
The author would like to thank Anthony Stonehouse, PhD for his technical support, critical review and medical writing support for the chapter.
In addition, Gregg Simonson, PhD and Amy Halseth, PhD provided valuable critique and suggestions for improvements and the author is indebted to both.

Contents

1. Introduction and Epidemiology of Type 2 Diabetes

Type 2 diabetes is an increasingly common disease, estimated to affect approximately 200 million individuals worldwide. Diabetes affects more than 7% of the US population, and it is estimated that children born in 2000 have a 33% lifetime risk of developing diabetes. The increased prevalence of type 2 diabetes is associated with increasing numbers of individuals with both microvascular and macrovascular complications—resulting in significant diabetes related morbidity and mortality. The health care and indirect costs (lost worker productivity) of type 2 diabetes in the United States in 2007 were estimated at more than $170 billion.[1] While estimates of the worldwide prevalence of diabetes vary, it is anticipated that by 2030, type 2 diabetes will affect approximately 365 million persons, or more than 5% of the worldwide population.[2] Interestingly, the highest rates of diabetes are expected to be clustered in developing regions, including South America, Africa, South Asia and the Asian Pacific rim.

There are a number of well-recognized factors that increase the risk of developing type 2 diabetes:

- Development of overweight problems and obesity

- Increasing adoption of a Western type diet and reductions in physical activity

- Family history of type 2 diabetes

- The presence of pre diabetes—including impaired glucose tolerance and/or impaired fasting glucose

- The presence of insulin resistance, conditions associated with insulin resistance (such as polycystic ovarian syndrome) and markers of the metabolic syndrome

- The presence of hypertension, dyslipidemia or both

- History of cardiovascular disease (CVD)

- High-risk population groups, including individuals of south Asian Indian, Hispanic, Native American and African descent

Individuals who develop type 2 diabetes are at a significantly increased risk for CVD.[3] Many classic cardiovascular risk factors cluster in individuals at risk for type 2 diabetes, including hypertension, dyslipidemia and insulin resistance—which can affect 50%-80% of individuals with type 2 diabetes. Treatment of both hypertension and dyslipidemia are central to the management of CVD risk in this population, the approach to which is detailed in later chapters in this manual. In addition, the management of overweight problems and obesity is receiving increasing attention, as it is readily apparent that higher rates of obesity contribute not only to the higher incidence of type 2 diabetes in children, adolescents and adults, but obesity further increases the risk of developing CVD.

Genetic markers have also been associated with the development of type 2 diabetes. The presence of specific alleles in genes that predict risk, such as polymorphisms in the peroxisome proliferator-activated receptor γ (PPARγ receptor),[4] are associated with an increase in the risk of type 2 diabetes. In addition, there are specific types of diabetes that are due to monogenic mutations, such as maturity onset diabetes of youth (MODY). However, the vast majority of patients have no single genetic marker, suggesting that type 2 diabetes is a polygenic disorder.

The lifetime risk of developing type 2 diabetes is significantly increased in first-degree relatives of those with type 2 diabetes, which highlights the polygenic but heritable nature of type 2 diabetes. Specifically, offspring of parents who both have type 2 diabetes are estimated to carry a lifetime risk of developing type 2 diabetes in excess of 70%, while those individuals with only 1 first-degree relative (parent, offspring or sibling) with type 2 diabetes have an estimated risk of between 30%-50%. Perhaps the most significant observation concerning the genetic nature of diabetes is the concordance in monozygotic twins, which is 70%-80% for type 2 diabetes,[5] compared to 50% for type 1 diabetes.

2. The Pathogenesis and Natural History of Pre-Diabetes and Type 2 Diabetes

The maintenance of normal glucose tolerance is dependent on a balance between β-cell secretory function (insulin secretion) and insulin sensitivity (insulin action).[6] Healthy individuals with normal glucose tolerance display a remarkable plasticity in β-cell secretory function, which can accommodate changes in insulin sensitivity of 5-to-7 fold.[7] In contrast, abnormalities in insulin sensitivity without compensatory changes in β-cell function result in abnormal glucose tolerance and are considered the core defects in the pathogenesis of type 2 diabetes.[8] However, it is increasingly recognized that other factors, such as insulin resistance, β-cell dysfunction, hyperglucagonemia, incretin hormones and hormones secreted by the adipocyte, contribute to the pathogenesis of type 2 diabetes.

Cell Dysfunction and Insulin Deficiency

Impaired β-cell secretory function (insulin deficiency) coupled with increased insulin requirements (insulin resistance) is widely accepted as a key physiologic defect contributing to the development of hyperglycemia in type 2 diabetes. Inadequate insulin secretory responses in the presence of significant insulin resistance results in early and progressive increases in plasma glucose, a simple relationship outlined in (Figure 1).

Numerous studies of β-cell secretory response, during the transition from normal to impaired glucose tolerance and type 2 diabetes, have demonstrated the central role of impaired β-cell response in the pathogenesis of hyperglycemia.[9] Impaired β-cell responsiveness is present many years before the onset of frank type 2 diabetes.[10] In detailed studies of individuals at risk for type 2 diabetes, progression from normal to impaired glucose tolerance has been associated with impairment in β-cell sensitivity to glucose.[11] Ferrannini and colleagues demonstrated that an impaired β-cell compensatory response to insulin resistance is present in patients with even modest abnormalities in post challenge glucose tolerance.[9] The same studies suggested that β-cell secretory response may decline by 50%-70% before the onset of impaired glucose tolerance or frank type 2 diabetes (Figure 2).[9,12]

In data from the United Kingdom Prospective Diabetes Study (UKPDS), investigators described a progressive loss of β-cell secretory function (as measured by the homeostasis model or HOMA-B) in the years immediately following the initial diagnosis of type 2 diabetes.[12] This progressive β-cell dysfunction occurred independent of the original treatment approach (either sulfonylurea, metformin or insulin).[13,14] These data suggested that the "natural history" of β-cell function was that of a progressive decline over time, and that this

Figure 1

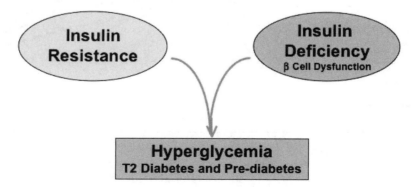

Pathophysiologic factors contributing to pre-diabetes and type 2 diabetes

Insulin resistance and insulin deficiency (β-cell dysfunction) are pathophysiologic factors contributing to hyperglycemia, pre-diabetes and, ultimately, type 2 diabetes.

decline contributes to a progressive deterioration in blood glucose. These data also support the clinical observation that many patients with long standing type 2 diabetes will ultimately require exogenous insulin therapy.

The pathogenesis and etiology of impaired β-cell secretory function has been studied extensively. It is well-known that longer intervals of hyperglycemia can result in a temporary decrease in insulin secretion. However, in healthy subjects, an increase in blood glucose results in a compensatory increase in both insulin synthesis and secretion. Moreover, as noted in the study by Ferrannini and colleagues, and shown schematically in Figure 3, individuals at risk for type 2 diabetes ultimately demonstrate an inability to meet the need for increased insulin secretion.[9] This decrease of insulin secretion in the setting of increased demand is the consequence of several pathophysiologic problems, including impaired glucose signaling of the β-cell, reduced insulin gene expression and a reduction in functional β cell mass. Studies by Butler and colleagues have shown that normoglycemic individuals with significant obesity (and hence insulin resistance) have an increase in β-cell mass, consistent with the chronic compensatory response to the demands placed on the β-cell.[15] Through a variety of mechanisms, including gluco and perhaps lipotoxicity, subjects at risk are unable to respond to increasing demands for insulin. This results not only in a decrease in insulin secretion, but again, as Butler and colleagues have demonstrated, individuals with type 2 diabetes ultimately have reductions in β-cell mass and function.[15]

Figure 4 provides a comprehensive description of the natural history of type 2 diabetes and outlines the role of insulin resistance and abnormal β-cell responsiveness seen in both pre diabetes and diabetes. Figure 4 highlights the initial compensatory hyperinsulinemia that develops in those with insulin resistance, yet also presents the relative

Figure 2

The progressive loss of β-cell function in UKPDS

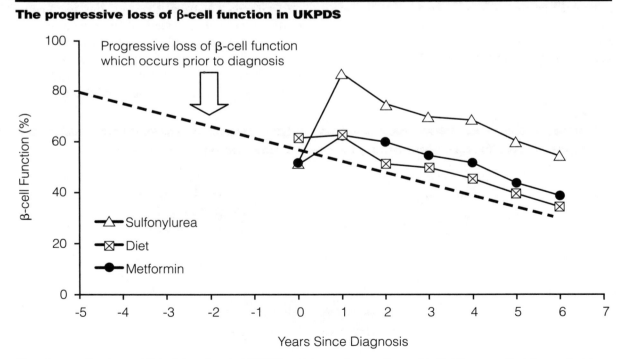

The progressive loss of β-cell function in UKPDS—observed regardless of initial therapeutic intervention in subjects with recently diagnosed type 2 diabetes.[12]

β-cell dysfunction described by Ferrannini and colleagues (Figure 3).[9] Even years before the onset of hyperglycemia, the core pathophysiologic defects of type 2 diabetes are present, with abnormal and deteriorating β-cell function and progressive or persistent insulin resistance giving rise to elevated postprandial glucose levels and later development of fasting hyperglycemia. This complex interplay, the role of impaired insulin secretion and the key elements of both hepatic and peripheral insulin resistance have been reviewed in detail in separate reports.[16]

A number of specific mechanisms are thought to contribute to β-cell dysfunction in type 2 diabetes. Hyperglycemia and increased intra islet and circulating free fatty acid (FFA) concentrations have been postulated to play key roles in the origins of impaired β-cell function. Acutely, hyperglycemia and increased FFA stimulate insulin secretion. However, chronic hyperglycemia impairs insulin secretion, insulin gene expression and insulin content.[17] In addition, elevated circulating FFAs contribute to impaired insulin action.[18,19] Several recent reviews provide additional detail on the role of lipids and lipotoxicity in the development of type 2 diabetes.

The Incretin Effect, Glucagon and Islet Dysfunction

The incretin effect has been described for many years and is the result of an observation that enhanced insulin release occurs following an oral glucose load, as compared to an isoglycemic intravenous glucose challenge.[20] The incretin hor-

Figure 3

Cell function in normal IGT, and diabetic subjects

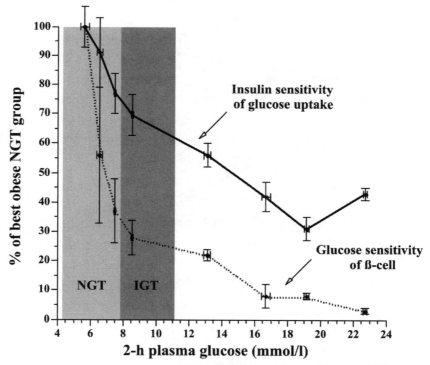

Plot of β-cell glucose sensitivity and insulin sensitivity against 2-h plasma glucose during oral glucose tolerance testing in obese NGT tertiles, IGT and T2DM quartiles. Data here are expressed as percent of the healthy obese NGT group in groups matched for body mass index.[9]

Ferrannini E, et al. β-Cell function in subjects spanning the range from normal glucose tolerance to overt diabetes: a new analysis. J Clin Endocrinol Metab. 2005; 90:493-500. Copyright 2005, The Endocrine Society.

mones—glucagon like peptide 1 (GLP 1) and gastric insulinotropic polypeptide (GIP)—secreted by the gut in response to the presence of food, were identified as being responsible for the incretin effect. Incretin hormones, particularly GLP-1, play a central role in enhancing insulin secretion, suppressing glucagon release, regulating gastric emptying and controlling food intake.[20]

The specific contribution of these defects in incretin action to the development of type 2 diabetes is poorly understood.[20] A number of investigators have suggested that either reduced concentrations of incretin hormones (principally GLP-1) or impaired incretin action (for both GLP-1 and GIP) contribute to the incretin "defect" observed in type 2 diabetes.

This decline in the incretin effect is illustrated graphically in the lower portion of the *natural history* image shown in Figure 4. While this defect remains a theoretical contributor, it is included to underscore the known importance of these gut peptides in glucose homeostasis, and supports the potential role of incretin based therapies for the treatment of type 2 diabetes. Whether the incretin "defect" is a central pathophysiologic contributor to hyperglycemia or simply the result of chronic hyperglycemia or other factors remains uncertain.[20]

Regardless of their role in of incretin hormones in the pathophysiology of type 2 diabetes, the pharmacologic application of incretin based therapies has emerged as a unique and useful tool—improv-

Figure 4

The natural history of type 2 diabetes.

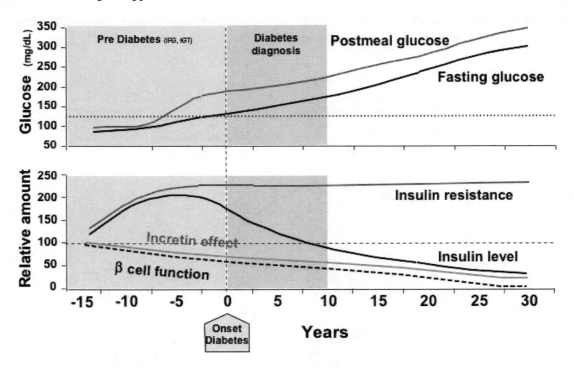

Figurative representation of the changes in plasma glucose concentration, insulin level, insulin resistance, β–cell function and incretin action in pre-diabetes and type 2 diabetes. The development of insulin resistance, early compensatory hyperinsulinemia and β-cell functional response are shown over many years — and highlight the interaction of these factors as well as incretin hormone action in the progression from normal glucose tolerance, to pre diabetes to type 2 diabetes.

ing glycemic control and, in some cases, β-cell function. GLP-1 receptor agonists and dipeptidyl peptidase 4 inhibitors (agents that bind to and inhibit the activity of the key peptidase involved in GLP-1 metabolism) have both been shown to lower plasma glucose, by means of enhanced insulin secretion and suppression of excess glucagon secretion.[20] In addition, GLP-1 receptor agonists delay gastric emptying and can decrease food intake and reduce body weight. These therapies, and their role in the management of type 2 diabetes, are reviewed in the following chapter.

While the incretin hormones GLP-1 and GIP have been the focus of significant attention, other peptides, including glucagon, glicentin and oxyntomodulin, have been shown (or postulated) to play a role in the regulation of energy balance and metabolism. Glicentin is a hormone released in response to digestion of food in the gut, and is secreted from pancreatic α cells and gut L cells. Glicentin has been shown to have insulinotropic actions in dogs, increases insulin release from the pancreas, and appears to inhibit gastric acid secretion and slow gastric emptying. Despite this complex set of actions in animals, little human data is available, and the role of glicentin in either the pathophysiology of type 2 diabetes or in clinical management remains uncertain.

Similarly, oxyntomodulin is a peptide hormone produced by the oxyntic (fundic) cells of the colon, and is known to suppress appetite. The mechanism of action of oxyntomodulin is not well understood, although it can bind to both the GLP 1 and glucagon receptor. The role of oxyntomodulin in type 2 diabetes or obesity is currently unknown.

Glucagon is a key contributor to hyperglycemia, in both type 1 and type 2 diabetes. Elevated plasma glucagon concentrations were first demonstrated in patients with type 2 diabetes in the early 1970s.[21] Moreover, in type 2 diabetes, glucagon excess is a major contributor to increased hepatic glucose output in the setting of insulin deficiency and insulin resistance.[22] The cause of this glucagon excess is poorly characterized, but may be the consequence of abnormal signalling from the impaired beta cell. Regardless, the capacity of traditional diabetes therapies (including insulin) to suppress excess

glucagon is quite limited; it is now receiving renewed attention with the new availability of incretin based therapies and amylin analogs. Both GLP-1 and amylin are unique in their capacity to significantly suppress excess glucagon, particularly in the postprandial state. Other therapeutic approaches that block the glucagon receptor have been explored in preclinical research, however, to date only 1 agent has been reported to have favorable effects in clinical trials.[23] In the years ahead, drugs that inhibit glucagon secretion or block the glucagon receptor are likely to be important components of treatment for patients with type 2 diabetes.

Insulin Resistance, the Liver and the Adipocyte

Insulin resistance is present in the vast majority (~80%) of individuals with type 2 diabetes, and in up to two-thirds of those with impaired glucose tolerance.[24] Insulin resistance in type 2 diabetes is characterized by a decreased ability of muscle, adipose tissue and liver to respond to both physiologic and supraphysiologic insulin concentrations. Insulin resistance at the level of the liver contributes to fasting hyperglycemia, and is a key target of several therapies for type 2 diabetes, including metformin, the thiazolidinediones and basal insulin.[16] Insulin resistance in muscle results in impaired glucose disposal, particularly in the postprandial state.[16] Finally, adipose tissue (particularly visceral fat) may not only be insulin-resistant, but excess lipolysis (and the resultant increase in circulating FFA) can contribute to the development and maintenance of insulin resistance and, also, islet dysfunction.

Detailed measurements of insulin action are accomplished via a variety of techniques, including simple measures of fasting plasma glucose and insulin (eg, the homeostasis model or HOMA S), intravenous glucose tolerance testing with mathematical modeling (frequently sampled intravenous glucose tolerance testing [FSIVGTT]) and hyperinsulinemic euglycemic clamp techniques.[16] Details on the techniques used for assessing insulin action have been reviewed carefully elsewhere.[16]

Insulin sensitivity varies manifold among healthy

Figure 5

Probable contributors to pre-diabetes and type 2 diabetes

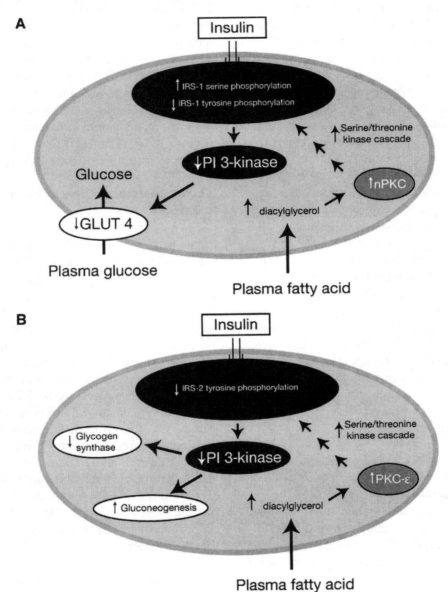

The mechanism of fatty acid-induced insulin resistance in muscle (A) and liver (B). GLUT 4 (glucose transporter 4); IRS (insulin receptor substrate); PI 3 kinase (phosphatidylinositol 3 kinase); nPKC (novel protein kinase C).

Reprinted from Peterson KF, Shulman GE. Am J Med. 2006; 119:10S–16S., with permission from Elsevier.

individuals and generally decreases with age. However (as shown in Figure 4), individuals at risk for diabetes, with pre diabetes and with frank type 2 diabetes generally have significant insulin resistance. Insulin resistance likely develops years before the onset of hyperglycemia. As with β cell dysfunction, the mechanisms involved in the development of insulin resistance are many and varied, and include a number of contributing factors, including:

• Decreased glucose uptake in muscle, due to reduction of muscle volume, and/or impaired insulin receptor signaling

• Increased abdominal visceral fat and/or increase in total fat mass, resulting in changes in specific adipocytokine concentrations (such as increases in tumor necrosis factor alpha, interleukin 1 and reductions in adiponectin)

• Hyperglycemia and/or elevated circulating and intracellular FFA

• The effect of other drugs or conditions that may increase insulin resistance (eg, glucocorticoids)

Figure 6

Changes in acute insulin response (AIR) relative to changes in insulin sensitivity

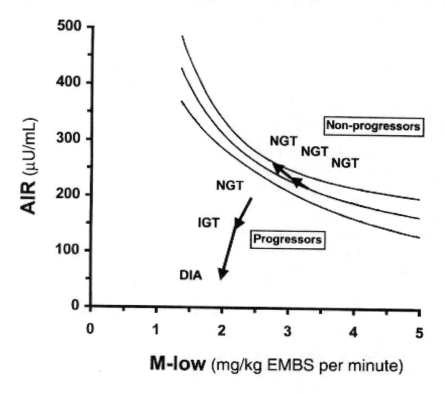

Changes in acute insulin response (AIR) relative to changes in insulin sensitivity (M-low) in Pima Indian subjects in whom glucose tolerance deteriorated from normal (NGT) to impaired (IGT) to diabetes (DIA) (progressors), and in subjects who retained NGT (non progressors). Lines represent the prediction line and the lower and upper limits of the 95% confidence interval of the regression between AIR and M low as derived from a reference population of 277 subjects from this community with NGT.[11]

Reprinted from Weyer C, et al. The natural history of insulin secretory dysfunction and insulin resistance in the pathogenesis of type 2 diabetes mellitus. J Clin Invest. 1999; 104:787 794., with permission.

3. Conclusion

As noted above, abnormal fatty acid metabolism may be both a cause and a consequence of the pathophysiologic defects of type 2 diabetes. Excess total fat mass and increased visceral adiposity are associated with the development of insulin resistance. A schematic representation of many of the probable contributors, including increased FFA concentrations, is provided in Figure 5 and has been previously reviewed in detail by Shulman and colleagues.[25]

There are other genetic and cellular factors that may contribute to the development of insulin resistance. Evidence for this genetic risk is demonstrated both by the heritable nature of type 2 diabetes and the observation that groups such as the Pima Indian population (with a lifetime risk of diabetes of ~40%-50%) develop significant insulin resistance well before the onset of diabetes. The progression from normal glucose tolerance to type 2 diabetes is associated with a decline in β-cell secretory function, in the setting of this persistent or worsening insulin resistance.[11]

Interestingly, not all individuals at risk or all individuals with significant insulin resistance will develop hyperglycemia. Robust compensatory β-cell responses that accommodate for persistent or worsening insulin resistance can prevent progression to type 2 diabetes. Indeed, the majority of individuals with significant obesity (and insulin resistance) do not develop type 2 diabetes (Figure 6).[11] The observations in Pima Indians, those with obesity and many other groups underscore the key role of these combined pathophysiologic defects in the development of type 2 diabetes.[11]

Our current understanding of the natural history of type 2 diabetes provides a framework for the clinical management of our patients, with management approaches focused on the treatment of the core pathophysiologic defects of diabetes. A proposed approach to the pharmacologic and lifestyle/nutritional management of type 2 diabetes, and the role of specific combination therapies is outlined in the following 2 chapters.

This brief overview on the epidemiology, pathogenesis and natural history of type 2 diabetes is designed to provide both a high-level scientific overview and a clinical perspective. Our understanding of the pathogenesis and natural history of type 2 diabetes helps set the stage for the approach to management, and can help guide the use of specific pharmacologic and non-pharmacologic therapies for our patients with type 2 diabetes. Given the growing epidemic of type 2 diabetes, a better understanding of the pathophysiology of this disorder is essential and should permit more effective treatment approaches to be employed. Specifically targeting the known pathophysiologic defects of insulin resistance and insulin deficiency, while also addressing other potentially important factors, such as the incretin defect, and yet-to-be discovered pathophysiologic contributors, is critical if good glycemic control is to be both achieved and sustained. The subsequent chapters detailing an approach to both non pharmacologic and lifestyle/nutritional treatment options will provide even greater insight into the many approaches that can be employed for patients with type 2 diabetes.

4. References

1. National Diabetes Fact Sheet 2007. American Diabetes Association, Inc. Available at http://www.cdc.gov/diabetes/pubs/pdf/ndfs_2007.pdf. Accessed on June 1, 2009.

2. Prevalence of Diabetes Worldwide: Country and Regional Data. World Health Organization. Available at http://www.who.int/diabetes/facts/world_figures/en/. Accessed on June 1, 2009.

3. Haffner SM, Stern MP, Hazuda HP, Mitchell BD, Patterson JK. Cardiovascular risk factors in confirmed prediabetic individuals: does the clock for coronary heart disease start ticking before the onset of clinical diabetes? *JAMA*. 1990;263:2893-2898.

4. Altshuler D, Hirschhorn JN, Klannemark M, et al. The common PPAR Pro12Ala polymorphism is associated with decreased risk of type 2 diabetes. *Nature Genetics*. 2000;26:76-80.

5. Medici F, Hawa M, Ianari A, Pyke DA, Leslie RD. Concordance rate for type II diabetes mellitus in monozygotic twins: actuarial analysis. *Diabetologia*. 1999;42:125-127.

6. Gagliardino JJ. Physiological endocrine control of energy homeostasis and postprandial blood glucose levels. *Eur Rev Med Pharmacol Sci*. 2005;9:75-92.

7. Ferrannini E, Natali A, Bell P, Cavallo-Perin P, Lalic N, Mingrone G. Insulin resistance and hypersecretion in obesity. *J Clin Invest*. 1997;100:1166-1173.

8. DeFronzo RA. Pathogenesis of type 2 diabetes mellitus: metabolic and molecular implications for identifying diabetes genes. *Diabetes*. 1997;5:117-269.

9. Ferrannini E, Gastaldelli A, Miyazaki Y, Matsuda M, Mari A, DeFronzo RA. β Cell function in subjects spanning the range from normal glucose tolerance to overt diabetes: a new analysis. *J Clin Endocrinol Metab*. 2005;90:493-500.

10. Utzschneider KM, Prigeon RL, Faulenbach MV, et al. Oral disposition index predicts the development of future diabetes above and beyond fasting and 2 h glucose levels. *Diabetes Care*. 2009;32:335-341.

11. Weyer C, Bogardus C, Mott DM, Pratley RE. The natural history of insulin secretory dysfunction and insulin resistance in the pathogenesis of type 2 diabetes mellitus. *J Clin Invest*. 1999;104:787-794.

12. UK Prospective Diabetes Study Group. Overview of 6 years' therapy of type II diabetes: a progressive disease (UKPDS 16). *Diabetes*. 1995;44:1249-1258.

13. UK Prospective Diabetes Study Group. Intensive blood glucose control with sulphonylureas or insulin compared with conventional treatment and risk of complications in patients with type 2 diabetes (UKPDS 33). *Lancet*. 1998;352:837-853.

14. UK Prospective Diabetes Study Group. Effect of intensive blood glucose control with metformin on complications in overweight patients with type 2 diabetes (UKPDS 34). *Lancet*. 1998;352:854-865.

15. Butler AE, Janson J, Bonner-Weir S, Ritzel R, Rizza RA, Butler PC. β-cell deficit and increased β-cell apoptosis in humans with type 2 diabetes. *Diabetes*. 2003;52:102-110.

16. Adbul Ghani MA, Tripathy D, DeFronzo RA. Contributions of β cell dysfunction and insulin resistance to the pathogenesis of impaired glucose tolerance and impaired fasting glucose. *Diabetes Care*. 2006; 29:1130-1139.

17. Poitout V, Robertson RP. Minireview: Secondary β cell failure in type 2 diabetes—a convergence of glucotoxicity and lipotoxicity. *Endocrinology*. 2002;143:339-342.

18. Prentki M. Glucotoxicity, lipotoxicity and pancreatic β cell failure: a role for malonyl CoA, PPAR α and altered lipid partitioning. *Can J Diabetes Care*. 2001;25:36-46.

19. Boden G, Chen X. Effects of fat on glucose uptake and utilization in patients with NIDDM. *J Clin Invest*. 1995;96:1261-1268.

20. Nauck MA, Drucker DJ. The incretin system: glucagon-like peptide 1 receptor agonists and dipeptidyl peptidase 4 inhibitors in type 2 diabetes. *Lancet*. 2006; 368:1696-1705.

21. Unger RH. Glucagon physiology and pathophysiology in the light of new advances. *Diabetologia*. 1985;28:574-578.

22. Raskin P, Unger RH. Hyperglucagonemia and its suppression; importance in the metabolic control of diabetes. *N Engl J Med*. 1978;299:433-436.

23. Petersen KF, Sullivan JT. Effects of a novel glucagon receptor antagonist (Bay 27 9955) on glucagon stimulated glucose production in humans. *Diabetologia*. 2001;44:2018-2024.

24. Bonora E, Kiechl S, Willeit J, et al. Prevalence of insulin resistance in metabolic disorders: The Bruneck Study. *Diabetes*. 1998;47:1643 1649.

25. Peterson KF, Shulman GI. Molecular mechanisms of insulin resistance in humans and their potential links with mitochondrial dysfunction. *Am J Med*. 2006;119:10S-16S.

Chapter 3: Microvascular Complications of Diabetes: Retinopathy and Nephropathy

Carol Hatch Wysham, MD

Contents

1. Introduction

The characteristic microvascular complications of diabetes mellitus – retinopathy, nephropathy and neuropathy – continue to cause substantial morbidity in patients with type 1 and type 2 diabetes. Diabetes remains the most common cause of new cases of end-stage renal disease (ESRD) and blindness among adults, and diabetes increases the risk of amputation by approximately 15-fold. From 1980 to 2002, the incidence of ESRD has increased over 5-fold: much of this attributable to the rapid growth of nephropathy in type 2 diabetes patients. The morbidity, mortality and health care costs of nephropathy make it critical for clinicians to effectively screen for, prevent, diagnose and treat nephropathy in its early stages, and to slow progression of established diabetic nephropathy. Diabetic retinopathy is the most common microvascular complication of diabetes mellitus and results in more than 5000 new cases of blindness each year.

Over the past 2 decades, considerable evidence has amassed; clearly establishing the relationship between elevated blood glucose and the risk of microvascular complications. More importantly, landmark studies, including the Diabetes Control and Complications Trial (DCCT)[1] and the United Kingdom Prospective Diabetes Study (UKPDS), have shown that intensive blood glucose control significantly reduces the risk for the development of these complications.

Pathobiology of Retinopathy and Nephropathy in Diabetes

While animal and experimental data have suggested an important interplay between vascular risk factors, human studies suggest that hyperglycemia *per se* is central to the pathogenesis of the microvascular complications of diabetes. The general features of the damage to the glucose sensitive tissues (capillary endothelial cells in the retina and to the mesagnial cells in the renal glomerulus) by hyperglycemia are shown in Figure 1. Detail on the pathobiology of neuropathy and foot lesions are detailed in subsequent chapters in this manual.

It is hypothesized that hyperglycemia damages these tissues via 4 mechanisms:

• Increased flux through the polyol pathway

• Increased production of AGE precursors

• Activation of protein kinase-C

• Increased activity through the hexosamine pathway

Figure 2 summarizes how these pathways are linked in the pathogenesis of hyperglycemia-induced tissue damage. Intracellular hyperglycemia causes an increase in mitochondrial superoxide, resulting in increased levels of reactive oxygen species. These, in turn, cause strand breaks in DNA, activating the enzyme poly (DP-ribose) polymerase (PARP) which decreases activity of glyceraldehyde-3 phosphate dehydrogenase (GAPDH) and increases glycolytic metabolites.

Specific pathogenetic mechanisms contributing to the development of retinopathy include small vessel pericyte loss; a crucial step as these tissues maintain the integrity between the vascular endothelial cells lining the retinal vessels. Damage to these cells results in increased vascular permeability, due in great part to loss of the supportive function to the vascular endothelial cells. In DR, there is a preferential loss of pericytes, followed by subsequent loss of vascular endothelial cell function. Thickening of basement membranes also develops, and this can lead to abnormal functioning of retinal vessels.

Finally, increased oxidative damage occurs in the setting of chronic hyperglycemia, and the production of oxygen-free radicals may cause direct damage to retinal endothelium.

Figure 1

General features of hyperglycemia-induced tissue damage

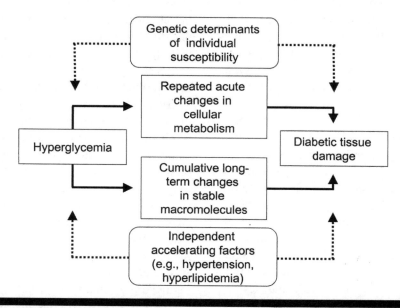

Brownlee M. Diabetes 2005; 54:1615-1625

Figure 2

Mitochondrial overproduction of superoxide activates four major pathways of hyperglycemic damage by inhibiting GAPDH

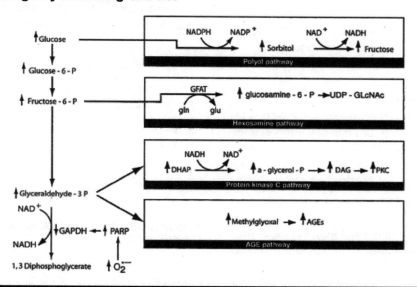

Brownlee M: Biochemistry and molecular cell biology of diabetic complications. Nature. 414:813-820,2001.

2. Glycemic Control and Microvascular Risk

The risk of both retinopathy and nephropathy are closely linked to chronic hyperglycemia, and the benefits of intensive control in reducing this risk are now well-established. Both the DCCT[1] and UKPDS have demonstrated that intensive blood glucose control significantly reduces the risk of these complications. The landmark DCCT trial was conceived and designed as a long-term, multi-center trial to address the question as to whether intensive insulin treatment in type 1 diabetes can significantly reduce the risk of development, or progression, of microvascular complication. A total of 1441 subjects were randomized to inten-sive insulin therapy (multiple daily injections or pump therapy) with target A1C <6.05%, targeting fasting glucose levels of 70-120 mg/dl pre-meal and <180 post-meal as compared to conventional therapy with 2 or more insulin injections daily; designed to limit symptoms of hyperglycemia and reduce the risk of hypoglycemia. As noted in the review of Gilliam and Hirsch, type 1 diabetes patients who received intensive therapy compared with conventional therapy experienced a 76% reduction in the risk of new onset and progressive retinopathy, a 39% risk reduction for the develop-ment of microalbuminuria, a 54% reduction for albuminuria and a 60% reduction for clinical neu-ropathy (see Chapter 1, Figure 11).

Furthermore, there was a highly significant, grad-ed relationship between mean A1C and risk of each of the microvascular complications (Figure 3).

Following completion of the DCCT trial, subjects continued in a post-interventional, follow-up study known as Epidemiology of Diabetes Interventions and Complications (EDIC). This long-term, open-ended assessment permitted investigators to assess the potential impact, risk and benefits of the initial intervention. In addition, cardiovascular risk and CVD events could be captured, with the hope that additional follow-up may shed light on the impact of intensive vs. conventional therapy on the rate of CVD events in those with type 1 diabetes.

Those in the conventional group were taught the principals of intensive insulin therapy, and all sub-jects received diabetes care from their community providers. The patients were seen at the research site annually. A1C values in both groups were similar shortly after the conclusion of DCCT, averaging approximately 8.0%. Even with several years of similar glycemic control following the initial intervention, the risk of microvascular com-plications was significantly lower in those origi-nally randomized to intensive therapy.[2] This obser-vation suggested the presence of a *legacy effect* (also termed *metabolic memory*) from the initial interval of intensive *glycemic control* on the risk of microvascular complications. The underlying mechanisms for this metabolic memory are not completely understood, but may reflect ongoing protection of tissues from even short periods of improved glycemic control, and/or significant, irreversible structural and functional tissue changes due to hyperglycemia in those treated with conventional therapy. Based in great part on the outcomes of DCCT, guidelines from the American Diabetes Association recommend treat-ing hyperglycemia with an A1C goal of <7% (or as low as possible, without unacceptable hypo-glycemia),[3] although these targets must be individ-ualized based on an individual's relative risk/benefit.

Figure 3

Relative risk of progression of diabetic complications as a function of mean A_{1C}*

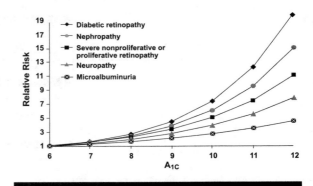

Based on DCCT data

Sklyer J. Endocrinol Metab Clin North Am. *1996;25:243*

DCCT firmly established the importance of glycemic control in reduction of risk for microvascular complications in type 1 diabetes, but questions remained about extrapolating the observations from DCCT to people with type 2 diabetes. The UKPDS study was designed to test the hypothesis that targeting normal glucose levels early in type 2 diabetes would reduce the risk, for both microvascular and macrovascular complications in patients with type 2 diabetes.[4,5] A total of 4075 subjects with newly diagnosed type 2 diabetes were randomly assigned to intensive (goal fasting plasma glucose <6 mmol/L) or conventional (best possible FPG with diet) treatment strategies. The intensive therapy arm was further subdivided into groups treated with initial sulfonylurea or insulin therapy. Additionally, 753 overweight subjects were randomized between intensive therapy with metformin and conventional therapy. Glycemic control was similar, regardless of the approach to intensive therapy throughout the 10 years of study. Although glycemic control in both groups deteriorated over time, significantly lower blood glucose values (with an approximately 0.9% difference in A1C) were maintained throughout the study. Compared to the conventional group, intensive therapy was associated with a 25% risk reduction in microvascular endpoint, a 12% reduction in risk for any diabetes-related endpoint and a 21% reduction in risk for death caused by diabetes. Although risk for myocardial infarction was reduced by 16%, this did not reach statistical significance in the main study.[4] However, in the overweight subjects, intensive therapy with metformin was associated with a 39% reduction of risk for MI, a 32% reduction of risk for any diabetes endpoint and a 36% reduction of risk for death, when compared to the conventionally treated subjects.[5]

As in the DCCT/EDIC studies, the UKPDS investigators continued to follow the subjects in an open-ended observation period following the end of the intervention period. While being cared for by their primary care providers, the A1C values declined in those individuals initially assigned to the conventional treatment arm, and the median A1C values in both groups was similar. Despite this observation, the reduction in risk of microvascular complications, myocardial infarction and mortality was seen in those individuals originally treated with the more intensive strategy, and this difference was evidenced up to 10 years post-intervention.[6] The results of UKPDS and its long-term follow-up are consistent with the observations of DCCT/EDIC. The findings of these 2 long-term studies suggest that, to ensure best outcomes in both type 1 and type 2 diabetes, more intensive glucose control should be considered as early in the course of disease as possible.

3. The Role of Hypertension and Dyslipidemia in Complications Management

Both hypertension and dyslipidemia occur commonly in individuals with type 1 and type 2 diabetes, and these 2 conditions contribute significantly to the risk for CVD. Hypertension may affect up to 30% of people with type 1 DM and can also contribute to a risk of progressive microvascular complications, and may herald the onset of nephropathy. More than two-thirds of people with type 2 DM have elevated blood pressure, and this condition often predates the diagnosis of hyperglycemia, as part of the metabolic complications of visceral obesity. In the UKPDS blood pressure study, tight blood pressure control (<150/85) vs. less tight control (<180/85) was associated with a 37% reduction in microvascular complications, which included a 34% reduced risk of progression of DR and 47% reduction in risk for visual deterioration.[7] These results have been replicated in several studies. In type 1, treatment of hypertension has been associated with reduction in risk for progression of nephropathy in multiple

studies, however, definite reduction in risk for retinopathy is lacking. More detailed discussions on the management of hypertension in diabetes is included in the summary of Chapter 9 in this manual.

Dyslipidemia is common in type 2 DM, and is characterized by the presence of elevated triglycerides, low HDL-cholesterol and small dense LDL-cholesterol. Lipids levels in well-controlled Type 1 diabetes are similar to the general population. Poor glycemic control is often associated with increased triglycerides and slightly increased LDL-cholesterol in both type 1 and type 2 diabetes.[3] Several studies have confirmed the relationship between elevated lipids and increased prevalence of diabetic retinopathy and nephropathy, however, there is little convincing evidence that lipid-lowering therapies alter the course of these microvascular complications. A sub study of the FIELD study demonstrated a 34% reduction in

Figure 4

Relative risk of the development or progression of nephropathy, retinopathy, and autonomic and peripheral neuropathy during the average follow-up of 7.8 years in the intensive-therapy group, as compared with the conventional-therapy group

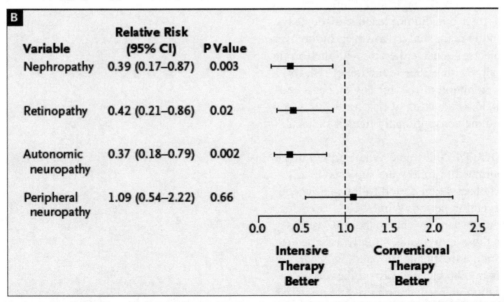

Gaede P, Vedel P, Larsen N, et al. N Engl J Med. *2003;348:383-393.*

the composite endpoint of macular edema, a 2-step progression of retinopathy and laser therapy in patients receiving fenofibrate.[8] Small studies evaluating the effects of HMG-CoA reductase inhibitors have revealed conflicting results, but are suggestive of a slowing rate of decline in GFR in patients with diabetes. More detailed evidence and the approach to the management of dyslipidemia in diabetes is provided in Chapter 10.

Multiple Risk Factor Intervention

The effect of aggressive treatment of hyperglycemia, hypertension and hyperlipidemia on microvascular and macrovascular endpoints has been studied in high-risk patients with nephropathy and elevated CVD risk. The STENO-2 trial randomized 160 subjects with type 2 diabetes and microalbuminuria; subjects received either intensive or standard control of all diabetes vascular risk factors, including hypertension, dyslipidemia and hyperglycemia. After a mean follow-up of 7.8 years, the risk for development of retinopathy and nephropathy were each reduced by 60%, (Figure 4) suggesting that multi-risk factor intervention is of benefit in these high-risk populations.[9] These beneficial effects were maintained 5 years after the end of the intervention, but given the size of the study it was not feasible to evaluate the relative effects of the treatment of the individual risk factors.[10]

With this background on both pathogenesis and the established benefits of intensive glycemic (and multi-risk factor) control, we will now look more specifically at the clinical features, and screening and management of retinopathy and nephropathy in patients with diabetes.

Diabetic retinopathy (DR) results in approximately 6000 new cases of blindness each year, making it the leading cause of blindness affecting adults under the age of 65. After 20 years of diabetes, 95% of people with type 1 and 60% of those with type 2 diabetes will have some degree of retinopathy (Figure 5). Changes consistent with DR develop before the clinical diagnosis of DM is evident, and have been described in 7.9% of patients with impaired glucose intolerance that were enrolled in the diabetes prevention trial.[11]

Vascular changes in diabetic retinopathy are caused by insults to the arterioles, capillaries and venules, that result in increased vascular permeability, basement membrane thickening and reduction in the blood flow to the retina. At the microscopic level, hyperglycemia-induced loss of pericytes leads to the loss of vascular endothelial cell function, which in turn results in increased vascular permeability.

Clinically, diabetic retinopathy generally progresses from mild nonproliferative (NPDR), characterized by increased vascular permeability, to more severe changes of NPDR, characterized by vascular closure. Proliferative diabetic retinopathy (PDR) is characterized by hypoxia-induced formation of new blood vessels in the retinal area and on the surface of the vitreous.

Clinical features of NPDR (see Figure 6)

Microaneurysms appear as small dots along the weakened retinal capillaries. They occasionally are associated with retinal edema, due to leakage of serum.

Retinal Hemorrhages appear as red dots, blots or flame shapes, and are generally not contiguous with blood vessels.

Hard Exudates represent lipid deposits within the retina and appear as yellow lesions with distinct edges.

Figure 5

The majority of patients with immune-mediated DM will develop DR after 20 years

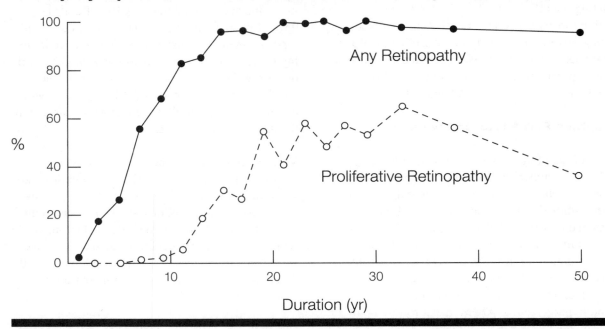

Any Retinopathy

Proliferative Retinopathy

%

Duration (yr)

Figure 6

Clinical Features of NPDR

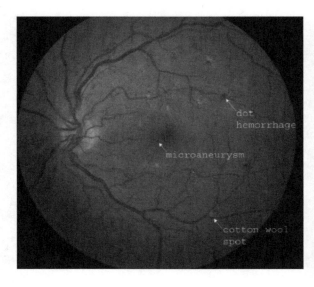

dot hemorrhage

microaneurysm

cotton wool spot

Figure 7

Clinical Features of PDR

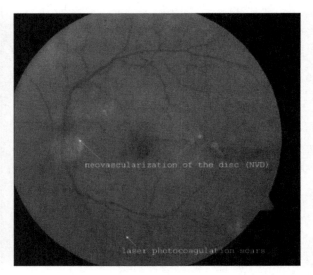

neovascularization of the disc (NVD)

laser photocoagulation scars

Cotton Wool Spots represent areas of retinal ischemia, due to the blockage of axoplasmic flow in the superficial retinal nerve fiber layer. They appear as white, soft-edged spots and tend to be transient.

Venous Beading is another manifestation of retinal hypoxia and consists of focal dilations of the retinal veins.

Intraretinal Microvascular Abnormalities (IRMA) are dilated, tortuous capillaries that are formed when blood flow in adjacent capillaries is severely compromised.

Clinical Features of PDR (see Figure 7)

Neovascularization represents the formation of new blood vessels in response to retinal ischemia and elevated levels of vascular endothelial growth factor (VEGF).

Preretinal Hemorrhages include blood found within the vitreous or between the vitreous and the retina.

Fibrovascular Proliferation is a late stage of PDR and represents areas of neovascularization that have contracted. This can result in detachment of the retina, if it causes traction on the underlying retina.

Diabetic Macular Edema (DME) occurs when fluid leaks into the intraretinal layer of the macula. DME is the most frequent cause of visual loss in patients with NPDR. When fluid collects in the region of the macula, patients may lose some or all of their central vision. DME can be found in association with NPDR or PDR, and is felt to be due to direct leakage from microaneurysms, as well as to the increase in vascular permeability.

Screening for Diabetic Retinopathy

Ophthalmoscopy, through a dilated pupil, is the preferred screening method for DR. Undilated examinations by primary care physicians have a 49% error rate for diagnosis of proliferative retinopathy.[13] The guidelines for screening for DR are outlined in Table 2.

Prevention and Management of Diabetic Retinopathy

As noted above, intensive glycemic control is central to the clinical effort to reduce the risk of diabetic retinopathy. Once a diagnosis of diabetic retinopathy has been made, strict control of multiple risk factors, especially hyperglycemia and hypertension, is critical to prevent progression of DR. Patients with macular edema, severe NPDR or any PDR require prompt care of an experienced ophthalmologist specializing in retinal diseases. Additionally, ancillary testing is often indicated to assess severity of NPDR and direct appropriate treatment and follow-up (Table 1). Fluorescein angiography (FA) is performed by rapid sequence photography of the retina, following the intravenous injection of sodium fluorescein. It is useful in detection of early vascular changes, macular ischemia and macular edema. Many ophthalmologists will use it to help guide treatment for laser photocoagulation. Optical Coherence Tomography (OCT) provides a cross-sectional image of the retina, and is used in patients with macular edema to detect changes in thickness of the macular region and to monitor treatment of DME.

Laser Photocoagulation
Panretinal photocoagulation (PRP) is performed as treatment for neovascularization. By directing 1000-2000 burns to areas of ischemic retina, oxygen demand to that area is reduced, thereby reducing levels of VEGF and the drive for neovascularization. Optimally, this will decrease growth of the abnormal vessels. The Diabetic Retinopathy Study (DRS) demonstrated that PRP treatment of PDR reduced severe visual loss by 50%.[15] Potentially, those treated with PRP may experience a slight loss of central vision, constricted peripheral vision and reduced adaptation to the dark.[14]

Focal or Grid Laser Photocoagulation was found effective in treating DME and reducing the risk of severe visual loss by 50%, when studied in the Early Treatment Diabetic Retinopathy Study (ETDRS).[16] When DME is due to multiple leaking microaneurysms, focal laser treatment is administered. If DME is more diffuse, a grid laser photocoagulation is performed.

Table 1

International Clinical Diabetic Retinopathy Severity Scale[12]

Proposed Disease Severity	Findings on Dilated Ophthalmoscopy
No apparent retinopathy	No abnormalities
Mild NPDR	Microaneurysms only
Moderate NPDR	More than microaneurysms, including hard exudates, cotton wool spots, but less than severe NPDR
Severe NPDR	Any of the following: • More than 20 intraretinal hemorrhages in each of 4 quadrants • Definite venous beading in 2 quadrants • Prominent IRMA in 1 quadrant
PDR	1 or more of the following: • Neovascularization • Vitreous/preretinal hemorrhage

---

Table 2

Ophthalmoscopy Screening Intervals for Patients with Diagnosis of DR 14

Diabetes Diagnosed	First Exam	Follow-Up
Type 1	5 years after onset	Yearly
Type 2	At time of diagnosis	Yearly
Prior to pregnancy (type1 or type 2)	Prior to conception or early in the first trimester	Physician discretion pending results of first exam

---

Table 3 summarizes the follow-up and treatment of patients who carry the diagnosis of DR.

Surgical Treatment

Tractional retinal detachment is an indication for surgical intervention. Additionally, vitrectomy is indicated for severe visual loss due to non-resolving vitreous hemorrhage.

Future Directions

There is ongoing research into medical therapies for prevention and treatment of diabetic retinopathy. Many of these proposed therapies focus on attempts to inhibit one of the pathways outlined in Figure 2. Thus far, the results of studies evaluating antiplatelet agents, aldose reductase inhibitors and protein kinase C inhibitors have been disappointing. There does appears to be a role of intravitreal steroid injection for treatment of diffuse DME that has been unresponsive to grid laser therapy. Compared to those treated with placebo, patients treated with intravitreal steroids had twice the chance of improvement in visual acuity. However, there was a high incidence of cataracts and increased intraocular pressure.[17] There is considerable interest in the evaluation of agents that suppress VEGF for the treatment of DR. 3 agents are under evaluation. Results of early RCT of Pegaptanib in 172 patients with DME suggest improvement in visual acuity, macular thickness and the need for laser treatment. Retrospective analysis of the 16 eyes with PDR showed regression of neovascularization.[18] Though not licensed for intraocular use, another anti-VEGF agent, bevacizumab (Avastin™), is approved for colorectal cancer and appears to have efficacy comparable to pegaptanib. A trial comparing the efficacy of laser treatment, intravitreal bevacizumab and combined therapy is ongoing.

Table 3

Management Recommendations for Patients with Diagnosis of DR

Severity of Retinopathy	Presence of Clinically Signifigant Macular Edema	Follow-Up (Months)	Panretinal Laser Photocoagulation	Focal Laser
Normal or minimal NPDR	No	12	No	None
Mild to moderate NPDR	No	6-12	No	None
	Yes	2-4	No	Usually
Severe NDPR	No	2-4	Consider	No
	Yes	2-4	Consider	Usually
Non-high-risk PDR	No	2-4	Consider	No
	Yes	2-4	Consider	Usually
High-risk PDR	No	3-4	Usually	No
	Yes	3-4	Usually	Usually

5. Diabetic Nephropathy

The incidence of diabetic nephropathy (DN) has risen dramatically over the past 3 decades. Diabetes is now the most common single cause of ESRD/ESKD in the U.S. and Europe, accounting for about 50% of new cases. This increase has been driven primarily by the increase in prevalence of type 2 diabetes. Approximately 20%-40% of patients with type 1 or type 2 diabetes will develop nephropathy, a small fraction of which will go on to develop ESRD. However, compared to non-Hispanic Caucasians, Native Americans, Hispanics and African Americans are at disproportionately high risk for developing diabetic nephropathy (Figure 8).

Uncontrolled hyperglycemia is the primary driver for the development of DN, though only a minority of patients with diabetes will develop it. As reviewed earlier in this chapter, hyperglycemia likely impacts glomerular structures through its impact on oxidative stress, AGE, PKC and sorbitol pathways. Some of the other potential risk factors for development of diabetic nephropathy are shown in Figure 9. Of these, genetics and hypertension are likely the most important.

The glomerular changes in diabetic glomerulopathy are illustrated in Figure 10. On the right, there is increase in mesangial matrix, thickening of the glomerular basement membrane and loss of podocytes. Mesangial expansion results in decreased filtration surface area and reduced GFR. Decreased podocyte density results in loss of structural barrier, leading to increased permeability to albumin. As these changes progress, urinary albumin excretion increases and increased intraglomerular pressure develops. Figure 11 is a schematic for the development of glomerular injury in DN.

Classically, it is thought that diabetic nephropathy progresses in a predictable fashion. The earliest feature is glomerular hyperperfusion, accompanied by increased glomerular capillary pressure and hyperfiltration, primarily driven by hyperglycemia. In those at risk for nephropathy, an excess urinary excretion of albumin ensues. Without medical intervention, a person who develops microalbuminuria (30-300 mg/24 hours or 30-300 mg/g creatinine) has about a 50% risk for pro-

gression to overt proteinuria (albumin secretion greater than 300 mg in 24 hours or >300 mg/g creatinine). A gradual decline in GFR generally follows the onset of overt proteinuria. However, it has been recognized that a substantial number of diabetic patients with renal insufficiency are normoalbuminuric. Using an eGFR <60 as definition for renal insufficiency, up to 20% of people with diabetic kidney disease may be normoalbuminuric, even after excluding those on agents impacting the RAS. These individuals appear to be at lower risk for ESRD and death than those with elevated albumin excretion.[19] Figure 12 is an historical view of the progression of DN in type 1 diabetes. Kidney disease rarely presents within 5 years of diagnosis. The peak incidence occurs between 5-15 years and starts to decline after 20 years. Type 2 diabetes has a more variable course. These patients may present with albuminuria, in part due to long duration of undiagnosed hyperglycemia, hypertension or atherosclerosis.

Screening for Diabetic Nephropathy

A test for the presence of albuminuria, as well as a serum creatinine test(with estimation of GFR), should be performed upon diagnosis of type 2 diabetes, starting 5 years after the diagnosis of type 1 diabetes and yearly thereafter. Albumin levels can be measured, either by a timed (4-or-24 hour) collection or by measurement of an albumin/creatinine ratio on a random spot collection. Generally, the latter is preferred, due to convenience in the outpatient setting. Microalbuminuria

Table 4

Causes of Transient Elevation in Urinary Albumin Excretion

- Short term hyperglycemia
- Exercise
- Urinary tract infections
- Marked hypertension
- Heart failure
- Acute febrile illness
- Pregnancy

Figure 8

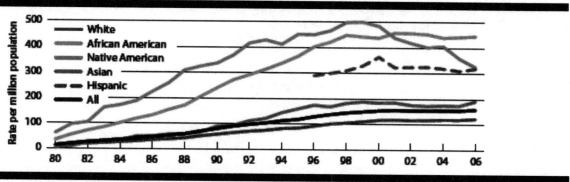

Source: *United States Renal Data Service; www.usrds.org*

Figure 9

Putative promoters for progression of diabetic neuropathy

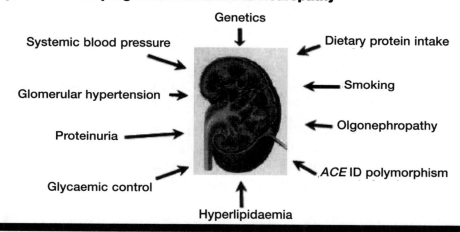

Modified from Rossing P. Prediction, progression and prevention of diabetic nephropathy. The Minkowski Lecture 2005. Diabetologia 2006;49:11-19

Figure 10

Glomerular changes in diabetic glomerulopathy

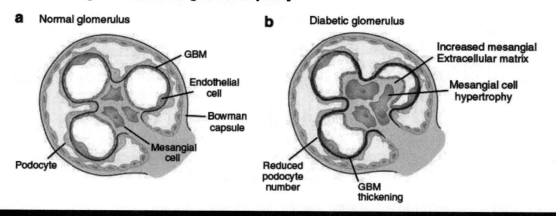

Jefferson JA, Shankland SU, Pichler RH. Kidney International *2008; 74:22-36*

Figure 11

Development of glomerular injury in DN

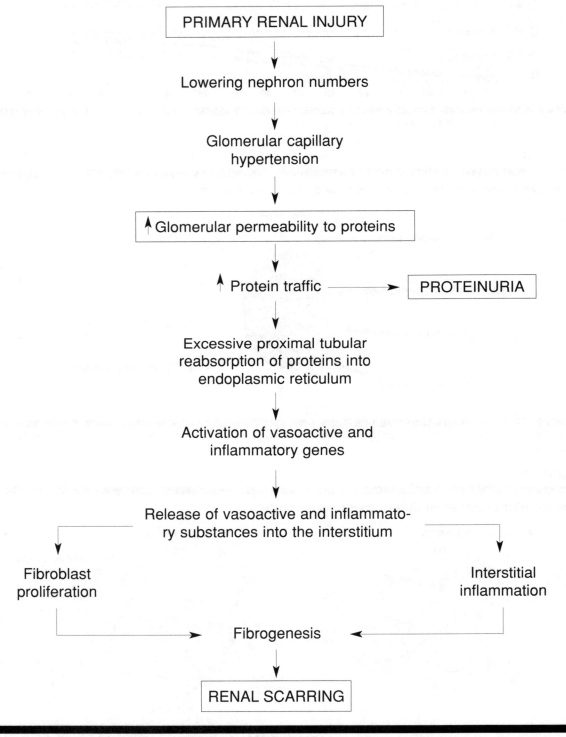

Ruggenenti P, Remuzzi G. Ann Rev of Medicine 2000; 51:315-327

Figure 12

Graphic representation of the natural history of diabetic glomerulosclerosis

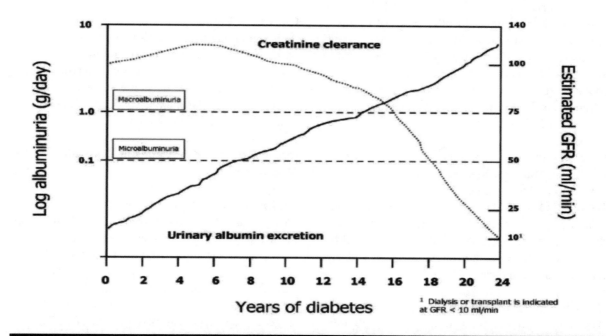

is diagnosed when albumin level reaches 30 mg/g cr, and overt proteinuria is diagnosed when urinary albumin excretion reaches 300 mg/gr CR. Routine urinary dipstick tests are not sensitive enough to use to screen for microalbuminuria, although rapid screening can now be accomplished with dipstick tests that detect microalbuminuria: a test that must be confirmed with a laboratory determination. Urinary albumin excretion can be affected by several conditions (Table 4). For this reason, all abnormal microalbumin levels should generally be repeated in 3 months, before diagnosing a patient with microalbuminuria.

Management of Early Diabetic Nephropathy

Glycemic Control

As noted earlier, optimal glycemic management is paramount to prevent the microvascular complications of diabetes, including DN. As reviewed earlier, intensive glycemic control has been associated with a marked reduction in the development of albuminuria. Additionally, both the DCCT study

and the UKPDS demonstrated the importance of achieving good control as quickly as possible.

Blood Pressure Control

Hypertension is a risk factor for the development and progression of DN. In patients with type 1 diabetes, hypertension generally heralds the onset of microalbuminuria. In contrast, hypertension is present upon diagnosis in a substantial percentage of patients with type 2 diabetes.

Animal studies showed that lowering the intra-glomerular pressure was associated with reduced albumin excretion, and was protective of renal function. Early studies in humans showed a reduction in rate of fall of GFR, when BP was controlled in patients with diabetic nephropathy. The landmark study of Lewis et al demonstrated that an antihypertensive regimen that included the angiotensin-converting enzyme inhibitor (ACE-I), captopril, was associated with a marked reduction in risk of doubling of the baseline creatinine level.[20] Similar results have been demonstrated in patients with type 2 diabetes, using angiotensin receptor blockers (ARB). Many studies have subsequently shown that treatment with ACE-I or ARB reduces proteinuria, and these classes of drugs are used interchangeably. Further reduction in proteinuria with combined ACE-I/ARB treatment has been reported.[21] Both classes of agents lead to an increase in serum creatinine and a modest decrease in GFR of 10%-20%. As compared to ACE-I, ARB has the advantage of lack of cough as a side effect, and appears to be associated with a lower risk for hyperkalemia, but has the disadvantage of increased cost.

Current guidelines recommend ACE-I or ARB as first-line therapy for hypertension in patients with DN, with additional agents as needed to achieve BP <130/80. Considering the very strong association of proteinuria with the progression of kidney disease, it is recommended that ACE-I or ARB be used in all patients with proteinuria, even with normal blood pressures.

Dietary Protein Restriction
After animal studies showed that urinary albumin excretion could be reduced with a low protein diet, a human study, the Modification of Diet in Renal Disease (MDRD), was carried out. There were no differences in outcome between those randomized to the low protein diet and those to no protein restriction.[22] Currently, patients with diabetic nephropathy should be encouraged consume no more than 30% of their calories from protein.

Control of Lipids
Although, numerous small studies suggest that lipid control might improve renal outcomes in patients with DN,[23] current recommendations for treatment of lipids are the same as those for diabetes without nephropathy. These recommendations are detailed in Chapter 10.

Management of Advancing Diabetic Nephropathy

All patients should have an estimated GFR calculated, using either the Cockcroft-Gault formula or the MDRD equation. Kidney disease has been divided into 5 stages, based upon the GFR (Figure 13). At stage 3, the complications of kidney disease, such as anemia and renal osteodystrophy begin to appear, particularly in those with DN. By stage 4, preparation for management of ESRD should begin. Referral to nephrology should occur no later than early stage 4.

Figure 13

Chronic kidney disease stages defined by GFR

CKD* Stage	Description	GFR* (mL/min/1.73 m²)
Stage 1	Kidney damage with normal or ↑ GFR	≥90
Stage 2	Kidney damage with mild ↓ GFR	60-89
Stage 3	Moderate ↓ GFR	30-59
Stage 4	Severe ↓ GFR	15-29
Stage 5	Kidney failure	<15 or dialysis

CKD = chronic kidney disease; GFR = glomerular filtration rate
Source: National Kidney Foundation. K/DOQI Clinical Practice Guidelines for Chronic Kidney Disease: Evaluation, Classification and Stratification, 2002.

6. Conclusion

Management of Anemia

In chronic kidney disease, hemoglobin levels decrease as GFR falls below 60 ml/min. Epidemiologic studies suggest that anemia is a risk factor for the progression of DN, however, there is no evidence that treatment of anemia is associated with slowed progression. Regardless, treatment of anemia in CKD improves survival, decreases morbidity and enhances quality of life. Annual screening for anemia should begin when the GFR falls below 60 ml/min. If present, patients should be treated with iron, followed by epoetin alfa, as needed.

Renal Osteodystrophy

Beginning with stage 3 kidney disease, parathyroid hormone, calcium, phosphorus and vitamin D levels should be monitored yearly. Increased PTH levels should be treated to targets established by the National Kidney Foundation at http://www.kidney.org/professionals/KDOQI/guidelines_bone/index.htm

Medication Adjustment

For patients with DN, there is no consensus as to the appropriate time to stop metformin. Most would agree that risk for lactic acidosis is very low when eGFR remains above 50 ml/min. Below that, a careful balancing of risk of lactic acidosis with the likely deterioration in glucose control should occur. NSAIDS should be avoided, when possible. Other medications commonly used in patients with diabetes that may require dose adjustments include: allopurinol, antibiotics, antivirals, antifungals, fibrates, lovastatin, simvastatin, gabapentin, H^2 blockers and antihistamines.

Although DN and DR continue to be associated with considerable morbidity, aggressive control of conventional risk factors for vascular disease, including hyperglycemia, hyperlipidemia, hypertension and smoking has resulted in a significant reduction in risk, as demonstrated in the STENO-2 study in patients with T2DM. Danish researchers have demonstrated a marked reduction in risk for DN and DR over time (Figure 14A & 14Bb). They evaluated the 20-year incidence of DN and DR, according to the date of diagnosis, in 600 subjects with type 1 diabetes. The cumulative incidence of DN in those diagnosed in the years 1965-1970 was 31.1%, compared to 13.7% in those diagnosed 1980-1984. The cumulative incidence of DR was reduced to a similar degree, 31.2% to 12.5%, respectively. Those diagnosed later had antihypertensives started earlier in the course of their disease, had lower BP and A1C levels, and fewer were actively smoking. These data lend strong support to the importance of addressing all of the known risk factors for complications of diabetes in all of our patients with diabetes.

Figure 14A

Cumulative incidence of diabetic nephropathy

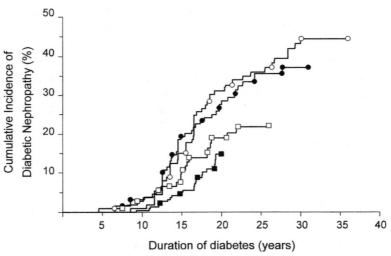

Cumulative incidence of diabetic nephropathy in 600 type 1 diabetic patients with onset of diabetes from 1965 to 1969 (n = 113, group A [ ]), 1970 to 1974 (n = 130, group B [●]), 1975 to 1979 (n = 113, group C [ ]), and 1979 to 1984 (n = 244, group D [ ]). P < 0.001, log-rank test, pooled over strata. Not all patients in group D have yet been followed for 20 years. For pairwise log-rank test over strata after 20 years of diabetes, see results.

Figure 14B

Cumulative incidence of proliferative retinopathy

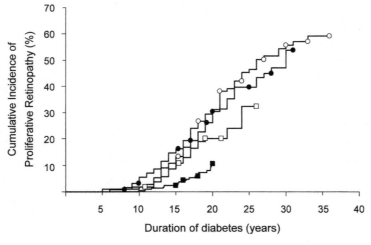

Cumulative incidence of proliferative retinopathy in 600 type 1 diabetic patients with onset of diabetes from 1965 to 1969 (n = 113, group A [ ]), 1970 to 1974 (n = 130, group B [●]), 1975 to 1979 (n = 113, group C [ ]), and 1979 to 1984 (n = 244, group D [ ]). P < 0.001, log-rank test, pooled over strata. Not all patients in group D have yet been followed for 20 years. For pairwise log-rank test over strata after 20 years of diabetes, see results.

7. References

1. The Diabetes Control and Complications Trial Research Group. The effect of intensive treatment of diabetes on the development and progression of long term complications in insulin dependent diabetes mellitus. *N Engl J Med*. 1993;329:977-986.

2. Writing Group for the Diabetes Control and Complications Trial/Epidemiology of Diabetes Intervention and Complications Research Group. Sustained effect of intensive treatment of type 1 diabetes mellitus on development and progression of diabetic nephropathy. *JAMA*. 2003;290:2159-2167.

3. Standards of Medical Care in Diabetes. *Diabetes Care*. 2009;32:S13-S61.

4. UK Prospective Diabetes Study (UKPDS) Group. Intensive blood-glucose control with sulphonylureas or insulin compared with conventional treatment and risk of complications in patients with type 2 diabetes (UKPDS 33). *Lancet*. 1998;352:837-853.

5. UK Prospective Diabetes Study (UKPDS) Group. Effect of intensive blood-glucose control with metformin on complications in overweight patients with type 2 diabetes. (UKPDS 34). *Lancet*. 1998:352:854-865.

6. Holman RR, Paul SK, Bethal MA, et al. 10-year follow-up of intensive control of type 2 diabetes. *N Engl J Med*. 2008;359:1577-1589.

7. UK Prospective Diabetes Study (UKPDS) Group. Tight blood pressure control and risk of macrovascular and microvascular complications in type 2 diabetes: (UKPDS 38). *BMJ*. 1999;318:708-713.

8. Keech AC, Mitchell P, Summanen PA. Effect of fenofibrate on need for laser treatment for diabetic retinopathy. *Lancet*. 2007;370:1687-1697.

9. Gaede P, Vedel P, Larsen N, et al. Multifactorial intervention and cardiovascular disease in patients with type 2 diabetes. *N Engl J Med*. 2003;348:383-393.

10. Gaede P, Lund-Anderson H, Parving HH, Pederson O. Multifactorial intervention on mortality in type 2 diabetes. *N Engl J Med*. 2008;358:580-591.

11. Diabetes Prevention Program Research Group. The prevalence of retinopathy in impaired glucose tolerance and recent onset diabetes in the diabetes prevention program. *Diab Med*. 2007;24:137-144.

12. Wilkinson CP, Ferris FL 3rd, Kelin RE, et al for the Global Diabetic Retinopathy Project Group. Proposed international clinical diabetic retinopathy and diabetic macular edema disease severity scales. *Ophthalmology*. 2003;110:1677-1682.

13. Sussman EJ, Tsiaras WG, Soper KA. Diagnosis of diabetic eye disease. *JAMA*. 1982:247:3231-3234.

14. American Academy of Ophthalmology Retina Panel, Preferred Practice Patterns Committee. Diabetic retinopathy. Presented at: American Academy of Opthalmology 2003 Annual Meeting; November 15-18, 2003; Anaheim, CA.

15. Photocoagulation treatment of proliferative diabetic retinopathy: the second report of diabetic retinopathy study findings. *Ophthalmology*. 1978;85(1):82-106.

16. Early Treatment Diabetic Retinopathy Study Research Group. Treatment technique and clinical guidelines for photocoagulation of diabetic macular edema. ETDRS report 2. *Ophthalmology*.1987;94:761-774.

17. Cunningham ET, Wysham chapter figures.zipAdamis AP, Altaweel M, et al for the Macugen Diabetic Retinopathy Study Group. A phase II randomized double-masked trial of pegaptanib, an anti-vascular endothelial growth factor aptamer, for diabetic macular edema. *Ophthalmology*. 2005;112:1747-1757.

18. Adamis AP Altaweel M, Bressler NM, et al for the Macugen Diabetic Retinopathy Study Group. Changes in retinal neovascularization after pegaptanib (Macugen) therapy in diabetic individuals. *Ophthalmology*. 2006;113:23-28.

19. Rigalleua V, Lasseur C, Raffaitin C, et al. Normoalbuminuric renal insufficiency in diabetic patients. *Diabetes Care*. 2007;30:2034-2039.

20. Lewis EJ, Hunsicker LG, Clarke WR, et al. Renoprotective effect of the angiotensin-converting enzyme inhibition on diabetic nephropathy. *N Engl J Med*. 2001;345:861-869.

21. Jacobsen P, Anderson S, Rossing K, Jensen BR, Parving H-H. Dual blockade of the rennin-angiotensin system versus maximal recommended dose of ACE inhibition in diabetic nephropathy. *Kidney International*. 2003;63:1874

22. Klahr S, Levey AS, Beck GJ, et al. The effects of dietay protein restriction and blood-pressure control on progression of chronic renal disease. *N Engl J Med*. 1994;330:877-884.

23. Chen H-C, Guh J-Y, Chang J-M, Hsieh M-C, Shin S-J, Lai Y-H. Role of lipid control in diabetic nephropathy. *Kidney Int*. 2005;67:S60-S62.

Chapter 4: Diabetic Neuropathy/ The Diabetic Foot

Andrew JM Boulton, MD, DSc (Hon), FRCP
Agbor Ndip, MD

Contents

Chapter 4A:
Diabetic Neuropathy

Andrew JM Boulton, MD, DSc (Hon), FRCP
Agbor Ndip, MD

Contents

1. Introduction

History

Although the history of diabetic neuropathy can be traced as far back as that of diabetes, it was not until the 18th century that Western scientists started studying the complications of diabetes with the recognition of neuropathy as a common complication and the subject of scientific interest and systematic studies. Marshall de Calvi, a French physician, was the first to correctly identify the relationship between diabetes and the nervous system. His works were supported by those of Althaus, who further emphasized the nocturnal character of the pain in 1884. But it is Frederick William Pavy, the 19th century British physician to whom credit is given for first describing neuropathic symptoms and associating these with diabetes. Pavy also pointed out that the onset of neuropathic symptoms may precede those of clinical diabetes. Later, Charcot extended these observations as well as described the neuroarthropathy that is now named after him. Davies-Pryce, a resident surgeon of Nottingham Dispensary in England, was the first to describe the micro- and macroscopic changes in the peripheral nerves of people with diabetes and to recognize the link between "diabetic neuritis and perforating foot ulcers". The awareness of neuropathy as a common diabetes complication was such that in the late 19th century, Purdy was able to assert; *"It is rare to meet with a case of diabetes in which there is not more or less nervous disturbance."*

Definition

Diabetic neuropathy (DN) is a term used to describe a variety of affections of the nervous system caused by diabetes. The multifaceted nature of diabetic neuropathies has made it difficult to accurately define the condition. Nevertheless, members of an international consensus meeting on the outpatient diagnosis and management of DN agreed on a simple definition of DN as "the presence of symptoms and/or signs of peripheral nerve dysfunction in people with diabetes after the exclusion of other causes".[1] They emphasized that a diagnosis of DN cannot be made without a careful clinical examination, as the absence of symptoms does not mean the absence of neuropathy – asymptomatic neuropathy being common. It should be highlighted that DN is a diagnosis of exclusion, as non-diabetic causes of neuropathy are not uncommon in people with diabetes. This is exemplified by the Rochester Diabetic Neuropathy Study, in which up to 10% of peripheral neuropathy in diabetic patients was deemed to be of non-diabetic causation.[2]

However, for research, epidemiologic and clinical trial purposes, a more detailed definition that includes subclinical neuropathy is required.[3] The San Antonio Consensus defined diabetic neuropathy as "a demonstrable disorder either clinically evident or subclinical, occurring in the setting of diabetes without nondiabetic causes, including manifestations in the somatic and/or autonomic parts of the peripheral nervous system."[4] This chapter will focus on the epidemiology, etiology, diagnosis and management of diabetic somatic peripheral sensorimotor neuropathy.

2. Epidemiology and Classification

Although it can be argued that DN is probably the most common long-term complication of diabetes, it is difficult to assign an accurate prevalence for a variety of reasons including: 1.) an inconsistency in the definition and diagnostic criteria; 2.) differences in the characteristics of the study population (clinic-vs.- population based); 3.) failure to determine non-diabetic causes; and, 4.) the inherent heterogeneity in the clinical presentation of diabetic neuropathies. In fact, the prevalence of diabetic neuropathy has variously been reported to vary from 10%-100%.[5]

Just as diabetes can affect almost any organ of the body, diabetic neuropathy can involve any part of the nervous system and includes the central nervous system and both autonomic and somatic components of the peripheral nervous system. Several classification systems for diabetic neuropathies have been proposed based on presumed etiology, topographical features or disease pathogenesis. However, the mechanistic link between putative etiological factors and the development of neuropathy is complex and less well understood. Perhaps the most useful systems for the practicing physician are those based on clinical manifestations. Table 1 presents 3 systems of clinical classification as suggested in the 2005 American Diabetes Association (ADA) statement.[6] However, this chapter will focus on diabetic peripheral sensorimotor neuropathy which is well characterized, and has the potential to affect quality of life and lead to deleterious lower limb complications.

Table 1

Three Classification Systems for Diabetic Neuropathies

A: Clinical Classification of DNs

Polyneuropathy **Mononeuropathy**

Polyneuropathy	Mononeuropathy
• Sensory - Acute Sensory - Chronic sensorimotor	• Isolated peripheral
• Autonomic - Cardiovasculare - Gastrointestinal - Genitourinary - Other	• Mononeuritis multiplex • Truncal
• Proximal Motor (amyotrophy)	
• Truncal	

B: Patterns of Neuropathy in Diabetes

- Length-dependent diabetic polyneuropathy
- Distal symmetrical sensory polyneuropathy
- Large fiber neuropathy
- Painful symmetrical polyneuropathhy
- Autonomic neuropathies
- Focal and multifocal neuroathies
- Cranial neuropathies
- Limb neuropathies
- Truncal neuropathies
- Non-diabetic neuropathies more common in diabetes
- Pressure palsies
- Acquired inflammatory demyelinating polyneuropathy

continued

Table 1 (continued)

Three Classification Systems for Diabetic Neuropathies

C: Classification of DN

- Rapidly reverseible
- Hyperglycemic neuropathy
- Generalized symmetrical polyneuropathies
- Sensorimotor (chronic)
- Acute sensory
- Autonomic
- Focal and multifocal neuropathies
- Carnial
- Thracolumber radiculoneuropathy
- Focal limb
- Proximal motor (amyotrophy)
- Superimposed chronic inflammatory demyelinating neuropathy

3. Pathophysiology of Diabetic Neuropathies

As with other chronic complications of diabetes, various pathogenetic mechanisms have been implicated in the development of DN. The identification of key mechanistic pathways holds promise for developing novel therapeutic agents that modulate these pathways and, consequently, offer a treatment modality for DN. Such newer agents have had variable results but, most importantly, have confirmed and underpinned the multifactorial nature of the etiopathogenesis of DN. Notwithstanding, some of the commonly accepted mechanisms include:

- Hyperglycaemia (increased polyol pathway, non-enzymatic glycosylation, deficiency in nerve growth factors)

- Nerve ischemia (macro/microangiopathy, hypertension oxidative stress)

- Impaired insulin signaling,

- Inflammation

- Genetic factors

- Altered metabolism of fatty acids and carnitine

Hyperglycemia

Evidence that hyperglycemia can lead to DN is both direct and indirect. 2 landmark studies, the Diabetes Complications and Control Trial (DCCT) and the UK Prospective Diabetes Study (UKPDS), have shown that intensive therapy and improved blood glucose control reduce the incidence and slow the progression of diabetic neuropathy.[8-10] These benefits are well established in type 1 diabetes but less well in type 2 diabetes. The Steno 2 trial, which involved tight glycemic control in type 2 diabetes, failed to show any benefit in neuropathy outcomes in those on the more intensive multidisciplinary intervention group compared to those on standard care.[11] Nevertheless, the severity of neuropathy is related to the degree of hyperglycemia[12] the neuropathy associated with impaired glucose tolerance (IGT) being lesser than that associated with newly diagnosed diabetes.[13]

Mechanistically, various pathways have been implicated in hyperglycemia-induced nerve damage. These can be broadly summarized into 2 prevailing concepts, namely, vascular and neurochemical.[14]

The Vascular Concept

This concept maintains that hyperglycemia-induced endothelial dysfunction results in reduced nerve blood flow (NBF), vascular reactivity and endoneural hypoxia, thus causing functional and structural changes in the nerve.[15] The endothelial changes in the vasa nervorum have been attributed to increased aldose reductase activity, non-enzymatic glycation and glycoxidation, activation of protein kinase C, oxidative-nitrosative stress and changes in arachidonic acid and prostaglandin metabolism.[15] More recently, other mechanisms have been implicated and include:

- Decreased expression of the vanilloid receptor 1 in vasa nervorum[16]

- Increased production of angiotensin (AT) II and activation of the AT1-receptor[17]

- Activation of poly (ADP-ribose) polymerase-1 (PARP)[18], nuclear factor-$\varkappa$B (NF-$\varkappa$B)[19] and cyclooxygenase-2 (COX-2)[20]

The Neurochemical Concept

This concept essentially rests on the premise that the same mechanisms involved in the vascular theory are not exclusive to the endothelium of vasa nervorum but may also affect the neural elements of the peripheral nervous system (PNS), such as Schwann cells, spinal cord oligodendrocytes and dorsal root ganglion neurons. It further proposes that other pathobiochemical abnormalities can directly affect the nerve cell, namely:

- Metabolic derangements (down regulation of Na+K+ATP-ase activity[21]; changes in fatty acid and phospholipid metabolism[22])

- Impaired secretion of nerve growth factors[23]

- Abnormal signal transduction[24]

- Mitochondrial dysfunction and premature apoptosis of dorsal root ganglion (DRG) and Schwann cells[25]

Disturbances of Fatty Acid and Lipid Metabolism

Diabetes is associated with abnormal FFA metabolism and can cause disturbances in the desaturation of gamma-linolenic acid (GLA), resulting in reduced production of vasodilatory compounds with a consequent decrease in nerve blood flow.[26] Treatment with gamma-linolenic acid has been shown to improve nerve function in diabetes.[27] Carnitine deficiency has been found in patients with microvascular complications of diabetes, including neuropathy. In streptozotocin-induced diabetic rats, carnitine deficiency has been associated with hyperactivation of polyol pathway, while in human studies, replacement therapy with Acetyl- L-carnitine has been shown to improve painful neuropathy symptoms.[28]

Impaired Insulin Signaling and C-peptide Action

Impaired insulin/C-peptide action has emerged as a prominent factor in the pathogenesis of the microvascular complications in type 1 diabetes. Putative mechanisms in causation of DN include altered Na+K+ATPase activity, nerve growth factors and nerve cell apoptosis. It is well documented that neuropathy in both experimental and human studies differs in type 1 and type 2 diabetes. The neuropathy in type 1 diabetes shows a more rapid progression with more severe functional and structural changes.[29] Such differences are accounted for by impaired insulin action and signal transduction in type 1 diabetes, whereas hyperglycemia per se contributes equally to neuropathy in the 2 types of diabetes. There are 2 types of insulin receptors – type A (IR-A) and type B (IR-B). Glucose metabolism is regulated by insulin via IR-B. However, the central and peripheral nervous systems contain more IR-A than IR-B, but at normal serum insulin levels, the insulin affinities of both these receptors are similar. Thus, it is very possible that correction of insulin levels in treatments for type 1 diabetes or insulin-sensitizing therapy in the case of type 2 diabetes, not only corrects glucose metabolism but also has independent effects on the function of peripheral nervous system.[30] As a corollary, since defects in insulin action predates disordered glucose metabolism (including hyperglycemia) in type 2 diabetes, it is probable that insulin signaling/receptor defects may well explain the occurrence of neuropathy in pre-diabetes. In addition, some studies in type 1 diabetic patients suggest a salutary effect of C-peptide replacement in the prevention and amelioration of diabetic neuropathy[31] although these data are limited.

Inflammation

There is also evidence, albeit limited, that suggest subclinical inflammation is associated with and perhaps causative of DN and neuropathic impairments. However, this association appears rather specific, as only certain immune mediators are involved. In a recent study, high levels of C-reactive protein and interleukin-6 were found to be consistently associated with DPN, high MNSI (Michigan Neuropathy Screening Instrument) score and specific neuropathic deficits, whereas some inverse associations were seen for interleukin-18.[32] High serum TNF-α level has also been associated with the presence of DN in humans,[33,] while in experimental diabetes, increased expression of NF-kappa B in diabetic sciatic endothelial cells and Schwann cells of limbs was subjected to ischemia-reperfusion injury.[34]

Hypertension

Various studies have confirmed the association of hypertension and diabetic sensory neuropathy. It is thought that the presence of hypertension, by favoring the onset and progression of atherosclerosis with consequent peripheral nerve ischemia, contributes to the onset of neuropathy in diabetes.[35] The benefits of hypertension management are well established for the prevention of cardiovascular, renal and retinal complications of diabetes, and these same standards should be applied for both the prevention and management of DN.

4. Diagnosis of Diabetic Sensorimotor Neuropathy

Clinical Presentation

Distal Sensory Neuropathy
- Most common of all the diabetic neuropathies

- Extremely variable, can range from severely painful (positive symptoms) to completely painless

Painful symptoms
- Diffuse symmetrical disorder

- Mainly affects the feet and lower legs in a stocking distribution

- Occasionally involves the hands in a glove distribution

- Mostly, symptoms are gradual (chronic), but may be acute

  #### - Chronic sensory symptoms
- Onset is insidious and symptoms are intermittent in early stages,

- As disease progresses, motor dysfunction (small muscle wasting: sensorimotor neuropathy occurs)

  #### - Acute sensory symptoms
- May occur after a period of severe metabolic instability or a sudden improvement of control ("insulin neuritis")[36]

- Symptoms are usually severe, while QST may be normal

- Painful symptoms are usually difficult for the patient to describe

- Typically, patient may describe: burning pain; stabbing and shooting sensations uncomfortable temperature sensations paresthesias hyperesthesias and allodynia

- Symptoms fluctuate with time but tend to be extremely uncomfortable, distressing and prone to nocturnal exacerbation

- The bedclothes may irritate the feet, such that the patient sleeps without them, with feet hanging over the sides of the bed (bedclothes hyperesthesias)

Painless Symptoms

- Usually mild or "negative symptoms"

- Decreased pain sensation

- Deadness and numbness

- May present with an insensitive foot ulcer[36]

- Postural instability

  - Only recently recognized as a manifestation

  - Falls and unsteadiness (disturbances in proprioception) are common

  - Often result in depression[38]

  - Studies have confirmed that neuropathic patients sway more when quantitatively assessed with Romberg's test[39]

Table 2

Painful and non-painful Manifestations of Diabetic Sensorimotor Neuropathy

Motor	Sensory	
	Non-painful	Painful
Weakness	Thick	Prickling
Small muscle wasting	Stiff	Tingling
	Asleep	Knife-like
	Throbbing	Like electric shock
		Squeezing
	Formication (ants crawling)	Constriction
	Like walking on cotton Hurting	Loss of balance
		Burning
		Freezing
		Throbbing
		Allodynia
		Hyperalgesia

It should be noted that some patients can have painless neuropathy but periodically experience spontaneous pain, making patients confused as to how to clearly describe their symptoms. This is the so-called painful painless foot and in such patients, "eliciting the presence of pain can be painstaking"

Although neuropathic symptoms are predominantly sensory, in many cases the signs are both sensory and motor, with minor degrees of small muscle wasting and occasionally weakness (hence the term sensorimotor neuropathy). The ankle reflex is usually reduced or absent, and the skin in the dorsal and especially plantar surfaces may be dry and cracking, owing to associated sympathetic autonomic dysfunction. The sympathetic dysfunction may result in increased A-V shunting, distended dorsal foot veins and a warm foot. There may be a foot deformity due to loss of interosseous muscles resulting in abnormal forces.

Small-Fiber Neuropathy

Some authorities believe that there exists a specific small-fiber neuropathy with neuropathic pain, sometimes together with autonomic dysfunction but few signs. However, this shares many similarities with the acute sensory neuropathy, but symptoms tend to be more persistent. It is believed to represent an early stage in the development of chronic sensorimotor neuropathy.

These painful sensory neuropathies should not be confused with hyperglycemic neuropathy, which may occur in newly diagnosed patients and is characterized by rapidly reversible abnormalities of nerve function and, occasionally, transient symptoms.

Psychological Aspects of Diabetic Peripheral Neuropathy

Diabetic neuropathy can cause devastating effects on psychosocial functioning and quality of life.[40] Depression and anxiety are the most commonly recognized psychosocial maladaptation in patients with diabetic neuropathy[41] and clinicians must recognize them as these can affect adherence and outcome. Any underlying psychosocial disorder must

be taken into consideration when therapeutic strategies are being considered. Pain associated with DN may have a substantial impact on the quality of life, particularly by causing considerable interference in sleep and enjoyment of life.[42] Despite this significant impact, in one survey 39% of the diabetic patients had no treatment for their neuropathic pain.[43]

Clinical Course of Chronic Distal Sensory Neuropathy

- Unpredictable

- Varies with each patient

- Symptoms wax and wane but persist for years

- Improvement in symptoms does not always equate with parallel improvement in nerve function or QST

Controversy persists as to which sensory modality is first affected, although it is generally accepted that small-fiber dysfunction is present early in the course of neuropathy. Nonetheless, it remains clear that there is gradual loss of nerve function in diabetic patients that is more rapid than that in age-matched non-diabetic subjects. This rate of loss is related to the level of glycemic control.[44-46] One consequence of this progressive loss of nerve function is an increasing risk of insensitive foot ulceration.[47]

Differential Diagnosis of Diabetic Sensory Neuropathy

The diagnosis of diabetic neuropathy is essentially clinical and rarely is recourse made to further investigations. However, diabetic neuropathy remains a diagnosis of exclusion; therefore, the presentation of neuropathic symptoms in a patient with diabetes does not obviate the need to rule-out other non diabetes-related causes of neuropathy. Conversely, the absence of specific symptoms cannot be taken as the absence of diabetic neuropathy. It is not uncommon for the same patient to have 2 or more aetiologies for neuropathy. In the United States, diabetes and alcoholism are the 2 most common causes of peripheral neuropathy. The following should be considered in differential diagnosis of peripheral neuropathy:

- Alcoholism

- Hereditary

- Toxic, drugs eg, isoniazid, chemotherapy, anti-rejection agents (tacrolimus)

- Metabolic eg, diabetes, porphyria, hypocalcemia, amyloidosis, myxoedema

- Infections eg, HIV, syphilis, leprosy

- Inflammatory eg, CIDP (chronic inflammatory demyelinating polyradiculoneuropathy) CIDP, vasculitis

- Ischemic and disorders

- Paraneoplastic disorders and malignancies, eg, bronchogenic carcinoma

A thorough clinical history and physical examination can provide invaluable pointers to possible underlying conditions. The patient history should include an assessment of quality of life including mood, physical and social functioning and social support. The detailed characteristics and factors associated to the pain most be elucidated bearing in mind that some patients may be unable to communicate unusual sensations.

Assessment of Diabetic Neuropathy

Assessment scales - symptoms
Various assessment tools have been designed either as questionnaires or scales to help the clinician characterize neuropathic pain. The following section will describe some of the most widely used tools.

Visual Analogue Scale (VAS) and Verbal Descriptor Scale (VDS)
These are simple self-reported scales and provide a unidirectional means of assessing pain. The VAS uses a 10-cm visual analogue scale, while the VDS is based on a 5-point verbal rating. They

may be used to follow a patient's response to treatment.

Likert scales
Patients are asked to rate their response to a statement from 1 to 5 where 1 indicates "strongly agree" 5 indicates strongly disagree and, 3 indicates 'neither agree nor disagree'. For instance, patients may be asked to rate the statement pain interferes with my life on a daily basis"

Other assessment tools include: the McGill pain questionnaire, brief pain inventory, neuropathic pain scale, NeuroQoL (neuropathy quality of life), Michigan neuropathy screening instrument (MNSI) and the neuropathy symptom score (NSS).

Assessment of sensory and motor function - signs
A complete physical examination should include a systematic and meticulous test for the different sensory modalities. All assessments are done with the patient supine and with their eyes closed to eliminate visual bias. The following are usually included in the examination:

Monofilament
The standard 10-g Semmes-Weinstein monofilament is design to buckle at a force of 10-g when applied perpendicular to the skin surface briskly, such that the nylon filament bows. It is the most widely used device in clinical practice in the assessment of diabetic neuropathy.[48] It is also a good predictor of foot ulcer risk.[49,50] Not all monofilaments supplied by different companies buckle at this force and each clinician should identify reliable suppliers.

Heat/Cold discrimination
This is assessed using a neurotherm which is a rod with one end being plastic (feels normal or hot) and the other end made of metal (cold). Alternatively, the base of a tuning fork is immersed alternately in a beaker of ice/warm water for testing cold/hot sensation respectively.

Pinprick
A neurotip is a suitably designed pin with a sharp and a blunt end. It is applied on the dorsum of the foot proximal to the toenail.

Tuning fork

The standard 128Hz tuning fork is used to assess vibration sensation. It is typically applied to the apex of the big toe.

Vibration perception threshold (VPT)

This is assessed using a neurothesiometre (powered by a rechargeable battery) or a biothesiometer (needs current source). A VPT >25V is generally considered as evidence of the presence of sensory neuropathy and a risk factor for foot ulceration.

Deep tendon reflex

Deep tendon reflex (DTR) can either be present (normal), preseny after reinforcement (Jendrassik maneuver) (abnormal) or completely absent (abnormal). It is assessed using a suitable tendon hammer and when used to evaluate the neuropathy disability score, the ankle reflex is the preferred site for testing.

The Modified Neuropathy Disability Score (NDS)

A composite score known as the neuropathy disability score has been proposed to grade the severity of neuropathy based on the testing of four modalities. An NDS score 3-5 is considered mild neuropathy; 6-8 moderate neuropathy and 9-10 severe neuropathy.[51]

Quantitative Sensory Testing

The term Quantitative Sensory Testing (QST) has been assigned to testing protocols that aim to give more precise determination of perception threshold for different sensations. Vibration (Aδ fibers), thermal (Aß-fibers) and pain (C-fibers and Aß-fibers) thresholds have been proven to be able to detect sub clinical neuropathy in diabetic patients. The QST has been found to be safe and effective. It is however limited by the individual's attention, motivation and cooperation as well as age, sex, body mass, smoking and alcohol consumption. It is not recommended as a sole criterion for defining diabetic neuropathy.

Ancillary investigations

This section discusses some ancillary investigations used in evaluate diabetic peripheral neuropathy. It should be emphasized that they are usually for research purposes and are not routinely performed in the clinical assessment of patients except in specific entities of neuropathy.

Table 3

The Modified Neuropathy Disability Score

		Score	Right	Left
Sensory score				
	Vibration sense 128Hz tuning fork at apex of the hallux	Normal=0		
	Temperature Perception on the dorsum of the foot	Reduced/abnormal=1		
	Pinprick			
Reflex score	**Ankle reflex**	Present=0 Present with reinforcement=1 Absent=2		
NDS total out of 10				

Electrophysiology

This is a specialist tool used in the investigation of diabetic neuropathies. In distal sensorimotor neuropathy, they provide a measure of the following:

- Nerve conduction velocity (NCV)

- Peak amplitudes, area and duration (sensory and motor nerves)

- F-waves

- Distribution of velocities

- Excitability

Although reliable, electrophysiologic testing is not routinely required nor recommended in the diagnosis of diabetic neuropathy. It may be used to detect sub clinical neuropathy, evaluate the extent of nerve dysfunction and in the diagnosis of specific entities like entrapment neuropathies (carpal tunnel syndrome). Electrophysiologic tests can also be used as surrogate end points in interventional studies of nerve function. The estimated loss of NCV due to diabetic neuropathy is approximately 0.5m per second per year.[52] In a 10-year follow-up study of patients with newly diagnosed type 2 diabetes, the sural nerve showed the largest NCV deficit (3.9 ms-1) followed by the peroneal nerve (3.0 ms-1).[53]

Skin Punch Biopsy

A skin biopsy is used to assess small dermal nerve fibers that are not amenable to electrophysiologic evaluation.[54] Although invasive, it only uses 3-mm of skin that is subsequently analyzed by immunohistochemical staining. It is mostly performed in research settings and is not recommended for the routine clinical assessment of neuropathy.

Other Surrogates Markers

Recently, some researchers have developed corneal confocal microscopy (CCM) as a technique in assessing nerve damage *in vivo*.[55,56] CCM measures corneal nerve fiber length, nerve fiber density, nerve branch density and corneal nerve tortuosity.[57] It offers the advantage that it is non-invasive, hence iterative, and can therefore be used to follow response to treatment. CCM measures correlates well with electrophysiologic and morphologic nerve assessment. Longer term studies are ongoing that would determine their utility in clinical evaluation of neuropathy.[58]

5. Treatment of Diabetic Peripheral Neuropathy

Aims

Management of diabetic peripheral sensorimotor neuropathy should aim to:

- Prevent disease progression and thus forestalling further nerve damage,

- Providing symptomatic relief, including adequate pain management

- Preventing neuropathic complications (foot lesions/ulcers and Charcot neuroarthropathy [Ch 4B])

A detailed discussion with the patient and in some cases, other family members, is essential and should focus on the following key points.

- Dispel misconceptions and allay fears. Some patients with neuropathy believe that because their feet are warm, they are less likely to develop ulcers (warm means good). In addition, some symptoms may be overlooked by patients or they may not associate this with neuropathy. Patients with insensate feet need to be reassured that foot ulceration and/or amputation are not inevitable provided appropriate preventive foot care measures are taken

- Manage patient expectations. Therapeutic objectives should be realistic and the clinician should not be enticed into promising instant/complete pain relief. Clinical response to certain agents is not always instantly observable. It should be made clear to the patient that, while all means will be employed to control symptoms, response to specific therapy is unpredictable and varied

- Reiterating the opportunity for optimum and stable metabolic control. There is plenty of evidence linking hyperglycaemia to the development and progression of diabetic neuropathy. Also, blood glucose flux (sudden changes in blood glucose control) has been associated with the development of neuropathic pain.[59] This can occur after starting insulin (insulin neuritis)[60,61] or following a successful pancreas transplant. For these reasons, we underline the need for an optimal as well as a stable glycemic control in the management of neuropathy and neuropathic pain. The gain from such optimum control is not limited to likely improvements in neuropathy but may actually help slow the progression of other diabetic complications in general

Pharmacological Therapy for Managing Diabetic Sensory Neuropathy

In general, the treatment of DN must be tailored to individual patients and should take into consideration the specific clinical features, as well as associated comorbidities. For instance, a patient with neuropathic pain and co-existing depression or anxiety may benefit from a neuropathic agent that is either anti-depressive or anxiolytic. Side effects are common and care must be taken when prescribing certain agents to elderly people (anti-cholinergic effect), heavy machinery workers (sedative effect) or those with renal impairment (toxicity, dose modification). Two broad categories of treatment can be considered: 1.), those that target the underlying pathogenetic mechanism of DN and 2.), those that provide symptomatic/pain relief

Therapeutic modalities based on the pathogenesis of DN

Almost every pathway involved in the pathogenesis of DN has been explored in an effort to find novel therapeutic approaches. The advantage of such an approach is that as glycemic control for most patients is not expected to be optimal; these therapies might be effective even in individuals with poor glycemic control through their action on specific etiopathogenic pathways. However, while some have shown initial promise, the overall results have been varied and mixed. Although the following warrant specific mention, none is available or licensed for use in DN in the U.S.

- Protein kinase C (PKC) inhibitors

- Anti-oxidants, eg, γ - linolenic acid (GLA)

- Vasodilators, eg, ACE inhibitors,

- Aldose reductase inhibitors (ARIs) and

- C-peptide.

- Nerve growth factors eg vascular endothelial growth factor (VEGF).

Therapeutic modalities for symptom (pain) relief

It is essential to review the pathways involved in generating, transmitting and perceiving the sensa-

Figure 1

Different mechanisms of pain and possible treatments: Pain targets[62]

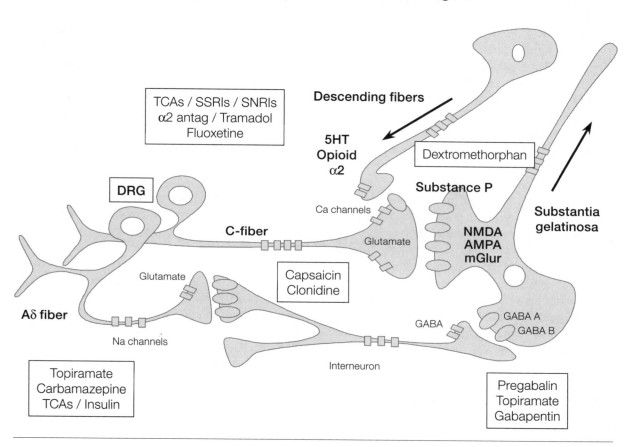

C-fibers are modulated by sympathetic input with spontaneous firing of different neurotransmitters to the dorsal root ganglia (DRG), spinal cord and cerebral cortex. Sympathetic blockers (clonidine) and depletion of axonal SP used by C-fibers as their neurotransmitter (capsaicin) may improve pain. In contrast, Aδ fibers utilize NA+ channels for their conduction and agents that inhibit Na+ exchange, such as antiepileptic drugs, tricyclic antidepressants and insulin, may ameliorate this form of pain. Anticonvulsants (carbamazepine, gabapentin, pregabalin, topiramate) potentiate GABA activity, inhibit Na+ and Ca channels and inhibit NMDA and AMPA receptors. Dextromethorphan blocks NMDA receptors in the spinal cord. TCA, SSRIs and SNRIs inhibit serotonin and norepinephrine reuptake, enhancing their effect in endogenous pain-inhibitory systems in the brain. Abbreviations: SP: substance P; TCA: tricyclic antidepressants; SSRIs: selective serotonin reuptake inhibitors; SNRIs: serotonin and norepinephrine reuptake inhibitors; NMDA: N-methyl-D-aspartate; AMPA: amino-3-hydroxy-5-methyl-4-isoxazole propionic acid; GABA: gamma-aminobutyric acid

tion of neuropathic pain in other to be able to gain an understanding of the different treatment options. The schema in Figure 1 provides a simple illustration of the neuronal mechanisms involved in pain and the potential treatments available to approach these specific targets.[62]

Tricyclic antidepressants (TCAs): Tricyclics have been used for the treatment of neuropathic pain for approximately 3 decades but most studies assessing their efficacy were conducted in the 1980s and 1990s and did not meet FDA regulatory standards. Hence, although most local and international guidelines recommend their use in DN, they are not FDA-approved for this specific use (off-license indication). In general, tricyclics have been replaced as first-line agents in the U.S. as a result of the higher frequency of adverse events as compared to other agents. However, when tolerated, they are efficacious in treatment of neuropathic pain and this has been confirmed in randomized trials. They have different potencies and are either noradrenalin reuptake inhibitors (NRIs, eg, nortriptyline and desipramine), or both noradrenalin and serotonin reuptake inhibitors (NSRIs, eg, clomipramine).[63] TCAs have a good dose-response relationship with relief of neuropathic pain occurring before their anti-depressive effects.[64] Adverse side effects are common and dose-related. Hence, dose titration is essential, starting from the smallest dose and increasing up until desired pain relief or development of adverse effects. Their affinity for muscarinic receptors is responsible for the typical atropine-like side effects of dry mouth, blurred vision, constipation, urine retention, recumbent tachycardia and memory impairment, which is especially relevant in the elderly, where delirium can result even from therapeutic doses. In a recent cost utility analysis of common first-line agents, desipramine (100 mg/day) was found to be more cost-effective than gabapentin or pregabalin for treating painful diabetic neuropathy; its cost-effectiveness was similar to duloxetine (60 mg/day).[65] TCAs are transported in blood protein-bound and metabolized via the CYP450 pathway and thus have the potential of interacting with drugs such as beta-blockers, levothyroxine and statins.[66]

Selective serotonin-reuptake inhibitors (SSRIs): The effect of SSRIs on neuropathic pain is mediated via beta-2 adrenoceptor activation resulting in a blocking of the reuptake of the neurotransmitter amines, serotonin (5-hydroxytryptophane, 5-HT) and/or noradrenalin.[67,68] Thus concomitant use of beta-adrenoceptor antagonists (beta-blockers) can reduce the efficacy of SSRIs. Duloxetine is the most commonly used SSRI in the treatment of DN and has both analgesic and major antidepressant effects. Duloxetine and venlafaxine are mainly SSRIs with minimal noradrenalin reuptake inhibition. Duloxetine is effective, generally well tolerated even by elderly patients,[69] has a simple dosage and these properties are likely to enhance patient compliance.[70] Nausea is a common side effect reported by 10% of individuals.[71] Other SSRIs used in the treatment of neuropathic pain include paroxetine and citalopram.

Anticonvulsants: Anticonvulsant therapies are now widely used for symptomatic management of painful neuropathies. Their primary mechanism of action includes calcium channel blockade, sodium channel blockade, GABA activity and antagonism of glutamate at N-methyl-D-aspartate (NMDA) receptors or α-amino-3-hydroxy-5-methyl-4-isoxazole propionic acid (AMPA).[72] Pregabalin is an $\alpha 2$-δ ligand similar to γ-amino butyric acid (GABA) whilst gabapentin is a GABA analogue. GABA modulates the influx of calcium at presynaptic voltage-sensitive calcium channels,[73] resulting in a decrease in the release of several neurotransmitters, including glutamate and norepinephrine. The anticonvulsants have relatively lesser drug interactions and side effects. The newer one's like pregabalin, gabapentin, and lamotrigine, have fewer side effects and are now being used in lieu of carbamazepine. In the U.S.A., gabapentin and pregabalin are licensed for use in neuropathic pain and carbamazepine in trigeminal neuralgia. In general, anticonvulsants are efficacious and have a more favorable side effect profile compared to TCAs. The main adverse effects reported with pregabalin in studies are dizziness, somnolence and peripheral edema.[74] Pain and sleep improvements noted with pregabalin are dose-related: the greatest and quickest effects noted in patients treated with 600 mg QD.[75] Pregabalin also has anxiolytic properties and this is of potential benefit in patients with anxiety states. Pregabalin, lamotrigine and gabapentin have no interaction with CYP450 pathway hence are unlikely to have major drug interaction. Carbamazepine in contrast, is metabolized in the liver via CYP450 pathway and thus can affect the metabolism of drugs commonly co-prescribed in diabetes, such as gliclazide, glimepiride, bisoprolol, atorvastatin and simvastatin.[66]

Opioids

Opioids are mostly used as adjuncts in the treatment of painful neuropathy. Their concomitant use with anticonvulsants may achieve better pain relief at lower doses, hence mitigating the occurrence of side effects. The coadministration of prolonged-release oxycodone in patients on existing gabapentin therapy has been shown to improve pain relief and to reduce sleep disturbance without exacerbating of opiate-induced side effects.[76] Similarly, the combination of gabapentin and morphine has been shown to achieve better analgesia at lower doses of each drug than either as a single agent.[77] This apparent synergism between anticonvulsants and opiates is not limited to gabapentin. A recent open-label, prospective, multicenter study also showed that combining pregabalin with prolonged-release oxycodone was safer and more effective than either drug alone.[78] Tramadol is a central opioid analgesic that is occasionally used in the treatment of neuropathic pain, although its efficacy has not been established in randomized studies.

Anti-arrhythmic drugs: occasionally, the anti-arrhythmic drug, mexiletine is used in the treatment of DN.

Topical treatment and physical therapy

Topical capsaicin, isosorbide dinitrate spray, lidocaine and transdermal clonidine have on occasion been shown to improve neuropathic pain in limited studies.

Table 4 summarizes the different treatment options for the management of painful diabetic neuropathy.

Table 4

Treatment Options for painful diabetic neuropathy (Adapted from McQuay et al, Zeigler and Dobecki et al)[79-81]

Compound/ measure	Starting dose	Dose per day	Remarks	Side Effects	NNT
Optimal diabetes control					
Diet, OAD,insulin	-	individual	Aim: HbA1C≤6.5%	-	-
Pathogenetically oriented					
α-Lipoic acid (thioctic acid)[b]		600 mg IV. infusion	Duration: 3 weeks Not available in U.S.		6.3
		1200-1800 mg orally	Good safety profile Not available in U.S.		
Symptomatic treatment					
Tricyclic anitdepressants (TAC)					
Amitriptyline[b]	10–25 mg	(10-) 25-150 mg	NNMH: 15	++++	2.1
Desipramine[b]		(10-) 25-150 mg	NNMH: 24	++++	2.2/3.2
Imipramine[b]		(10-) 25-150 mg	CRR	++++	1.3/2.4/3.0
Clomipramine[b]		(10-) 25-150 mg	NNMH: 8.7		2.1
Nortriptyline[b]		(10-) 25-150 mg	plus Fluphenazine		1.2 d
SSNRI					
Duloxetine[a]	60 mg	60-120 mg	NNT 120 mg, 60 mg	++	5.3, 4.9

Table 4 (continued)

Treatment Options for Painful Diabetic Neuropathy (Adapted from McQuay et al, Zeigler and Dobecki et al)[79-81]

Compound/ measure	Starting dose	Dose per day	Remarks	Side Effects	NNT
SSRIs					
Paroxetine		40		+++	
Citalopram		40		+++	
Anticonvulsants					
Carbamazepine[a]	100 mg b.i.d.	200-800		+++	
Gabapentin[a]	300 mg nocte (100 mg in elderly)	900-3600 mg	High doses	++	
Pregabalin[a]	75mg nocte or BID. (less in renal impairment)	300-600 mg	NNT 600 mg, 300 mg	++	
Weak opioids					
Tramadol[b]	50 mg	50-400 mg	NNMH: 7.8	+++	
Local treatment					
Capsaicin (0.025%) cream		QID. Topically	Max. duration: 6-8 weeks		
Strong opioids					

(continued)

Table 4

Treatment Options for Painful Diabetic Neuropathy (Adapted from McQuay et al, Zeigler and Dobecki et al)[79-81]

	Compound/ measure	Starting dose	Dose per day	Remarks	Side Effects	NNT
Pain resistant to standard pharmacotherapy	Oxycodone[b]			Add-on treatment	+++	
	Electrical spinal cord stimulation (ESCS)			Invasive, specialist required		
Physical therapy	TENS, medical gymnasts				No AE	
	Balneotherapy, relaxation therapy					
	Acupuncture				No AE	
	Psychological support			Uncontrolled study		

[a] Available and licensed (FDA-approved) for use in neuropathic pain in the U.S..
[b] Available in U.S. but off-label (only used in some specialized centers)
OAD, oral antidiabetic drugs; CRR, concentration-response relationship; NNMH, number needed for major harm; TENS, transcutaneous electrical nerve stimulation; AE, adverse events; SSRI, Selective serotonin reuptake inhibitors; SSNRI, selective serotonin norepinephrine reuptake inhibitors.

6. Complications of Diabetic Peripheral Neuropathy

Apart from being a complication of diabetes, peripheral neuropathy is also a risk factor for other diabetes complications. Two notable complications of peripheral neuropathy in diabetes are Charcot neuroarthropathy and neuropathic (painless) foot ulceration/amputation and these are discussed in the next chapter.

7. Conclusion

Diabetic neuropathy is a common complication of diabetes. Its clinical presentation is multifaceted, as is its etiopathogenesis. The clinical picture ranges from painless symptoms to sometimes debilitating pain and occasionally psychosocial maladaptation may result in symptoms of anxiety and/or depression. The diagnosis of DN is purely clinical and rests on the ability to obtain a good medical history, coupled with simple sensory and/or motor neuron tests. The complex dimensions of DN must be borne in mind when considering management options. Optimum metabolic (glycemic) control is perhaps the most effective option that targets the underlying pathology. As new research unravels the underlying mechanism, novel therapies are emerging. However, their use is limited by the lack of long-term data. Until such data are available, symptomatic, should be used to improve patients' quality of life.

DN constitutes a substantial risk of adverse lower limb complications, including foot ulcerations, infection, amputation and the redoubtable Charcot neuroarthropathy. Thus, systematic and early screening for diabetic neuropathy is mandatory and necessary in all diabetic patients.

8. References

1. Boulton AJM, Gries FA, Jervell JA. Guidelines for the diagnosis and outpatient management of diabetic peripheral neuropathy. *Diabet Med*. 1998;15:508–514.

2. Dyck PJ, Katz KM, Karnes JL, et al. The prevalence by staged severity of various types of diabetic neuropathy, retinopathy and nephropathy in a population-based cohort: the Rochester Diabetic Neuropathy Study. *Neurology*. 1993;43:817–824.

3. Dyck PJ, Melton J, O'Brien PC, et al: Approaches to improve epidemiological studies of diabetic neuropathy. *Diabetes*. 1997;46:S5–S8.

4. Consensus statement. Report and recommendations of the San Antonio conference on diabetic neuropathy. *Diabetes Care*. 1988;11:592–597.

5. Ziegler D. Diagnosis staging and epidemiology of diabetic peripheral neuropathy. *Diab Nutr Metab*. 1994;7:342-348.

6. Boulton AJ, Vinik AI, Arezzo JC, et al for the American Diabetes Association. Diabetic neuropathies: a statement by the American Diabetes Association. *Diabetes Care*. 2005;28(4):956-962.

7. Boulton AJM, Malik RA, Arezzo JC, et al. Diabetic somatic neuropathies. *Diabetes Care*. 2004;27:1458-1486.

8. Writing Team for the Diabetes Control and Complications Trial/Epidemiology of Diabetes Interventions and Complications Research Group. Effect of intensive therapy on the microvascular complications of type 1 diabetes mellitus. *JAMA*. 2002;287:2563–2569

9. Stratton I., Adler AI, Neil H, et al. Association of glycaemia with macrovascular and microvascular complications of type 2 diabetes (UKPDS 35): prospective observational study. *BMJ*. 2000;321:405–412.

10. Boulton A. Lowering the risk of neuropathy, foot ulcers and amputations. *Diabetes Med*. 1998;15:S57–S59.

11. Gaede P, Vedel P, Larsen N, Jensen GV, Parving HH, Pedersen O. Multifactorial intervention and cardiovascular disease in patients with type 2 diabetes. *N Engl J Med*. 2003;348:383–393.

12. Partanen J, Niskanen L, Lehtinen J, Mervaala E, Siitonen O, Uusitupa M. Natural history of peripheral neuropathy in patients with non-insulin dependent diabetes. *New Engl J Med*. 1995;333:39–84.

13. American Diabetes Association: Proceedings of a consensus development conference on standardized measures in diabetic neuropathy. *Diabetes Care*. 1992;15:1079–1107.

14. Obrosova IG. Diabetes and the peripheral nerve. *Biochim Biophys Acta*.(2008); epub ahead of print.

15. Cameron N, Eaton SE, Cotter MA, Tesfaye S. Vascular factors and metabolic interactions in the pathogenesis of diabetic neuropathy. *Diabetologia*. 2001;44,1973–1988.

16. Davidson EP, Coppey LJ, Yorek MA. Activity and expression of the vanilloid receptor 1 (TRPV1) is altered by long-term diabetes in epineurial arterioles of the rat sciatic nerve, *Diab Met Res Rev*. 2006;22:211–219.

17. Coppey LJ, Davidson EP, Rinehart TW, et al, Angiotensin converting enzyme (ACE) inhibitor or angiotensin II receptor antagonist (ARB) attenuate diabetic neuropathy in streptozotocin-diabetic rats. *Diabetes*. 2006;55:341–348.

18. Obrosova IG, Li F, Abatan O, et al. Role of poly(ADP-ribose) polymerase activation in diabetic neuropathy. *Diabetes*. 2004;53:711–720.

19. Cameron NE, Cotter MA. Pro-inflammatory mechanisms in diabetic neuropathy: focus on the nuclear factor kappa B pathway. *Curr. Drug Targets*. 2008;9:60–67.

20. Pop-Busui R, Marinescu V, Van Huysen C, et al. Dissection of metabolic, vascular, and nerve conduction interrelationships in experimental diabetic neuropathy by cyclooxygenase inhibition and acetyl-L-carnitine administration. *Diabetes*. 2002;51:2619–2628

21. Sima AA, Sugimoto K. Experimental diabetic neuropathy: an update. *Diabetologia*. 1999;42:773–788.

22. Kuruvilla R, Eichberg J. Depletion of phospholipid arachidonoyl-containing molecular species in a human Schwann cell line grown in elevated glucose and their restoration by an aldose reductase inhibitor. *J. Neurochem*. 1998;71:775–783.

23. Tomlinson DR, Gardiner NJ. Glucose neurotoxicity. Nat. Rev. *Neurosci*. 2008;9:36–45.

24. Purves T, Middlemas A, Agthong S, et al. A role for mitogen-activated protein kinases in the etiology ofdiabetic neuropathy. *FASEB J*. 2001;15:2508–2514.

25. Russell JW, Sullivan KA, Windebank AJ, Herrmann DN, Feldman EL. Neurons undergo apoptosis in animal and cell culture models of diabetes. *Neurobiol. Dis*. 1999;6:347–363.

26. Horrobin DF. Gamma linolenic acid. *Rev Contemp Phacother*. 1990;1:1-41.

27. Malik RA. Pathology and pathogenesis of diabetic neuropathy. *Diabetic Med*. 1999;7:253 – 260

28. Evans JD, Jacobs TF, Evans EW. Role of acetyl-L-carnitine in the treatment of diabetic peripheral neuropathy. *Ann Pharmacother*. 2008;42(11):1686-1691.

29. Sima AA. The heterogeneity of diabetic neuropathy. *Front Biosci*. 2008 1;13:4809-4816.

30. Dobretsov M, Romanovsky D, Stimers JR. Early diabetic neuropathy: triggers and mechanisms. *World J Gastroenterol*. 2007;13:175-191

31. Hills CE, Brunskill NJ. Cellular and physiological effects of C-peptide. *Clin Sci (Lond)*. 2009;116:565-574.

32. Herder C, Lankisch M, Ziegler D, et al. Subclinical Inflammation and Diabetic Polyneuropathy: MONICA/KORA Survey F3 (Augsburg/Germany). *Diabetes Care*. 2009; epub ahead of print.

33. González-Clemente JM, Mauricio D, Richart C, Broch M, Caixàs A, Megia A, Giménez-Palop O, Simón I, Martínez-Riquelme A, Giménez-Pérez G, Vendrell J. Diabetic neuropathy is associated with activation of the TNF-alpha system in subjects with type 1 diabetes mellitus. *Clin Endocrinol (Oxf)*. 2005;63:525-529.

34. Wang Y, Schmeichel AM, Iida H, Schmelzer JD, Low PA. Enhanced inflammatory response via activation of NF-kappaB in acute experimental diabetic neuropathy subjected to ischemia-reperfusion injury. *J Neurol Sci*. 2006;247:47-52.

35. Jarmuzewska EA, Ghidoni A, Mangoni AA. Hypertension and sensorimotor peripheral neuropathy in type 2 diabetes. *Eur Neurol*. 2007;57:91-95.

36. Caravat CM. Insulin neuritis. A case report. *Va Med Mo*. 1933;59:745–746.

37. Boulton AJM, Malik RA, Arezzo JC, Sosenko JM. Diabetic somatic neuropathy: Technical review. *Diabetes Care*. 2004;27:1458–1487.

38. Vileikyte L, Leventhal H, Gozalez JS, et al. Diabetic peripheral neuropathy and depressive symptoms: the association revisited. *Diabetes Care*. 2005;28:2378-2383

39. Katoulis EC, Ebdon-Parry M, Hollis S, et al. Postural instability in diabetic neuropathic patients at risk of foot ulceration. *Diabet Med*. 1997;14:296–300.

40. Vileikyte L. Diabetic foot ulcers: a quality of life issue. *Diabetes Metab Res Rev*. 2001; 17: 246-249.

41. Vileikyte L, Rubin RR, Leventhal H. Psychological aspects of diabetic neuropathic foot complications: an overview. *Diabetes Metab Res Rev*. 2004;20 (suppl 1):S13-8

42. Galer BS, Gianas A, Jensen MP. Painful diabetic neuropathy: epidemiology, pain description, and quality of life. *Diabetes Res Clin Pract*. 2000; 47: 123-128.

43. Daousi C, MacFarlane IA, Woodward A, Nurmikko TJ, Bundred PE, Benbow SJ. Chronic painful peripheral neuropathy in an urban community: a controlled comparison of people with and without diabetes. *Diabet Med*. 2004;21:976-982.

44. Diabetes Control of Complications Trial Research Group: The effect of intensive diabetes therapy on the development and progression of neuropathy. *Ann Intern Med*. 1995;122:561–568.

45. United Kingdom Prospective Diabetes Study: Intensive blood glucose control with sulphonylureas or insulin compared with conventional treatment and risk of complications in patients with type 2 diabetes. *Lancet*. 1998;352:837–853.

46. Martin CL, Albers J, Herman WH, et al. for the DCCT/EDIC Research Group. Neuropathy among the diabetes control and complications trial cohort 8 years after trial compeltion. *Diabetes Care*. 2006;29:340-344.

47. Abbott CA, Vileikyte L, Williamson S, Carrington AL, Boulton AJ. Multicenter study of the incidence of and predictive risk factors for diabetic neuropathic foot ulceration. *Diabetes Care*. 1998;21:1071–1074.

48. Valk GD, de Sonnaville JJ, van Houtum WH, et al. The assessment of diabetic polyneuropathy in daily practice: reproducibility and validity of Semmes-Weinstein monofilaments and clinical neurological examination. *Muscle Nerve*. 1997;20:116–118.

49. Mayfield JA, Sugarman JR. The use of Semmes-Weinstein monofilament and other threshold tests for preventing foot ulceration and amputation in people with diabetes. *J Fam Pract*. 2000;49:517–529.

50. Abbott CA, Carrington AL, Ashe H, et al. The North-West Diabetes Foot Care Study: incidence of, and risk factors for, new diabetic foot ulceration in a community-based patient cohort. *Diabet Med*. 2002;19(5):377-384.

51. Young MJ, Boulton AJ, Macleod AF, Williams DR, Sonksen PH. A multicentre study of the prevalence of diabetic peripheral neuropathy in the United Kingdom hospital clinic population. *Diabetologia*. 1993;36:150–154.

52. Arezzo JC. The use of electrophysiology for the assessment of diabetic neuropathy. *Neurosci Res Comm*. 1997;21:13–22.

53. Partanen J, Niskanen L, Lehtinen J, Mervaala E, Siitonen O, Uusitupa M. Natural history of peripheral neuropathy in patients with non-insulin dependent diabetes. *New Engl J Med*. 1995;333:39–84.

54. Hirai A, Yasuda H, Joko M, Maeda T, Kikkawa R. Evaluation of diabetic neuropathy through the quantitation of cutaneous nerves. *J Neurol Sci*. 2000;172:55–62.

55. Malik RA, Kallinikos P, Abbott CA, et al. Corneal confocal microscopy: A non-invasive surrogate of nerve fibre damage and repair in diabetic patients. *Diabetologia*. 2003;46:683–688.

56. Kallinikos P, Berhanu M, O'Donnell C, Boulton AJ, Efron N, Malik RA. Corneal nerve tortuosity in diabetic patients with neuropathy. *Invest Ophthalmol Vis Sci*. 2004;45:418–422.

57. Kallinikos P, Berhanu M, O'Donnell C, Boulton AJ, Efron N, Malik RA. Corneal nerve tortuosity in diabetic patients with neuropathy. *Invest Ophthalmol Vis Sci*. 2004;45(2):418-422.

58. Mehra S, Tavakoli M, Kallinikos PA, Efron N, Boulton AJ, Augustine T, Malik RA. Corneal confocal microscopy detects early nerve regeneration after pancreas transplantation in patients with type 1 diabetes. *Diabetes Care*. 2007;30(10):2608-2612.

59. Oyibo SO, Prasad YD, Jackson NJ, Jude EB, Boulton AJ. The relationship between blood glucose excursions and painful diabetic peripheral neuropathy: a pilot study. *Diabet Med*. 2002;19:870-873

60. Caravat CM. Insulin neuritis. A case report. *Va Med Mo*. 2002;1933;59:745–746, 1933.

61. Wilson JL, Sokol DK, Smith LH, Snook RJ, Waguespack SG, Kincaid JC. Acute painful neuropathy (insulin neuritis) in a boy following rapid glycemic control for type 1 diabetes mellitus. *J Child Neurol*. 2003;18:365–367.

62. Vinik A, Mehrabyan A. Diabetic neuropathies. *Med Clin of North Am*. 2004;88(4):947-999.

63. Gillman PK. Tricyclic antidepressant pharmacology and therapeutic drug interactions updated. *Br J Pharmacol*. 2007;151:737–748.

64. Sindrup SH, Gram LF, Skjold T, Frøland A, Beck-Nielsen H. Concentration-response relationship in imipramine treatment of diabetic neuropathy symptoms. *Clin Pharmacol Ther*. 1990;47(4):509-515.

65. O'Connor AB, Noyes K, Holloway RG. A cost-utility comparison of four first-line medications in painful diabetic neuropathy. *Pharmacoeconomics*. 2008;26(12):1045-1064.

66. Gore M, Sadosky A, Leslie D, Sheehan AH. Selecting an appropriate medication for treating neuropathic pain in patients with diabetes: a study using the U.K. and Germany Mediplus databases. *Pain Pract*. 2008;8(4):253-262.

67. Yalcin I, Choucair-Jaafar N, Benbouzid M, et al. beta(2)-adrenoceptors are critical for antidepressant treatment of neuropathic pain. *Ann Neurol*. 2009;65(2):218-225.

68. Yalcin I, Tessier LH, Petit-Demoulière N, et al. Beta(2)-adrenoceptors are essential for desipramine, venlafaxine or reboxetine action in neuropathic pain. *Neurobiol Dis*. 2009;33(3):386-94.

69. Wasan AD, Ossanna MJ, Raskin J, et al. Safety and efficacy of duloxetine in the treatment of diabetic peripheral neuropathic pain in older patients. *Curr Drug Saf*. 2009;4(1):22-29.

70. Giannopoulos S, Kosmidou M, Sarmas I, et al. Patient compliance with SSRIs and gabapentin in painful diabetic neuropathy. *Clin J Pain*. 2007;23(3):267-269.

71. Raskin J, Smith TR, Wong K, et al. Duloxetine versus routine care in the long-term management of diabetic peripheral neuropathic pain. *J Palliat Med*. 2006;9(1):29-40.

72. LaRoche SM, Helmers SL. The new antiepileptic drugs: scientific review. *JAMA*. 2004;291:605-614.

73. Stahl SM. Mechanism of action of alpha2delta ligands: Voltage sensitive calcium channel (VSCC) modulators. *J Clin Psychiatry*. 2004;65:1033-1034.

74. Hurley RW, Lesley MR, Adams MC, Brummett CM, Wu CL. Pregabalin as a treatment for painful diabetic peripheral neuropathy: a meta-analysis. *Reg Anesth Pain Med*. 2008;33(5):389-94.

75. Freeman R, Durso-Decruz E, Emir B. Efficacy, safety, and tolerability of pregabalin treatment for painful diabetic peripheral neuropathy: findings from seven randomized, controlled trials across a range of doses. *Diabetes Care*. 2008;31(7):1448-1454.

76. Hanna M, O'Brien C, Wilson MC. Prolonged-release oxycodone enhances the effects of existing gabapentin therapy in painful diabetic neuropathy patients. *Eur J Pain*. 2008;12(6):804-813.

77. Gilron I, Bailey JM, Tu D, Holden RR, Weaver DF, Houlden RL. Morphine, gabapentin, or their combination for neuropathic pain. *N Engl J Med*. (2005)31;352(13):1324-1334.

78. Gatti A, Sabato AF, Occhioni R, Colini Baldeschi G, Reale C. Controlled-release oxycodone and pregabalin in the treatment of neuropathic pain: results of a multicenter Italian study. *Eur Neurol*. 2009;61(3):129-137.

79. McQuay HJ, Tramèr M, Nye BA, Carroll D, Wiffen PJ, Moore RA. A systematic review of antidepressants in neuropathic pain. *Pain*. 1996;68:217-227.

80. Ziegler D. Painful diabetic neuropathy: treatment and future aspects. *Diabetes Metab Res Rev*. 2008;24 (suppl) 1:S52-S57.

81. Dobecki DA, Schocket SM, Wallace MS. Update on pharmacotherapy guidelines for the treatment of neuropathic pain. *Curr Pain Headache Rep*. 2006;10(3):185-190.

Chapter 4B:
The Diabetic Foot

Andrew JM Boulton, MD, DSc (Hon), FRCP

Contents

1. Scope of the Problem

Diabetic foot problems have been recognized as increasingly important in recent years, as they represent the commonest cause of hospital admission amongst diabetic patients in Western countries, are responsible for much morbidity, and even mortality, and are a major economic drain on the health care system. The global term "diabetic foot" is used to refer to a variety of pathologic conditions that might affect the feet of diabetic patients. Whereas neuropathy is a major contributory factor in the etiopathogenesis of foot ulceration and Charcot Neuroarthropathy (CN), it can all too often be implicated in the causal chain ultimately resulting in amputation. However, in recent years, neuroischemic and ischemic ulcers have become increasingly more common, possibly because neuropathic ulcers are easier to prevent.[1]

A number of facts also attest to the increasing importance of diabetic foot disease:

- Foot ulceration is common, affecting up to 25% of diabetic patients during their lifetime, and over 85% of lower limb amputations are preceded by foot ulcers: diabetes remains the commonest cause of non-traumatic amputation in Western countries.[2,3]

- Prevention is the first step towards solving diabetic foot problems. Although it was estimated in 2005 that a leg is lost to diabetes somewhere in the world every 30 seconds, the vast majority of these amputations should be preventable.

- Strategies aimed at preventing foot ulcers can be cost-effective and cost-saving, if increased education and effort are focused on those with recognized foot problems.

- Diabetes is now the commonest cause of CN in Western countries, another condition that should be generally preventable.[5]

- Recent data from the U.S. suggests that, in 2007, over $30 billion was spent by the health care system on the management of foot ulcers and amputations in people with diabetes.[6]

Epidemiology of Diabetic Foot Problems

Foot ulceration and amputation will be considered together in this section, as they are closely interrelated. A selection of epidemiologic data for diabetic foot ulceration and amputation, originating from studies from a number of different countries, is provided in Table 1. As can be seen in Table 1, reported frequencies of amputation and ulceration do vary considerably as a consequence of different diagnostic criteria used, as well as regional differences. However, diabetes remains a major cause of non-traumatic amputation across the world, with rates being as great as 15 times higher than in the non-diabetic population. It is not possible to do direct comparisons between studies and countries because of methodological issues and, additionally, surveys invariably include only patients with previously diagnosed diabetes, whereas in type 2 diabetes, foot problems may be a presenting feature. In the United Kingdom Prospective Diabetes Study, for example, 13% of patients had neuropathy at diagnosis of diabetes of sufficient severity to put them at major risk for foot problems.

2. Etiopathogenesis of Foot Ulceration and Amputations

A thorough understanding of the pathways that result in the development of foot lesions is essential if we are to be successful in reducing the high incidence of foot ulcers and ultimately amputations in diabetes. Ulceration does not occur spontaneously, rather, it is the combination of causative factors that result in the development of a lesion. A list of those factors which evidence has indicated increase the risk of developing a foot ulcer is provided in Table 2. A schematic diagram of the pathways to foot ulceration is displayed in Figure 1.

Sensorimotor neuropathy is very common in patients with diabetes, and it has been estimated that up to 50% of older type 2 patients have sensory loss of sufficient severity to put them at increased risk of developing foot problems. It must be remembered that many patients have insensitive feet at risk of ulceration, without experiencing any typical neuropathic symptoms. *Thus, the diagnosis of the "at risk neuropathic foot" can only be made after a careful clinical examination has been performed: history alone is insufficient.*

Peripheral vascular disease (PVD) is also more common in patients with diabetes, tends to occur at an earlier age and is more likely to involve dis-

Table 2

Factors Increasing Risk of Diabetic Foot Ulceration

Peripheral Neuropathy
- **Somatic**
- **Autonomic**

Peripheral Vascular Disease
Past history of foot ulcers
Other long-term complication
- **End-stage renal disease**
- Visual loss

Plantar Callus Foot Deformity

Edema
Ethnic background
Poor social background
Living alone
More common contributory factors shown in bold

Table 1

Epidemiology of Foot Ulceration and Amputation[7]

Country	Year	N	Prevalence (%)		Incidence (%)		Risk factors for foot ulcers (%)
			Ulcers	Amputation	Ulcers	Amputation	
Germany	2008	4778	0.8[a]	1.6	-		>40
Bahrain	2007	1477	5.9	-	-		45
UK	2002	9710	1.7	1.3	2.2		>50
Greece	2002	821	4.8	-	-		>50
Netherlands	1999	665	-	-	2.1	0.6	-
U.S.	1994	8965	-	-	2.0	0.3	-
UK	1994	821	1.4[a]	-			42

[a]Active ulcers: 5.4% past or current ulcer

tal vessels. As noted above, in recent years neuroischemic ulcers (in which the combination of neuropathy and PVD exists in the same patient) together with some form of trauma are becoming increasingly common in diabetic foot clinics.[1]

Whereas sensorimotor neuropathy and PVD are the main contributory factors in the pathway to foot ulceration, a number of other contributory factors are well-recognized. Sympathetic autonomic dysfunction of the lower limbs leads to reduced sweating, resulting in dry skin and, potentially, the build-up of a callus. Moreover, this sympathetic dysfunction results in increased blood flow to the foot in the absence of large vessel disease, resulting in the **warm foot.** It must be remembered that the warm, insensitive foot is just as much at risk for foot problems as the **cool foot** secondary to PVD.

It has been increasingly recognized in recent years that patients with end-stage renal disease (ESRD), particularly those on dialysis, have a much greater risk of developing foot lesions. Similarly, retinopathy (especially with disturbed vision) has been shown to increase the risk of foot lesions.

The foot deformities are also common in those patients at risk for foot ulcers, and are likely due to a combination of motor neuropathy, cheiroarthropathy (limited joint mobility) and altered gait patterns. The **high-risk** neuropathic foot often has clawing of the toes, prominent metatarsal heads, a high arch and small muscle wasting. Finally, there appear to be ethnic differences in the risk of developing a foot problem, with patients from India and sub-continental Asia, Hispanic Americans and native Americans being at increased risk over patients of European origin.

Pathways to Ulceration

It is most common that a combination of 2 or more risk factors ultimately contribute to the development of diabetic foot lesions. In a prospective study on the causation of foot ulceration, Reiber et al[8] identified a number of causal pathways, with the commonest triad of component causes being neuropathy, deformity and trauma (present in nearly 2 out of 3 incident foot ulcer cases). Edema and ischemia were also common component causes. Thus, the patient with insensi-

Figure 1

Pathways to diabetic foot ulceration

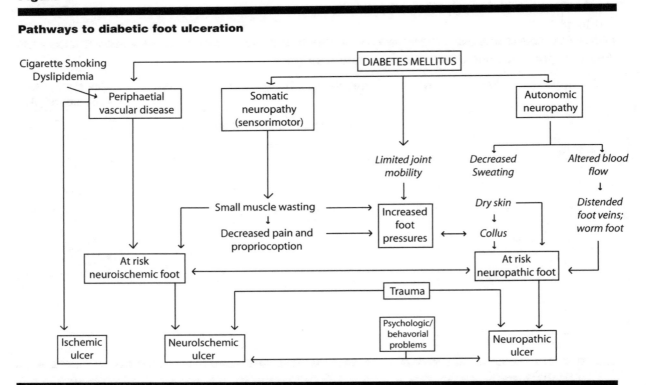

tivity secondary to neuropathy, claw toes and prominent metatarsal heads may develop an ulcer because of inappropriate footwear (commonest cause of trauma in the U.S.), which rubs against prominent parts of the foot and leads to ulceration that is not initially detected by the individual. In neuroischemic ulcers, the 3 component causes of ischemia, trauma and neuropathy are often seen in patients presenting with new lesions.

Table 3

Key Components of the Diabetic Foot Exam

Inspection

- **Evidence of past/present ulcers**
- **Foot shape?**

  prominent metatarsal heads/claw toes
  hallux valgus
  muscle wasting
  Charcot deformity

- Dermatological?
  callus
  erythema
  sweating

Neurological

- 10g monofilament at 4 sites on each foot, + 1 of the following
- Vibration using 128HZ tuning fork
- Pinprick sensation
- Ankle reflexes
- Vibration perception threshold

Vascular

- Foot pulses
- Ankle Brachial Pressure Index, if indicated

3. Screening and Prevention

As noted above, it has been stated that the vast majority of foot problems in diabetes are potentially preventable: the first step in prevention must be the identification of the *at-risk population.* It is now accepted that every patient with diabetes should be screened for major complications, including risk of foot ulcers, at least annually, and such a review can be carried out either in the primary care or hospital setting. A task force of the American Diabetes Association (ADA) recently addressed the question of what should be included for foot screening in the *comprehensive diabetic foot examination* (CDFE).[9] Wherever possible, recommendations were made according to evidence-based medicine, and emphasis was placed on a simple clinical examination, as up to 50% of foot ulcer patients have no history of any neuropathic or vascular symptoms. There is a strong evidence base to support the use of simple clinical tests as predictors of foot ulcers.[9,10] A summary of the key components of the CDFE is provided in Table 3. 2 simple clinical assessments, the 10 g pressure perception using the 10 g monofilament and 1 of 4 other tests was recommended for neuropathy, whereas foot pulse palpation remains the mainstay in the assessment of the peripheral vasculature. The ankle brachial index should also be tested in patients with diabetes over 50 years of age, if possible.[11]

Interventions for High-risk Patients

Any abnormality of the above screening tests would place a patient into a group at higher risk of ulceration, and potential interventions will be discussed under a number of sub-headings, the most important of which is education.

Education

A reduction in neuropathic foot problems will only be achieved if we remember that patients with insensitive feet have lost their warning signal — *pain* — that ordinarily brings the patient to their doctor. Thus, the care of the patient with no pain sensation or other peripheral sensations is a new challenge, for which we have little training. It is difficult for us to comprehend, for example, that an intelligent patient would buy and wear a pair of shoes 3 sizes too small and come to our clinic with an extensive shoe-induced ulcer. The explanation, however, is simple: with reduced sensation, a very tight fit stimulates the remaining pressure nerve endings and is then interpreted by the patient as a normal fit. In order to successfully reduce the risk of foot ulcers and amputations, we must realize that with the loss of pain there is also diminished motivation in the healing and, more importantly, the prevention of injury.

It may be for this reason that there is little evidence to actually support the use of preventative education in first foot ulcers in diabetes. Patients clearly need to be informed of the risk of having insensate feet, the need for regular self-inspection, foot hygiene and podiatry treatment and, additionally, they must be told what action to take in the event of an injury or the discovery of a foot ulcer. However, it has been shown that patients often possess distorted beliefs about neuropathy,[12] thinking that it is a circulatory problem and subsequently do not link foot ulcers and amputation. Thus, an educational program that focuses on reducing foot ulcers will be doomed to failure and, therefore, much work is required in the area of preventative education. Sadly, a recent study of a focused foot care education program in patients with a history of ulcers could find no evidence that such targeted education was associated with a reduced incidence of foot ulceration.[13]

Podiatry

Regular nail and skin care, callus trimming and education by a podiatrist are all essential in the management of the high-risk diabetic foot. Attempted self-care has been reported in several cases to cause ulceration and, similarly, self-care of calluses must be discouraged.

Footwear/Orthoses/Hosiery

Whereas inappropriate footwear is often a common cause of foot ulceration in insensitive feet, good footwear has been shown in more than 1 study to reduce the incidence of recurrent ulceration.[5,7]

amoxicillin/clavulanic acid combination (Augmentin®) or clindamycin.

Limb-threatening Infection

Patients with a limb-threatening infection generally display systemic systems and signs, and require hospitalization and parenteral antibiotics. Deep wound and blood cultures should be obtained, the circulation assessed with non-invasive studies and metabolic control should be optimized. Early surgical debridement is indicated in such cases and, as above, antibiotic regimens should be broad-spectrum until sensitivities are known. For such serious infections, a combination of clindamycin and ciprofloxacin, or flucloxacillin, ampicillin and metronidazole may be suitable.

An increasing concern with diabetic foot clinics is the identification and isolation of antibiotic-resistant pathogens, such as Methicillin-resistant Staphylococcus Aureus (MRSA). In most cases, such organisms are opportunistic colonizers rather than true pathogens, and are secondary to the often inappropriate use of long duration broad-spectrum antibiotics. Anti-MRSA specific therapies are rarely indicated.

Adjunctive Therapies

A number of adjunctive therapies, including growth factors, bioengineered skin substitutes and others have been studied in the last decade. However, there is little evidence to support their regular use in the management of diabetic foot lesions. Many of these have recently been reviewed by the international working group on the diabetic foot.[18] There is some evidence for the use of hyperbaric oxygen, but this is generally of benefit only in ischemic ulcers with infection, when there is no possibility of distal bypass or angioplasty. There is stronger evidence to support the use of negative pressure wound therapy (NPWT) using vacuum-assisted closure in the management of complex diabetic foot wounds.[2] Recent randomized, controlled trials suggest that this modality might lead to more rapid appearance of granulation tissue, with a lesser chance of recurrent ulceration or even amputation.[7]

Osteomyelitis

The diagnosis of osteomyelitis in the diabetic foot remains a significant clinical challenge. Several diagnostic tests have been recommended and, amongst these, *probing to bone* has been shown to have the greatest predictive value, whereas plain radiographs are insensitive in early states in the natural history of osteomyelitis. Whereas the diagnosis is ultimately made in most cases using a plain radiograph of the foot, magnetic resonance imaging (MRI) is playing an increasing role in the diagnosis, as it has high sensitivity. The most recent review on this topic suggests that a combination of clinical and laboratory findings can significantly improve diagnostic accuracy for osteomyelitis in the diabetic foot. Most helpful is the combination of ulcer depth with serum inflammatory markers.[19] Contrary to traditional teaching, it is increasingly recognized that some cases of localized osteomyelitis, particularly those not involving a joint space, can be managed by long-term antibiotic therapy. Despite this, localized bony resection after appropriate antibiotic therapy remains the most common approach to care. It is clear that further research is needed in this area, as the evidence base for diagnosis and management of osteomyelitis remains very limited.[20]

Ischemic Ulcers

Ulcers in which there is a major ischemic component are generally graded C or D (with or without infection) under the UT wound classification system. All patients presenting with foot ulcers in which any degree of ischemia is suspected should have a non-invasive vascular assessment and be considered for arteriography. In addition to offloading and the management of infection, patients with significant arterial lesions warrant assessment by vascular surgery, and bypass should be considered, if appropriate. In the presence of osteomyelitis (UT 3D), ischemia can significantly, adversely influence the outcome. If possible, procedures to improve arterial inflow should be carried out prior to any surgical treatment of osteomyelitis, and all patients should be on appropriate antibiotic therapy. There is reasonable evidence that patients with significant arterial impairment, as confirmed by a low transcutaneous oxygen tension (TCOT), may experience delayed healing and an increased risk of amputation.

CN was first described in the mid-19th century by Jean-Martin Charcot, a Parisian neurologist. In the Western world, diabetes is now the most common cause of this largely preventable and common clinical problem. An accepted definition of a Charcot joint is one in which there is simultaneous presence of bone and joint destruction, fragmentation and remodeling: this condition is generally a painless, progressive and destructive arthropathy.

Permissive features for the development of acute CN include: somatic and autonomic neuropathy, adequate arterial inflow and trauma, which is often unrecognized. Loss of pain and pressure sensation permits repetitive, minor trauma in a foot with sympathetic neuropathy and, consequently, increased skin and bone blood flow occurs. Although classically described as painless, up to 50% of patients with acute CN may experience non-specific discomfort in the affected foot. Typically, patients present with the warm swollen foot in the absence of skin breaks. Affected patients tend to be younger than is usual for the patient presenting with a foot ulcer and, although a history of trauma may be present, the trauma is rarely of sufficient severity to account for the abnormalities observed on clinical examination. Although characterized by increased local bone resorption, the exact cellular mechanisms contributing to acute CN remain poorly understood.[21] There has recently been interest in the potential of molecular mechanisms, including the receptor activator of nuclear factor Kappa B ligand (RANK-L) as a potential mediator of osteoclast formation and activation. Jeffcoate has hypothesized that the RANK-L/osteoprotegerin pathway may play an important part in the development of acute CN.[21] More recently, it has been reported that monocytes isolated from patients with CN, cultured in the presence of macrophage-colony stimulating factor, results in an increase in osteoclast formation when compared to healthy control subjects.[22] These observations suggest that RANK-L mediated osteoclastic resorption contributes to the development of acute CN.

Left untreated, patients continue to bear weight on the acute Charcot foot and bony destruction with remodeling occurs, leading in many cases to gross deformities. There is substantial evidence that

6. Conclusion

offloading the affected foot using TCC (as an example), is an effective means to reduce disease activity during this acute phase. Use of the cast should continue until swelling and hyperemia have resolved and the skin temperature differential is 1° C or less, at which time custom-molded shoes with appropriate insoles are indicated. Bisphosphonates, potent inhibitors of osteoclast activation, have been suggested as useful adjunctive therapy in reducing disease activity in acute CN in a randomized trial. However, further confirmation is needed and trials are ongoing.

The management of advanced CN with bony deformity requiring reconstructive surgery is beyond the scope of this chapter and the reader is referred to a recent review by Robinson et al for additional detail.[23]

Diabetic foot disease causes significant morbidity and is associated with increased mortality. It should be clear that the spectrum of diabetic foot problems requires the involvement of individuals from many specialties. The diabetic foot cannot be regarded as the sole responsibility of the diabetologist alone, and a number of reports in the past decade have promoted the benefits of multi-disciplinary management of the diabetic foot. There is increasing evidence from long-term studies that support the adoption of a multi-disciplinary approach, not only in the hospital, but in the community setting, and this approach is associated with a reduced incidence of foot complications.[24] There is substantial evidence that a sustained reduction in major amputations can be achieved and maintained over 20 years, and all these data suggest that an aggressive approach to screening and management of diabetic foot problems in the future is likely to be associated with improved outcomes.[25]

7. References

1. Gershater MA, Lödahl M, Myberg P, et al. Complexity of factors related to outcome of neuropathic and neuroischaemic/ischemic diabetic foot ulcers: a cohort study. *Diabetologia.* 2009;52:398-407.

2. Singh N, Armstrong DG, Lipsky BA. Preventing foot ulcers in patients with diabetes. JAMA. 2005;293:217-228.

3. Boulton AJM, Vileikyte L, Ragnarson-Tennvall G, Apelqvist J. The global burden of diabetic foot disease. *Lancet.* 2005;366:1719-1724.

4. Ragnarson-Tennvall G, Apelqvist J. Prevention of diabetes-related foot ulcers and amputations: a cost-utility analysis based on Markov model simulations. *Diabetologia.* 2001;44:2077-2087.

5. Boulton AJM. The Diabetic Foot: from art to science. The 18th Camillo Golgi lecture. *Diabetologia.* 2004;47:1343-1353.

6. Rogers LX, Lavery LA, Armstrong DG. The right to bear legs. *J Amer Podiat Med Assoc.* 2008;98:166-168.

7. Boulton AJM. Foot problems in people with diabetes. In:

8. Reiber GE, Vileikyte L, Boyko EJ, et al. Causal pathways for incident lower-extremity ulcers in patients with diabetes from two settings. *Diabetes Care.* 1999;22:157-162.

9. Boulton AJM, Armstrong DG, Albert SF, et al. Comprehensive foot examination and risk assessment. *Diabetes Care.* 2008;31:1679-1685.

10. Abbott CA, Carrington AL, Ashe H, et al. The North-West Daibetes Foot Care Study: incidence of, and risk factors for, new diabetic foot ulceration in a community-based patient cohort. *Diabetic Med.* 2002;19:377-384.

11. American Diabetes Association. Peripheral arterial disease in people with diabetes. *Diabetes Care.* 2003;26:3333-3341.

12. Vileikyte L. Psychosocial and behavioral aspects of diabetic foot lesions. *Curr Diab Rep.* 2008;8:119-125.

13. Lincoln NB, Radford KA, Game FL, Jeffcoate WJ. Education for secondary prevention of foot ulcers in people with diabetes: a randomised controlled trial. *Diabetologia.* 2008;51:1954-1961.

14. Lavery LA, Higgins KR, Lanctot DR, et al. Preventing diabetic foot ulcer recurrence in high-risk patients: use of temperature monitoring as a self-assessment tool. *Diabetes Care.* 2007;30:14-20.

15. Piaggesi A, Viacava P, Rizzo L, et al. Semi-quantitative analysis of the histopathological features of the neuropathic foot ulcers: effects of pressure relief. *Diabetes Care.* 2003;26:3123-3128.

16. Lipsky BA. New developments in diagnosing and treatment diabetic foot infections. *Diabet Metab Res Rev.* 2008;24(suppl 1):S66-S71.

17. Lipsky BA, Berendt AR, Deery HG, et al. IDSA guidelines; diagnosis and treatment of diabetic foot infections. *Clin Infect Dis.* 2004;39:885-910.

18. Jeffcoate WJ, Lipsky BA, Berendt AR, et al. Unresolved issues in the management of ulcers of the foot in diabetes. *Diabetic Med.* 2008;25:1380-1389.

19. Fleischer AE, Didyk AA, Woods JB, Burns SE, Wrobel JS, Armstrong DG. Combined clinical and laboratory testing improves diagnostic accuracy ofr osteomyelitis in the diabetic foot. *J Foot Ankle Surg.* 2009;48:39-46.

20. Berendt AR, Peters EJ, Bakker K, et al. Diabetic foot osteomyelitis: a progress report on diagnosis and a systematic review of treatment. *Diabet Metab Res Rev.* 2008;24(suppl 1):S145-S161.

21. Jeffcoate WJ. Charcot neuroarthropathy. *Diabet Metab Res Rev.* 2008;24(suppl 1):S62-S65.

22. Mabilleau G, Petrova NL, Edmonds ME, Sabokhar A. Increased osteoclastic activity in acute Charcot osteoarthropathy: the role of receptor activator of nuclear factor-kappa B ligand. *Diabetologia.* 2008;51:1035-1040.

23. Robinson AH, Pasapula C, Brodsky JW. Surgical aspects of the diabetic foot. *J Bone Joint Surg* BR. 2009;91:1-7.

24. Krishnan S, Nash F, Baker N, Fowler D, Rayman G. Reduction in diabetic amputations over 11 years in a defined UK population: benefits of multidisciplinary team work and continuous prospective audit. *Diabetes Care.* 2008;31:99-101.

25. Larsson J, Eneroth M, Apelqvist J, Stenström A. Sustained reduction in major amputations in diabetic patients: 628 amputations in 461 patients in a defined population over a 20-year period. *Acta Orthop.* 2008;79:665-673.

Chapter 5: Obesity and Diabetes: Implications for Management

Steven R. Smith, MD
Corby Martin, PhD
Peter Katzmarzyk, PhD
Timothy Church, MD

Contents

1. Introduction

In this chapter, we will review the basics of obesity management. After providing a global view of the obesity epidemic and a discussion of the evidence linking obesity to type 2 diabetes, we review the basics of assessment of the obese patient. This is followed by a discussion of behavior modification as a means to achieve a healthy diet and increased physical activity. Reduced calorie diets and exercise are the cornerstones of obesity management. As part of a stepped care approach, if lifestyle modification is unsuccessful, then drug therapy is indicated in many patients. Once considered a treatment of last resort, bariatric surgery is moving into the mainstream. Finally, we will discuss what people who are successful in the long-term at weight loss do to keep the pounds off.

2. Assessment of the Obese Patient

Obesity is a disease of excess adiposity beyond the normal range for a person's age and sex. State-of-the art laboratory techniques, such as dual energy x-ray absorptiometry (DXA), magnetic resonance imaging (MRI) and computed tomography (CT), are now available that can quantify the amount of adipose tissue, both at the level of the entire body (ie, fat mass, % body fat) as well as the amount of adipose tissue in specific body compartments (visceral abdominal, subcutaneous, etc.). However, these techniques have been proven to be largely impractical for widespread use in population surveys. Population studies generally rely on anthropometric markers of adiposity. The most widely used measures are the body mass index (BMI; kg/m^2) and waist circumference. The World Health Organization[1] has proposed categories of BMI of underweight (<18.5 kg/m^2), normal weight ($18.5\text{-}24.9$ kg/m^2), overweight (≥ 25 kg/m^2) and obesity (≥ 30 kg/m^2), which have been adopted by the US National Institutes of Health (NIH).[2] (Table 1, Table 2a, Table 2b, Table 3, Figure 1) Further, the NIH has recommended that waist circumference thresholds of 88 cm in women and 102 cm in men are indicative of increased obesity-related health risks.[2] Waist circumference is measured differentways around the world. The NIH recommends measuring waist circumference using an inelastic tape measure at the level of the superior border of the iliac crest. The patients should be standing comfortably with feet shoulder-width apart, and the measurement should be made at the end of normal expiration, being careful to keep the tape parallel with the floor.[2]

Table 2a

Obesity Class Definitions - I

Classification	Obesity Class	BMI kg/m^2
Underweight		<18.5
Normal		18.5–24.9
Overweight		25–29.9
Obesity	I	30.0-34.9
35.0–39.9	II	35.0-39.9
Extreme Obesity	III	≥40.0

Table 3

Obesity Class Definitions - II

Waist Circumference
- High risk:
  - * Men >102 cm (40 in)
  - * Women >88 cm (35 in)

Table 1

Measures of Obesity

Body Mass Index (BMI) describes relative weight for height

Calculation

= Weight (kg)/height (m^2)

= Weight (lbs)/height (in^2) x 703

Figure 1

BMI from height and weight

Height \ Weight (lbs)	120	130	140	150	160	170	180	190	200	210	220	230	240	250	260	270	280	290	300
5'0"	23	25	27	29	31	33	35	37	39	41	43	45	47	49	51	53	55	57	59
5'2"	22	24	26	27	29	31	33	35	37	38	40	42	44	46	48	49	51	53	55
5'4"	21	22	24	26	28	29	31	33	34	36	38	40	41	43	45	46	48	50	52
5'6"	19	21	23	24	26	27	29	31	32	34	36	37	39	40	42	44	45	47	49
5'8"	18	20	21	23	24	26	27	29	30	32	34	35	37	38	40	41	43	44	46
5'10"	17	19	20	22	23	24	26	27	29	30	32	33	35	36	37	39	40	42	43
6'0"	16	18	19	20	22	23	24	26	27	29	30	31	33	34	35	37	38	39	41
6'2"	15	17	18	19	21	22	23	24	26	27	28	30	31	32	33	35	36	37	39
6'4"	15	16	17	18	20	21	22	23	24	26	27	28	29	30	32	33	34	35	37

3. Epidemiology of Obesity and Type 2 Diabetes

It is currently estimated that more than 1.5 billion people worldwide are overweight,[3] and that the prevalence of type 2 diabetes is expected to increase from 171 million in 2000 to 366 million by 2030.[4] Obesity is a key indicator of a patient's risk of developing type 2 diabetes, as relative risk for type 2 diabetes increases substantially in overweight and obese men and women, by comparison to normal weight individuals.[5,6] The increasing burden of obesity, type 2 diabetes and associated cardiovascular disease threatens to overwhelm the health care systems of many developed and developing countries. A review of the worldwide epidemiology of obesity and type 2 diabetes is beyond the scope of this chapter; however we focus here on the recent trends that have occurred in the United States, a population which seems to be at the leading edge of the global epidemic.

Obesity

There are 2 main, ongoing population surveillance systems for obesity in the United States. The National Health and Nutrition Examination Survey (NHANES) collects measured height, weight (and BMI) and waist circumference data on a nationally representative sample of children, adolescents and adults on an ongoing basis. The Behavioral Risk Factor Surveillance System (BRFSS) collects self-reported height and weight (and BMI) data on a representative sample of the US adult population every 2 years. The BRFSS has a large enough sample size to allow for state-specific estimates of obesity prevalence; however, the smaller samples sizes in NHANES allows for the release of prevalence estimates at the national level only.

Both the NHANES and BRFSS have documented significant increases in the prevalence of the overweight and obese in the US population over recent decades. Figure 2 depicts the prevalence of obesity among adults from 1999-2004 in NHANES[5-9] and from 1991 to 2007 in the BRFSS.[8–13] Both series of surveys show dramatic increases in the prevalence of obesity over time. The higher prevalence of obesity in NHANES compared to the BRFSS is mainly the result of the method of data collection – heights and weights were directly measured in NHANES, whereas they were collected by

self-report in BRFSS, and adults tend to underreport their weight and overreport their height when participating in surveys that rely on responses to self-reported questionnaires.[14] The most recent data from NHANES indicate that over 34% of American adults are obese.[9]

There is also evidence that waist circumference is increasing over time in the U.S.[15,16] For example, the proportion of men and women with a waist circumference exceeding the NIH high-risk threshold (>102 cm in men and >88 cm in women) increased from 29.5% to 36.9% and from 46.7% to 55.1% between 1988-1994 and 1999-2000, respectively.[15] Further, there is also an indication that waist circumference may be increasing at a rate beyond that which would expected based on the increases in BMI.[17] These data suggest that, not only is the population becoming more obese, but it may also be becoming more abdominally obese over time.

There are very little data available on the incidence of obesity. However, the longitudinal design of the National Population Health Survey in Canada allows some insight into this issue. Among normal-weight adults 20-54 years of age in 1994-1995, 32% had become overweight by 2002-2003, and 23% of those who were overweight in 1994-1995 had become obese by 2002-2003.[18] These data highlight the progression of weight gain among normal-weight and overweight adults in the general population.

Type 2 Diabetes

The temporal trends in the prevalence of type 2 diabetes have paralleled the increases observed in obesity. In 1999-2002, the prevalence of diabetes among adults 20+ years of age was 9.3%; however, the prevalence of diagnosed diabetes was only 6.5%, as the remainder of the cases were undiagnosed until the time of the survey examination.[19] Between 1988-1994 and 1999-2002 in NHANES, the prevalence of diagnosed diabetes increased from 5.1% to 6.5%; however, the prevalence of undiagnosed diabetes remained stable (2.7% and 2.8%, respectively).[19] Data from the National Health Interview Survey indicates that the age-adjusted prevalence of diagnosed diabetes has increased from 2.5% in 1980 to 5.8% in 2006 (Figure 2 and Figure 3).[20]

The prevalence of diabetes represents a snap shot in time, as to the number of people with the disease at a given time. However, changes in prevalence over time can reflect either a change in the number of new cases (incidence), changes in the case-mortality rate or some combination of these 2 factors. A recent analysis of data from the BRFSS demonstrated that the incidence of diabetes in the U.S. increased, from 4.8 cases in 1000 persons in 1995-1997 to 9.1 cases in 1000 persons in 2005-2007.[21] The results from a population-based sample from Rochester, MN indicated that the total mortality burden associated with type 2 diabetes increased between 1970 to 1994, likely due to the rising incidence; however, mortality rates among those with type 2 diabetes declined by 13.8%.[22] An analysis of data from Ontario, Canada that examined multiple influences on type 2 diabetes demonstrated that the prevalence of type 2

Figure 2

Changes in the prevalence of obesity among US adults between 1999-2004 in the National Health and Nutrition Examination Survey and from 1991 to 2007 in the Behavioral Risk Factor Surveillance System

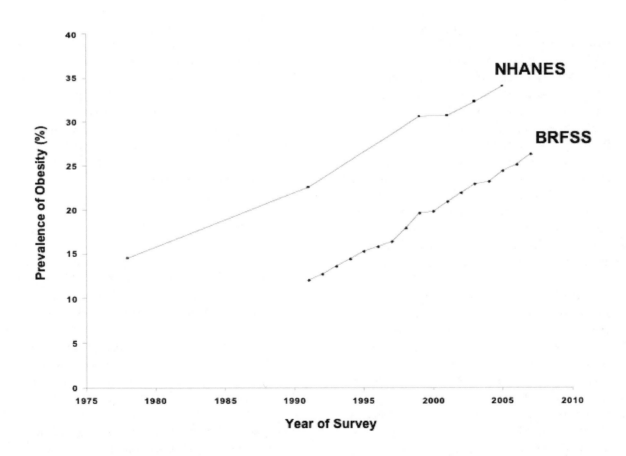

Figure 3

Changes in the age-adjusted prevalence of diabetes in the National Health Interview Survey from 1980 to 2006[18]

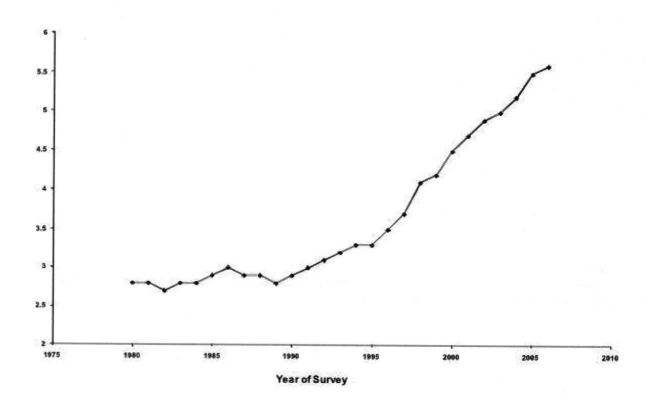

Year of Survey

diabetes increased, from 5.2% in 1995 to 8.8% in 2005; however, this increase was a function of an increase in the incidence rate from 6.6 cases in 1000 persons in 1997 to 8.2 cases in 1000 persons in 2003, and a reduction in the case mortality rate from 3.3 deaths in 1000 persons in 1995 to 1.9 deaths in 1000 persons in 2005.[23]

Epidemiology

The prevalence of both obesity and type 2 diabetes have both increased substantially over recent decades in the United States. Although data collection methods vary across different surveillance

systems, the results are consistent with respect to the temporal trends observed.

As with other chronic diseases, lifestyle modification is the cornerstone of obesity therapy. This stepped approach is appropriate and works well for other chronic diseases. The NHLBI treatment guidelines focus on the BMI and the presence of comorbidities, such as diabetes and hypertension.

Newer approaches, like the Edmonton obesity staging system, may supplant the more traditional NHLBI model.[24] This system adds to the current anthropometric (Table 2b) classification through staging, based on the presence and extent of comorbidities and functional limitations. The concept draws upon a growing body of literature that recognizes that some people with obesity are healthy and do not suffer the medical consequences of obesity, whereas many with lower BMIs have multiple comorbidities.

Population-based strategies may be implemented in the future, as was the case for smoking cessation programs, cholesterol reduction programs and dental cavities. Population level interventions could include additional efforts towards a healthy diet, but also modification of workplaces and cities to facilitate physical activity. Another tactic is to tax the foods which are unhealthy and subsidize foods that are healthy. To date, our political climate has not endorsed these population-level strategies, although that could change as the epidemic and costs associated with obesity and type 2 diabetes grow.

4. Treatment of Obesity

Overview (Table 4, Figure 4)

Who to treat and how?
Exercise and behavior/lifestyle modification are the cornerstones of treatment, and serve as a base for both pharmacotherapy and surgery.

Most patients who need to lose weight have made several attempts over their lifetime. As such, a careful history, which often finds multiple weight-loss attempts, is sufficient to move on toward more intensive interventions.

Benefits of modest weight loss
How much weight loss is enough? Modest weight loss on the order of 5%-10% of body weight is sufficient to produce beneficial effects on metabolism and prevent diabetes. (Figure 5)

Table 2b

Edmonton functional staging of obesity

Stage	Description
0	No apparent obesity-related risk factors (eg, blood pressure, serum lipids, fasting glucose, etc. within normal range), no physical symptoms, no psychopathology, no functional limitations and/or impairment of well being
1	Presence of obesity-related subclinical risk factors (eg, borderline hypertension, impaired fasting glucose, elevated liver enzymes, etc.), mild physical symptoms (eg, dyspnea on moderate exertion, occasional aches and pains, fatigue, etc.), mild psychopathology, mild functional limitations and/or mild impairment of well being
2	Presence of established obesity-related chronic disease (eg, hypertension, type 2 diabetes, sleep apnea, osteoarthritis, reflux disease, polycystic ovary syndrome, anxiety disorder, etc.), moderate limitations in activities of daily living and/or wellbeing
3	Established end-organ damage, such as myocardial infarction, heart failure, diabetic complications, incapacitating osteoarthritis, significant psychopathology, significant functional limitations and/or impairment of wellbeing
4	Severe (potentially end-stage) disabilities from obesity-related chronic diseases, severe disabling psychopathology, severe functional limitations and/or severe impairment of wellbeing

Table 4

Guide for Selecting Obesity Treatment

Treatment	BMI Category (kg/m²)				
	25–26.9	27–29.9	30–34.9	35–39.9	≥40
Diet, Exercise, Behavior Tx	+	+	+	+	+
Pharmacotherapy		*With co-morbidities*	+	+	+
Surgery				*With co-morbidities*	+

The Practical Guide: Identification, Evaluation, and Treatment of Overweight and Obesity in Adults. October 2000. NIH Publication No. 00-4084

Figure 4

Approaches to treatment of obesity

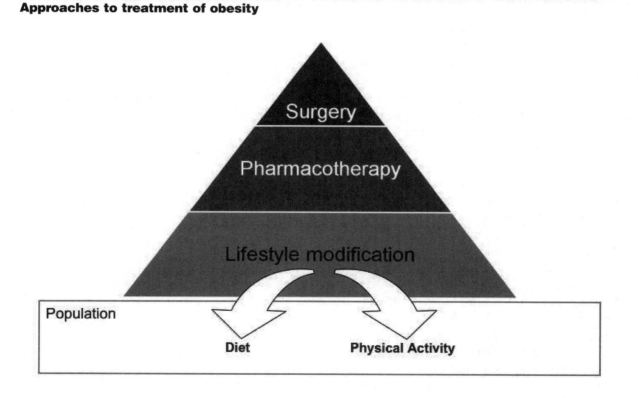

Figure 5

Weight loss prevents type 2 diabetes — the DPP

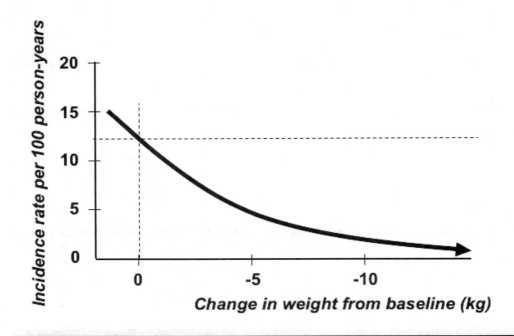

Redrawn from: Hamman, et al. Diabetes Care. 2006;29:2102-2107.

Rapid weight loss is discouraged, and the rapid loss of glycogen and water in the first few weeks of caloric burn is often misleading. Unfortunately, 5%-10% weight loss is not what most patients want. In fact, most patients have unrealistic expectations that cannot be met with available treatments. The exception to this rule is surgery, where most patients are satisfied with their weight loss. As newer drugs become available this may change, but for now we need to counsel our patients on what degree of weight loss is necessary for improved health, rather than cosmetic purposes.

Starting patients on a weight loss treatment

During the initiation of a weight loss treatment plan, patients should be counseled on a few key points. For example, many patients want a quick-fix and rapid weight loss. Early success with crash diets is often due to loss of glycogen and water, and is seldom sustained. A realistic target is 1-1.5 lbs per week; rates faster than this may increase the risk of gallstones. A multi-vitamin supplement is recommended. A discussion of the target weight encourages an open dialogue regarding realistic goals.

Exercise, Physical Activity and Weight Management

Regular physical activity has meaningful health benefits for individuals of any weight. For the purpose of general health, the goal should be at least 30 minutes per day, 5 or more days per week of moderate intensity activity ($\geq$150 minutes per week).[25] However, this amount of activity may not be enough to prevent weight gain in all individuals, leading many expert panels to recommend at least 60 minutes per day for the purpose of maintaining normal weight. For the purpose of weight loss, the combination of exercise and reduced caloric intake have been found to be more effective than either alone. The combination of reducing daily energy intake by 500-1000 calories (kcal), and a minimum of 150 minutes per week of exercise with the goal of increasing to 200-300 minutes per week ($\geq$2000 kcal) serves as a good foundation for developing an effective diet and exercise program.[26] Regular exercise has been identified as a key behavior in the prevention of weight regain after weight loss, and the available data suggests that to prevent weight regain it requires 300 or more minutes per week of moderate-intensity exercise.

Participation in exercise is not without risk, particularly in individuals with both occult and diagnosed chronic diseases. However, these risks can be minimized with a few basic steps, and the risk of serious events (ie, cardiac events) are rare when appropriate precautions are taken.[27] The most common risk of exercise is musculoskeletal injury with the risk increasing with excess weight, sedentary lifestyle, amount of exercise, intensity of exercise and participation in competitive sports. In order to minimize the risk of injury, the amount (volume) of daily activity should be increased gradually over time. Risk of serious events, such as sudden cardiac death or myocardial infarction, acutely increases with participation in higher intensity activities, both in individuals with diagnosed and occult heart disease. As a general rule, the risk of serious events associated with exercise sharply increases with exercise intensity and the number of medical conditions of the exerciser.

For most individuals, it is not necessary to undergo exercise stress testing or receive an extensive clinical examination prior to starting a moderate-intensity exercise program that includes a moderate rate of progression. However, individuals who wish to participate in higher intensity activities and/or those with existent CVD risk factors need physician clearance prior to participation, and in some cases this should include an exercise test. Since many overweight/obese individuals will qualify as moderate- or high-risk, they should seek clearance from their health care provider prior to starting an exercise program or increasing exercise intensity. It is particularly important for individuals with diabetes to make their health care team aware of new exercise and/or weight loss programs, because both of these activities usually result in the need to reduce diabetes medications or doses.

To summarize:

- For the purpose of general health, the goal should be at least 30 minutes per day, 5 or more days per week, of moderate intensity activity ($\geq$150 minutes per week).

- For the purpose of weight loss, the goals are to reduce daily energy intake by 500-1000 kcal and obtain a minimum of 150 minutes per week of exercise, with the goal of increasing to 200-300 minutes per week ($\geq$2000 kcal).

- For most individuals, it is not necessary to undergo exercise stress testing or receive an extensive clinical examination prior to starting a **moderate**-intensity exercise program that includes a **moderate** rate of progression.

- Individuals who wish to participate in higher intensity activities and/or those with existent CVD risk factors need physician clearance.

• For individuals with diabetes, participation in a new exercise and/or weight loss program typically results in the need to reduce diabetes medications or doses.

Behavioral Interventions

Lifestyle interventions and behavioral weight loss treatments typically span approximately 6 months and average 10% weight loss,[28] with clear benefits to the health of overweight or obese patients, with or without diseases such as diabetes. The Diabetes Prevention Program demonstrated that moderate weight loss can delay or prevent the onset of type 2 diabetes, with a lifestyle intervention for obesity reducing the risk of diabetes by 58%.[27, 29] Lifestyle interventions focus on modifying eating practices and increasing physical activity to produce an energy deficit. Behavior change is facilitated by techniques that rely on classical and operant conditioning principles. The cornerstones of effective interventions are a calorie-restricted diet, behavior therapy and increased physical activity. Over the past many years, effective components of weight loss treatment have been identified and are summarized herein.

Treatment delivery and goal setting
The duration and efficacy of treatment has increased since the 1970s. Greater weight loss is achieved with longer treatment, extended contact between patients and professionals, and group treatment, even if the patient prefers individual therapy.[30] The primary focus of treatment is the individual, but social support for behavior change is built by including spouses, family members and friends in treatment. Similarly, modification of the patient's environment is necessary to reinforce healthy eating and physical activity habits, and to discourage behaviors that sabotage weight loss efforts.

Patients ubiquitously desire a large amount of weight loss, which is highly improbable without an intervention such as bariatric surgery. Establishing realistic and attainable weight loss goals can reduce patients' dissatisfaction with the amount of weight they ultimately lose, but attempts to modify unrealistic weight loss goals are typically unsuccessful. Reasons for the persistent desire for a large and unrealistic weight loss could be the negative connotations associated with obesity and/or a history of discrimination. Obese people are frequently characterized by negative stereotypes (eg, lazy), and health care professionals are not immune to endorsing such stereotypes. Clinicians are encouraged to be sensitive to their own attitudes and biases, as well as the patient's history and social milieu.

Tools and Techniques to Promote Weight Loss

Over the past 40 years, a number of tools (or intervention techniques) have been developed, and their effect on weight loss and weight-loss maintenance has been systematically evaluated. A brief summary of these tools is included here.

Structured meal plans and nutrition education
Weight loss patients are prescribed a nutritionally adequate, calorie-restricted diet under the supervision of a dietitian. Meal plans that are highly structured and include portion-controlled foods or meal replacements are most effective at promoting weight loss.[31] Portion-controlled foods and meal replacements include: frozen entrees, nutrition shakes and bars. These foods are affordable, readily available and allow patients to easily eat healthy foods that meet the energy requirements of their diets. Patients simultaneously receive nutrition education and learn how to purchase and prepare healthy foods that will promote continued weight loss and long-term weight loss maintenance.

Self-monitoring and stimulus control
Patients record their food intake and physical activity using paper forms or electronic handheld diaries (eg, PDAs). This information is reviewed with the clinician and used to identify social, environmental or emotional cues to overeating or inactivity. Patients are also encouraged to keep a record of their daily body weights (or weights that are recorded at regular intervals, eg, every 3 days). Body weight data is viewed as an indicator of the patient's ability to adhere to the diet and exercise recommendations, which translate into an energy deficit that causes weight loss.

Figure 6

Behavior change (modification) techniques

- Make sure there is more than one color on your plate (red, green, yellow) and avoid brown and white

- Put your fork (or other utensil) down between bites

- Pause during your meal, talk, laugh, ask questions

- Always try to leave some food on your plate

- Keep tempting foods out of sight

- Shop from a shopping list, buying only what is on the list

- Remove serving dishes from the table while eating

- Leave the table as soon as you are done eating

- Serve and eat only 1 portion at a time

- Wait at least 5 minutes before going back for extra helpings

- Store foods in opaque containers, in the freezer when possible

- Go grocery shopping on a full stomach

- If you get an urge to eat, wait at least 5 minutes before eating, the urge may pass.

- Avoid eating while doing other activities, such as reading or watching the television

- Do nothing else while eating

- Buy foods that you must prepare in order to eat

- Have a list of alternative activities handy that you could do anytime you have the urge to eat

- Plan out your meals ahead of time

- Follow an eating schedule

- Keep healthy foods visible

- Identify high-risk situations and try to avoid them

- Avoid "automatic" eating, search for patterns in your eating, focusing on certain times of the day you are likely to eat, the amount of food that you eat, the foods that you choose to eat, and the places you eat. Be more conscious of these things, and try to avoid that "automatic" eating

- Take the time to enjoy the food you are eating, don't rush it

Certain situations or environments become associated with food intake or activity patterns, such as eating popcorn while watching a movie or being sedentary on the weekends. Stimulus control is used to limit the number of stimuli that are associated or "conditioned" with eating behavior and inactivity. Stimulus control recommendations include asking patients to eat at the same time and place in the absence of other stimuli such as television, slow their rate of eating and put utensils down between bites, eat on small plates and limit portion size, not have second servings and exercise on a regular schedule. Self-monitoring data can be used to identify situations or stimuli associated with food intake or inactivity.

Behavioral contracts and motivational interviewing

Behavior change is facilitated when behavioral contracts are used to clearly specify a behavioral goal, and the likelihood of the patient achieving the goal is increased if the patient is reinforced for success. Motivation is also facilitated by motivational interviewing, which has been found to facilitate glycemic control, weight loss and long-term weight loss maintenance among women diagnosed with type 2 diabetes.[32, 33]

Relapse prevention, problem-solving and booster treatments

Successful weight loss is followed by weight regain in the majority of patients. Long-term weight loss maintenance is possible, but very difficult for patients to achieve. Relapse prevention has been used to train patients to cope with high-risk situations and lapses, in an effort to prevent a return to previous behaviors that promote weight gain. Problem-solving training, however, is more effective at promoting weight loss maintenance than relapse prevention.[34] Problem-solving techniques train patients to actively address problems that threaten weight loss maintenance and to seek the support of professionals when needed. As noted earlier, longer treatment and extended contact with professionals is associated with greater weight loss and weight loss maintenance; therefore, booster treatments are encouraged, allowing patients to maintain contact with the clinician.

In summary, diet, behavior change and exercise

are effective at promoting meaningful weight loss that delays the onset of type 2 diabetes and improves health. Long-term weight loss maintenance is difficult, but longer treatment and continued contact with professionals promotes weight loss maintenance. A simple list of meal-time behavior modification strategies can be found in Figure 6.

Pharmacotherapy (Table 5)

Pharmacotherapy is appropriate when lifestyle modification is unsuccessful. Drugs are best *added on* to, rather than replacing, lifestyle modification. In general, pharmacotherapy is indicated only if lifestyle modification has been unsuccessful. This can be easily ascertained by taking a good history, as most patients have attempted weight loss through exercise and dieting on multiple occasions. Only a small percentage of patients are successful with a lifestyle-only approach, but those that are will not need pharmacotherapy. There may be situations where pharmacotherapy is indicated before trying lifestyle interventions, but the current literature is silent on this point. For example, patients who have difficulty exercising might find exercise easier after losing weight (as the initial loss of weight would relieve stress on knee and hip joints). Similarly, some patients have difficulty maintaining control over their dietary intake until they start a drug which helps control cravings and/or increases satiety. That drugs might help patients adhere to a lifestyle intervention program is an area where more data is needed.

Before starting new drugs, it is important to review other medications a patient is taking and, where possible, to stop or replace drugs that cause weight gain. For example, corticosteroids, beta blockers and newer antipsychotics can cause weight gain.

Screening for sleep apnea and/or depression is important, as these diagnoses can lead to weight gain and interfere with obesity therapy. Specifically, treating depression with anti-depressants that are weight-neutral or have modest weight loss effects should occur before starting an obesity treatment program. SSRIs, such as fluoxetine, have some effectiveness for weight

Table 5

Drugs approved by the FDA for treating obesity

Generic Name	DEA Schedule	Approved Use	Year Approved	Average weight loss[b]
Orlistat	None	Long term	1999	2.9kg[1]
Sibutramine	IV	Long term	1997	4.3kg[1]
Diethylpropion[a]	IV	Short term	1973	
Phentermine[a]	IV	Short term	1973	
Phendimetrazine[a]	III	Short term	1961	
Benzphetamine[a]	III	Short term	1960	

[a]Sympathomimetics
[b]Placebo-adjusted weight loss; see text for references

Table adapted from Yanovski SZ, Yanovski JA. N Engl J Med. 2002;346:591-602.
[1]From the meta-analysis by Rucker. BMJ. 2007;335;1194-1199.

loss. Unfortunately, the modest weight loss effects of SSRIs do not appear to be sustained over the long-term.[35] Wellbutrin™ (bupropion; SR 300–400 mg) was briefly tested as an anti-obesity drug.[36] Although bupropion is modestly effective for weight loss, it is not approved for the treatment of obesity. As such, buproprion is a good choice for milder forms of depression in obese patients.

When choosing/adjusting therapies for the treatment of diabetes it is important to recognize that insulin, sulfonylureas and thiazolidinediones all cause weight gain. Metformin produces a modest weight loss (1-2 kg) on average. Thiazolidinediones (TZDs: Actos™ , Avandia™) are well-known to increase both body fat and, in some patients, fluid retention and CHF. The effects of TZDs to increase food intake are probably via direct actions in the hypothalamus that increase appetite and decrease satiety. The effects of TZDs in increasing weight are not due to the formation of new adipocytes, as is frequently stated. This is important, as patients should be instructed to report changes in appetite and weight when starting these drugs, so that alternate therapies can be used early before large weight gains occur.

The GLP-1 analog Byetta™ (exenatide) and the amylin-mimetic Symlin™ (pramlintide) are injectable peptide drugs approved for treating diabetes; when used as indicated in the package insert they both have modest effects to reduce body weight. Many patients find this added benefit attractive. Before starting these drugs physicians should discuss the weight and appetite effects with patients, as a means to encourage greater adherence to a diet and lifestyle program.

There are only a few drugs that are approved for treating obesity. The sympathomimetics have been on the market the longest. These drugs are not approved for long-term use, and because they are controlled substances and are regulated by state laws to short-term use only (ie, 6-8 weeks maximum). Prescribers should check state laws carefully before using these drugs long-term. Phentermine is the most prescribed anti-obesity drug in the U.S.

Meridia™ (sibutramine) and Xenical™ (orlistat) are FDA-approved for long-term use. Sibutramine was approved by the FDA in 1997. It is a serotonin and noradrenaline reuptake inhibitor that reduces body weight by decreasing food intake, and it has a modest effect in increasing resting metabolism (increased caloric expenditure). Published efficacy and safety data extends out to 2 years, however, the SCOUT trial is exploring the hypothesis that *hard* cardiovascular endpoints, like MI, stroke and death, will be lower in sibutramine-treated patients. Weight loss with Meridia™ averages ~5% over placebo,[37] and sibutramine is also appropriate for weight loss maintenance, as shown in the STORM trial. When used in combination with a behavior therapy program, even more weight loss is seen. Importantly, HDL-C and triglycerides improve with long-term treatment. Given the mechanisms of action to block the reuptake of serotonin and norepinephrine, it should be anticipated that hypertension may become an adverse effect in a small percentage of patients. Sibutramine is dosed 10-15 mg/day, and can be taken with or without food.

Figure 7

─────────────────────────

Obesity surgery

Indications

BMI >40 kg/m2 or

1. BMI 35–39.9 kg/m2 and life-threatening cardiopulmonary disease, severe diabetes, or lifestyle impairment

2. Failure to achieve adequate weight loss with nonsurgical treatment

Contraindications

1. History of noncompliance with medical care

2. Certain psychiatric illnesses: personality disorder, uncontrolled depression, suicidal ideation, substance abuse

3. Unlikely to survive surgery

─────────────────────────

Reference — NIH Consensus Development Panel. Ann Intern Med. 1991;115:956.

Xenical™ (orlistat) is a pancreatic lipase inhibitor, which produces about 3% body weight loss on average.[35] A reduced-dose version is available OTC under the brand name Alli™. Xenical™ is safe, and an added bonus is data from the Xendos trial showing that Orlistat over 2 years can prevent or delay the development of type 2 diabetes.[38] Side effects include: fatty/oily stools in about a third of treated patients, increased defecation in about 20% of patients and other similar GI-related adverse events. These potential side effects should be included in the discussion with patients prior to initiation of therapy. Many patients don't experience these adverse effects, and the number and severity of GI adverse events tend to decrease over time. This is probably because patients learn to not consume high-fat foods. Loss of fat-soluble vitamins has been reported, and a multi-vitamin supplement with vitamins A and D is strongly recommended for patients taking Xenical™ or Alli™. Unfortunately, adding orlistat to sibutramine does not produce additional weight loss.

Obesity Surgery

Surgery is currently recommended after intensive lifestyle intervention is attempted. As the procedures become refined, there will certainly be a pressure downward in terms of the BMI cut-points for surgeries. The selection of patients for surgery is outlined in Figure 7. The choice of surgery is beyond the scope of this review, but the experience of the surgeon has a strong influence on the morbidity and mortality of the procedure, and thus, experience is very important.[39] An important milestone came with the recent publication of data from the Swedish Obese Subjects Study, showing that obesity surgery can reduce mortality.[40] This well-controlled data, along with the refinement of the surgical techniques and procedures, is leading very obese patients and their doctors to choose obesity surgery as a means to treat diabetes and other comorbidities. The effectiveness of these procedures for reversing diabetes approaches 80%[41] and 87% of patients are improved or reversed. Taken together, there is compelling clinical data to suggest that obesity surgery is medically effective and a good choice for many obese patients, especially when comorbidities such as type 2 diabetes are present.

Lessons from Successful Weight Loss Maintainers (Figure 8)

One thing to keep in mind is that, although few people are able to lose and maintain weight loss alone, there are several consistent features of people who are successful at weight loss long-term. Founded in 1994 by Drs James Hill and Rena Wing, the National Weight Control Registry collects data from successful losers in order to look at "what works" in the real world. People who have a minimum of 30 lbs. of weight loss for a minimum of 1 year have high physical activity levels and consume a low-fat diet.

Figure 8

Lessons from those who have succeeded in keeping weight off

Weight Loss Maintenance Strategies (NWCR)

- No similarity in how weight was lost

- Great similarity in how weight loss is being maintained

    * Low fat diet

    * Watching total calories

    * High daily levels of physical activity

    * Frequent self-monitoring

5. Conclusion

The obesity epidemic is not over; we are just now beginning to see the emergence of subsequent chronic diseases, such as type 2 diabetes. The costs associated with these diseases are staggering and are projected to become even greater in the future. Lifestyle intervention is the cornerstone of therapy. Behavior modification is more refined, and we now know that exercise is essential for general health and for weight maintenance. When used appropriately, drugs are an important second step. Although not applicable on a large scale, more and more patients are turning to obesity surgery. In the future, we may have more effective drugs that will reduce the need for surgery. In the interval, we can be effective in the clinic by using the tools we have, and by reinforcing a growing acknowledgement that the war against obesity is worth fighting.

6. References

1. World Health Organization. Obesity: Preventing and Managing the Global Epidemic. Report of a WHO Consultation on Obesity. Geneva, 1998.

2. NIH. Clinical Guidelines on the Identification, Evaluation, and Treatment of Overweight and Obesity in Adults--The Evidence Report. *Obes Res*. 1998;6(suppl 2):51S-209S.

3. Haslam DW, James WP. Obesity. *Lancet*. 2005;366:1197-1209.

4. Hossain P, Kawar B, El Nahas M. Obesity and diabetes in the developing world--a growing challenge. *N Engl J Med*. 2007;356:213-215.

5. Manson JE, Nathan DM, Krolewski AS, Stampfer MJ, Willett WC, Hennekens CH. A prospective study of exercise and incidence of diabetes among US male physicians. *JAMA*. 1992;268:63-67.

6. Rana JS, Li TY, Manson JE, Hu FB. Adiposity compared with physical inactivity and risk of type 2 diabetes in women. *Diabetes Care*. 2007;30:53-58.

7. Flegal KM, Carroll MD, Kuczmarski RJ, Johnson CL. Overweight and obesity in the United States: prevalence and trends, 1960-1994. *Int J Obes Relat Metab Disord*. 1998;22:39-47.

8. Ogden CL, Carroll MD, Curtin LR, McDowell MA, Tabak CJ, Flegal KM. Prevalence of overweight and obesity in the United States, 1999-2004. *JAMA*. 2006;295:1549-1555.

9. Ogden CL, Carroll MD, McDowell MA, Flegal KM. Obesity among adults in the United States - no change since 2003-2004. Hyattsville, MD: National Center for Health Statistics; 2007

10. CDC. Behavioral Risk Factor Surveillance System: 2008 statistics. Available at http://www.cdc.gov/BRFSS/. Accessed May 3, 2009.

11. Mokdad AH, Serdula MK, Dietz WH, Bowman BA, Marks JS, Koplan JP. The spread of the obesity epidemic in the United States, 1991-1998. *JAMA*. 1999;282:1519-1522.

12. Mokdad AH, Bowman BA, Ford ES, Vinicor F, Marks JS, Koplan JP. The continuing epidemics of obesity and diabetes in the United States. *JAMA*. 2001;286:1195-1200.

13. Mokdad AH, Ford ES, Bowman BA, et al. Prevalence of obesity, diabetes, and obesity-related health risk factors, 2001. *JAMA*. 2003;289:76-79.

14. Gorber SC, Tremblay M, Moher D, Gorber B. A comparison of direct vs. self-report measures for assessing height, weight and body mass index: a systematic review. *Obes Rev*. 2007;8:307-326.

15. Ford ES, Mokdad AH, Giles WH. Trends in waist circumference among U.S. adults. *Obes Res*. 2003;11:1223-1231.

16. Okosun IS, Choi ST, Boltri JM, et al. Trends of abdominal adiposity in white, black, and Mexican-American adults, 1988 to 2000. *Obes Res*. 2003;11:1010-1017.

17. Elobeid MA, Desmond RA, Thomas O, Keith SW, Allison DB: Waist circumference values are increasing beyond those expected from BMI increases. *Obesity (Silver Spring)*, 2007;15:2380-2383

18. Le Petit C, Berthelot JM. Obesity--a growing issue. *Health Rep*. 2006;17:43-50.

19. Cowie CC, Rust KF, Byrd-Holt DD, et al. Prevalence of diabetes and impaired fasting glucose in adults in the U.S. population: National Health And Nutrition Examination Survey 1999-2002. *Diabetes Care*. 2006;29:1263-1268.

20. CDC. U.S. Bureau of the Census, census of the population and population estimates. Data from the National Health Interview Survey. Data computed by the Division of Diabetes Translation, National Center for Chronic Disease Prevention and Health Promotion, Centers for Disease Control and Prevention. Available at http://www.cdc.gov/diabetes/statistics/prev/national/figage.htm. Accessed on May 3, 2009.

21. CDC. State-specific incidence of diabetes among adults--participating states, 1995-1997 and 2005-2007. *MMWR*. 2008;1169-1173.

22. Thomas RJ, Palumbo PJ, Melton LJ 3rd, et al. Trends in the mortality burden associated with diabetes mellitus: a population-based study in Rochester, Minn, 1970-1994. *Arch Intern Med*. 2003;163:445-451.

23. Lipscombe LL, Hux JE. Trends in diabetes prevalence, incidence, and mortality in Ontario, Canada 1995-2005: a population-based study. *Lancet* 2007;369:750-756.

24. Sharma AM, Kushner RF. A proposed clinical staging system for obesity. *Int J Obes (Lond)*. 2009;33:289-295.

25. US Department of Health and Human Services. Physical Activity Guidelines Advisory Committee Report 2008. Washington, DC: 2008.

26. Jakicic JM, Clark K, Coleman E, et al. American College of Sports Medicine position stand. Appropriate intervention strategies for weight loss and prevention of weight regain for adults. *Med Sci Sports Exerc*. 2001;33:2145-2156.

27. Haskell WL, Lee IM, Pate RR, et al. Physical activity and public health: updated recommendation for adults from the American College of Sports Medicine and the American Heart Association. *Med Sci Sports Exerc*. 2007;39:1423-1434.

28. Wadden TA, Butryn ML, Byrne KJ. Efficacy of lifestyle modification for long-term weight control. *Obes Res*. 2004;12 (suppl):151S-162S.

29. Knowler WC, Barrett-Connor E, Fowler SE, et al. Reduction in the incidence of type 2 diabetes with lifestyle intervention or metformin. *N Engl J Med*. 2002;346:393-403.

30. Renjilian DA, Perri MG, Nezu AM, McKelvey WF, Shermer RL, Anton SD. Individual versus group therapy for obesity: effects of matching participants to their treatment preferences. *J Consult Clin Psychol*. 2001;69:717-721.

31. Heymsfield SB, van Mierlo CA, van der Knaap HC, Heo M, Frier HI. Weight management using a meal replacement strategy: meta and pooling analysis from six studies. *Int J Obes Relat Metab Disord*. 2003;27:537-549.

32. West DS, DiLillo V, Bursac Z, Gore SA, Greene PG. Motivational interviewing improves weight loss in women with type 2 diabetes. *Diabetes Care*. 2007;30:1081-1087.

33. Miller WR, Rollnick S. Motivational interviewing: preparing people to change addictive behaviors. New York, NY: Guilford; 1991.

34. Perri MG, Nezu AM, McKelvey WF, Shermer RL, Renjilian DA, Viegener BJ. Relapse prevention training and problem-solving therapy in the long-term management of obesity. *J Consult Clin Psychol*. 2001;69:722-726.

35. Anderson JW, Greenway FL, Fujioka K, Gadde KM, McKenney J, O'Neil PM. Bupropion SR enhances weight loss: a 48-week double-blind, placebo- controlled trial. *Obes Res*. 2002;10:633-641.

36. Gray DS, Fujioka K, Devine W, Bray GA. A randomized double-blind clinical trial of fluoxetine in obese diabetics. *Int J Obes Relat Metab Disord*. 1992;16(suppl 4):S67-S72.

37. Padwal R, Li SK, Lau DC. Long-term pharmacotherapy for overweight and obesity: a systematic review and meta-analysis of randomized controlled trials. *Int J Obes Relat Metab Disord*. 2003;27:1437-1446.

38. Torgerson JS, Hauptman J, Boldrin MN, Sjostrom L. Xenical in the prevention of diabetes in obese subjects (XENDOS) study: a randomized study of orlistat as an adjunct to lifestyle changes for the prevention of type 2 diabetes in obese patients. *Diabetes Care*. 2004;27:155-161.

39. Flum DR, Salem L, Elrod JA, Dellinger EP, Cheadle A, Chan L. Early mortality among Medicare beneficiaries undergoing bariatric surgical procedures. *JAMA*. 2005;294:1903-1908.

40. Jacobson P, Torgerson JS, Sjostrom L, Bouchard C. Spouse resemblance in body mass index: effects on adult obesity prevalence in the offspring generation. *Am J Epidemiol*. 2007;165:101-108.

41. Buchwald H, Estok R, Fahrbach K, et al. Weight and type 2 diabetes after bariatric surgery: systematic review and meta-analysis. *Am J Med*. 2009;122:248-256.

Other resources:

The Practical Guide to the Identification, Evaluation, and Treatment of Overweight and Obesity in Adults. Available on NHLBI Web site: www.nhlbi.nih.gov and http://www.nhlbi.nih.gov/guidelines/obesity/ob_home.htm

Chapter 6: Diabetes Self-Management Education

Margaret Powers, PhD, RD, CDE
Diane Reader, MD

Contents

1. Introduction

Diabetes Self Management Education (DSME) is defined as the ongoing process of facilitating the knowledge, skill and ability necessary for diabetes self-care. Successful diabetes management is contingent upon many factors, including a patient's ability to understand the nature of the disease and how he or she can participate and enable the treatment plan. Thus, patient education is one of the most significant factors that can lead to a reduction in the morbidity and mortality associated with diabetes-related complications. The American Diabetes Association (ADA) Standards of Medical Care recommend that all people with diabetes should receive DSME, according to national standards, when their diabetes is diagnosed and as needed thereafter.

The National Standards for DSME are written to define quality diabetes education that can be implemented in diverse settings, and to facilitate improved health care outcomes. The national standards are reviewed periodically by a task force jointly convened by the ADA and the American Association of Diabetes Educators for appropriateness, relevance and scientific basis. A diabetes education program can become "recognized" as a quality program if it meets the national standards. There are over 3000 recognized programs for diabetes education at the date of this publication.

Each recognized program usually has a certified diabetes educator (CDE) as part of the program. Most large medical centers will have comprehensive programs that provide initial diabetes education, plus instruction for insulin use, continuous glucose monitoring and insulin pumps. Smaller clinics also have recognized programs, yet may have fewer CDEs and rely on other clinicians to support the program. The program CDEs are most often nurses, dietitians and pharmacists. If the program does not include a registered dietitian/CDE, most programs refer to a dietitian for medical nutrition therapy.

Referral to diabetes education is recommended for initial education, when medication changes are made, when a patient is struggling to improve glucose control or has an elevated A1C. Using an individual assessment with identification of desired outcomes, a plan will be developed using

educational, behavioral and psychological interventions with follow-up evaluation. Currently the Center for Medicare Services (CMS) provides reimbursement for 10 hours of DSME in the first year of diagnosis and for 2 hours annually thereafter. CMS also pays for 3 hours of medical nutrition therapy the first year and for 2 hours each year following. Private insurers will frequently pay for more education and medical nutrition therapy.

Behavior change is the unique outcome measurement for diabetes education. The American Association of Diabetes Educators (AADE) has summarized and categorized the self-care behaviors required for optimum diabetes self-management: the AADE 7 Self-Care Behaviors™. These 7 behaviors are:

- Healthy eating

- Being active

- Taking medication

- Monitoring

- Problem-solving

- Reducing risks

- Healthy coping

The Standards of Diabetes Education require that all diabetes education programs address these behaviors. Appendix A and B include information on accessing diabetes education programs and registered dietitians (many education programs include a registered dietitian), a referral form and a form for engaging patients in setting and tracking realistic self-care goals.

2. Medical Nutrition Therapy

Diabetes education engages patients in understanding and following their nutrition and medication therapies. A separate chapter is devoted to medication therapy; the rest of this chapter is devoted to nutrition therapy. The ADA recommends that registered dietitians provide medical nutrition therapy to patients with diabetes. Most health care professionals, however, are involved in providing some knowledge, skills and resources to help guide and support patients in making healthy food choices that are appropriate for their diabetes, just as they all support medication therapy. Thus, it is important that clinicians have an understanding of food plan strategies, methods, nutrition therapy recommendations and interventions throughout the continuum of type 2 diabetes.

This discussion focuses on pre-diabetes, early type 2 diabetes and established, longer duration type 2 diabetes. For each of these clinical stages, intervention recommendations are provided for the food plan, weight management, activity, diabetes education and support. Appendices are included that list diabetes resources, address frequently asked nutrition questions and identify diabetes education standards. Type 1 diabetes will not be specifically addressed, yet the general themes of individualization, therapy integration, resource provision and support also apply to this population.

Evidence for Medical Nutrition Therapy

Nutrition therapy is often referred to as the cornerstone of diabetes management and there is substantial evidence supporting its effectiveness in type 2 diabetes. Medical nutrition therapy can reduce A1C by 1%-2% and in the newly diagnosed patient may lower A1C by 3% or more. These outcomes are generally observed when trained registered dietitians (RDs) provide medical nutrition therapy (MNT). Yet, all health care professionals involved in diabetes care should be familiar with the basic principles of diabetes nutrition therapy in order to assess a patient's needs and successfully support the basic tenets of a diabetes food plan. Such an approach will permit clinicians to readily adjust nutrition or lifestyle recommendations for patients across the continuum of type 2 diabetes.

Goals of MNT

The overall goals for nutrition therapy for all individuals with diabetes are:

1. Achieve and maintain:

   - Blood glucose levels in the normal range or as close to normal as is safely possible

   - A lipid and lipoprotein profile that reduces the risk for vascular disease

   - Blood pressure levels in the normal range or as close to normal as is safely possible

2. To prevent, or at least slow, the rate of development of the chronic complications of diabetes by modifying nutrient intake and lifestyle

3. To address individual nutrition needs, taking into account personal and cultural preferences and willingness to change

4. To maintain the pleasure of eating by only limiting food choices when indicated by scientific evidence.

Providing MNT support for patients with type 2 diabetes includes:

   - Nutrition assessment and diagnosis

   - Nutrition recommendations and interventions

   - Monitoring and ongoing evaluation plan

The focus of nutrition therapy should be on the key areas above, and include instruction on carbohydrate intake and working with patients to match medication therapy to the patient's diet in an effort to achieve glycemic, lipid and blood pressure goals.

3. Food Planning Methods

Carbohydrate Counting

The primary food planning method used in the United States is carbohydrate counting. This is because there are many levels of carbohydrate counting, from very simple to very detailed guidelines that offer a spectrum of choices that can be advanced or changed as appropriate.

Carbohydrates are the primary food substance that raise postprandial blood glucose levels, so counting (managing or controlling) carbohydrate intake is key to controlling these glucose levels. Carbohydrate counting is a method to quantify and manage carbohydrate intake. In this food planning method, foods are portioned on the basis of their carbohydrate amount. 1 carbohydrate choice or serving contains about 15 grams of carbohydrate, 2 choices contain 30 grams of carbohydrate, etc (see Figure 1). Examples of 1 carbohydrate choice include: 1 small apple, 1 cup of milk, 1 slice of bread or 1 "fun size" candy bar.

Patients are guided as to how many choices they should have at their meals and snacks. Usually a range of choices is given, such as 2-3, 3-4, 4-5 choices per meal or even a wider range of 2-4 or 3-5. The range is based on a patient's usual eating pattern and what is a comfortable amount of carbohydrates to typically have day after day for a particular meal or snack. Monitoring and ongoing evaluation will determine if the range is appropriate (ie, fits the patient's eating pattern and results in meeting target blood glucose goals).

Table 1 provides general carbohydrate intake guidelines, although these are generalized and specific recommendations must be individualized. Individuals following a carbohydrate counting food plan need to understand: 1.) what foods contain carbohydrate; 2.) what serving size provides 15 grams of carbohydrate; and 3.) how many carbohydrate choices they should have at each meal and snack, if desired. Additionally, they need to know how to apply these guidelines in a variety of situations.

Patients are provided lists of food with corresponding portion sizes that equal ~15 grams of carbohydrate (range: 11-20 grams of carbohydrate). Figure 2 shows an example of a food list of carbohydrate choices. Patients who are being more precise with their carbohydrate intake often count specific grams of carbohydrate. For example, 1 cup of milk is 1 carbohydrate choice (15 grams of carb), yet it actually contains 12 grams of carb. To

Figure 1

Carbohydrate counting

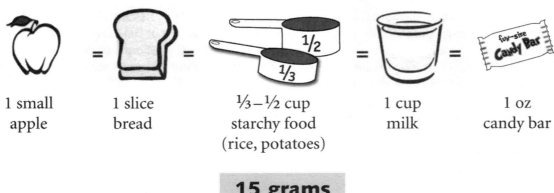

1 carbohydrate choice =

| 1 small apple | 1 slice bread | ⅓–½ cup starchy food (rice, potatoes) | 1 cup milk | 1 oz candy bar |

15 grams

Table 1

General Guidelines for Carbohydrate Intake per Meal

	Inactive, older or want to lose weigh	To maintain weight	Younger, active or need to gain weight
Meals - Women	2-3 carb choices 30-45 grams	3-4 carb choices 45-60 grams	4-5 carb choices 60-75 grams
Meals - Men	3-4 carb choices 45-60 grams	4-5 carb choices 60-75 grams	4-6 carb choices 60-90 grams
Snacks	0-1 carb choice	0-2 choices	1-2 carb choices
	0-15 grams	0-30 grams	15-30 grams

©2009 International Diabetes Center at Park Nicollet

Figure 2

Carbohydrate choices

Fruits/Fruit Juices	Carb Choices	Carb Grams
Berries (blueberries, raspberries, strawberries), 1 cup	1	14–20
Cherries, 12 (1 cup)	1	14
Fruit, canned, in light syrup or juice, ½ cup	1	15
Fruit (apple, banana, pear), whole, large	2	26–35
Fruit (kiwi, orange, peach, tangerine), whole, medium	1	11–16
Fruit (clementine, plum), whole, small, 2	1	16
Grapefruit, ½ large	1	13
Grapes, small, 17 (½ cup)	1	15
Juice (apple, grapefruit, orange, pineapple), ½ cup	1	11–17
Juice (cranberry, grape, prune), ⅓ cup	1	15
Melon (cantaloupe, honeydew, watermelon), 1 cup	1	11–16
Raisins, cran-raisins, other dried fruit, ¼ cup	2	26–32

be more precise, usually when one is dosing meal-time insulin, one would consider counting carbo-hydrate grams. That said, there are individuals on insulin who manage their diabetes extremely well by counting carbohydrate choices. Either group of patients would frequently use food labels to either count choices or grams. Food labels identify a serving size and the corresponding amount of car-bohydrate, making it fairly easy to incorporate a variety of foods into a food plan (see Figure 3).

Carbohydrate Counting for Mealtime Insulin Dosing

Some patients will benefit from mealtime insulin as diabetes advances and insulin is required. Table 2 describes 3 ways to determine the dosing of mealtime insulin. Although some patients can take set doses of mealtime (bolus) insulin, others will benefit from flexible dosing of their mealtime insulin, based on the anticipated amount of carbo-hydrates they plan to eat (Table 2 sections A and B show calculations for both of these situations).

Mealtime insulins include: aspart, glulisine, lispro and regular insulin. This insulin may be used in conjunction with a background (basal) insulin or with other diabetes medications at 1 or more meals. As endogenous insulin becomes more defi-cient, in the natural history of diabetes, back-ground and mealtime insulin is required through pre-mixed insulin or provided separately. When separate mealtime insulin is provided, an insulin-to-carbohydrate ratio is typically calculated.

An insulin-to-carb ratio is the most precise, as it matches the insulin dose to the food to be con-sumed. It is critical that patients using insulin-to-carbohydrate ratios with insulin injections or an insulin pump are able to accurately assess the car-bohydrate content of a wide variety of foods. Neglecting this important aspect of nutrition thera-py will result in miscalculating insulin doses, mak-ing it difficult to achieve glycemic goals.

In addition to evaluating an individual's ability to count carbohydrate choices or grams, the mealtime dose should be evaluated to determine if it is the correct amount with a set amount of carbohydrate. A general guideline to evaluate mealtime insulin

Figure 3

Nutrition facts example

Nutrition Facts
Serving Size 1 bar (36g)
Servings Per Package 6

Amount Per Serving

Calories 140   Calories from Fat 25

	%Daily Value*
Total Fat 3g	5%
Saturated Fat 0.5g	3%
Cholesterol 5mg	2%
Sodium 110mg	5%
Total Carbohydrate 27g	9%
Dietary Fiber 2g	4%
Sugars 9g	
Protein 2g	16%

Vitamin A 15%	•	Vitamin C 0%
Calcium 20%	•	Iron 10%

* Percent daily values are based on a 2,000 calorie diet. Your daily values may be higher or lower depending on your calorie needs:

	Calories:	2,000	2,500
Total Fat	Less than	65g	80g
Sat Fat	Less than	20g	25g
Cholesterol	Less than	300mg	300mg
Sodium	Less than	2400mg	2400mg
Total Carbohydrate		300g	375g
Dietary Fiber		25g	30g

Calories per gram:
Fat 9 • Carbohydrate 4 • Protein 4

dosing is that the 2 hour post-meal glucose level should be no higher than 40 mg/dL above pre-meal. For example, if the pre-meal glucose level is 120 mg/dl, the 2 hour post-meal glucose reading should be no greater than 160 md/dL. If it is sig-nificantly higher or drops below the pre-meal value, the mealtime dose or ratio needs to be adjusted. During the trial to assess the ratio, it is recommended to also record food intake and car-bohydrate count to ensure accuracy of carbohy-drate counting.

Table 2

Three Methods to Determine Mealtime Insulin (1st method is not a ratio) Insulin-to-Carbohydrate Ratio	
A. Basic Distribution	• 50% of total insulin is background or long-acting insulin
(Consistent carbohydrate intake with set doses of insulin)	• 50% of total insulin is mealtime divided by 3 meals = mealtime dose of insulin • Example: 60 units insulin per day; 30 units background and 30 units mealtime • 30/3 meals = 10 units insulin at each meal • Assumes consistent amount of carbohydrate intake at each meal
B. Insulin to carb ratio:	• 2 methods of calculation
Rule of 500	• 500 divided by the total daily dose of insulin = the number of grams of carbohydrate that one unit of rapid-acting covers. • Example: 500/30 units insulin = 16 grams of carbohydrate need 1 unit insulin
Based on Background Dose carb or 1:1 ratio	• About 15 units background uses 1 unit insulin per 15 grams • About 30 units background uses 2 units insulin per 15 grams carb or 2:1 ratio • About 45 units background uses 3 units insulin per 15 grams carb or 3:1 ratio

©2009 International Diabetes Center at Park Nicollet

Plate Method

The plate method uses a dinner serving plate to guide food choices (see Figures 4a and 4b). Depending on a patient's eating patterns, one is typically taught to fill either ¼ or ½ of their plate with carbohydrate foods, leaving ¼ for protein and ¼-½ for vegetables. The teaching materials help a patient to know which foods are carbohydrates and proteins. When used correctly, this method results in about 3-4 carbohydrate servings per meal.

Planned Menus

Planned menus provide the patient with specific food choices for meals and snacks throughout the day. Different meal options are provided to ensure a variety of food choices. This method is most effective when the example meals are based on an individual's eating pattern, and food likes and dislikes. It is used when a patient needs limited, specific, structured guidelines, such as when they are overwhelmed with the diagnosis of diabetes or other situations in their life, or they do not have the capacity for other methods. It guides a patient in maintaining a consistent carbohydrate intake without using the term *carbohydrate*.

This method is also used when a patient has a regular eating pattern that remains consistent from day to day. Just saying 'continue your current eating pattern' can leave some patients wondering what that specifically means. Providing written menus based on their patterns reinforces what the expectations are for meal size, composition and timing.

Table 3

Food Choices for People With Newly Diagnosed With Diabetes

Your food choices and eating habits are important when you have diabetes. The amount of food you eat may make a difference. Eating too much may cause your blood sugar (glucose) levels to go too high. Not eating enough may cause low blood glucose. Soon you meet with a dietitian to develop a food plan that will balance how you like to eat with taking care of your diabetes. Until then, here are some suggestions to help you get started.

- Eat 3 moderate-sized meals each day. It is important not to skip meals.
- Eat at about the same time each day.
- Include at least 2 of these foods at each meal (carbohydrates)

Bread, tortillas	Cereal
Rice, pasta, cereal	Fruit
Milk or yogurt	Starchy vegetables (peas, corn, potato, beans)

- If you like to snack, small snacks may be included. For example, you could have a piece of fruit, 4-6 crackers, 2 small cookies, ½ cup light ice-cream or 1 cup of milk. Let your dietitian or nurse know if you like to snack.
- Avoid regular soda pop and large glasses of fruit juice, sweetened tea or drink.
- Eat fewer foods or smaller portions of foods with added sugar such as desserts, candy or syrup.
- Limit your use of alcohol until you learn how to include it safely.
- Include a variety of healthy foods each day. Whole grains, fruits, vegetables, lean meats and low-fat dairy products all are nutritious choices.

Check with your health care provider to schedule a visit with an IDC dietitian and nurse educator to learn more about your diabetes treatment plan.

---

continued

Other Food Planning Methods

Patients may follow other food planning methods and be quite successful in managing their diabetes. The exchange food system is one such plan that has been used since the 1950s. Carbohydrate counting is based on the exchange system. The exchange system provides guidelines for carbohydrate intake as well as protein and fat; it recommends a specific number of choices from the individual carbohydrate groups (grains, milk, fruit, other), rather than consolidating all of them into 'carbohydrate choices' as with carbohydrate counting.

Others have successfully used some of the popular weight loss programs to manage their diabetes, such as WeightWatchers and the South Beach diet. An evaluation should be done to assess whether there are any safety questions that should be addressed prior to their use. Of special concern is the need to manage carbohydrate intake throughout the day to avoid hypo- or hyperglycemia. This is especially necessary when the patient is taking a hypoglycemic oral agent or insulin.

Initial General Eating Guidelines for Use by the Clinician

Initial general eating guidelines provide an overview of a diabetes food plan and introduce the patient to the basic tenets of a diabetes food plan. The basics are to: 1.) eat about the same amount of food at each meal and snack; 2.) eat at about the same time each day, and; 3.) avoid highly sugared foods. Often, these guidelines are provided to a patient when they are first diagnosed with type 2 diabetes and need guidance before they see a registered dietitian or receive diabetes self-manage-

Table 3 (continued)

	Sample Menu 1	Sample Menu 2
Breakfast Time _____	1/2 cup skim or 1% milk 3/4 cup cheerios (unsweetened cereal) 1 slice toast peanut butter 1.2 cup orange juice	1 English Muffin or 2 slices toast 1 flavored yogurt (light) 1 cup berries or small fruit Soft margarine or sugar-free jam coffee or tea
Snack (if desired)	orange	12 ounce coffee latte
Lunch Time _____	2 slices bread turkey 1 ounce pretzels or chips mayonnaise or soft margarine 1 cup skim milk	bowl of soup 5-6 crackers 1 small fruit side salad low-fat dressing diet soda pop
Snack (if desired)	1 granola bar	2 small cookies
Dinner Time _____	1 medium potato 1 small roll 1 cup skim or 1% milk chicken, pork, fish or beef dinner salad low-fat salad dressing soft margarine	1-1/2 cups casserole non-starchy vegetable (broccoli, carrots) 1 slice French bread soft margarine 1 glass ice tea
Snack (if desired)	3 cups popcorn	½ cup light ice cream

The foods listed below will have little effect on your blood sugars:

artificial sweeteners coffee, tea, diet soda	sugar-free popsicles or gelatin salad greens and non-starchy vegetables	condiments, 1 Tb. spices and seasonings

©2009 International Diabetes Center at Park Nicollet

ment education. An example of general eating guidelines is found in Table 3.

Treating Hypoglycemia: Key Nutrition Messages

All people who take hypoglycemic agents and insulin need to understand the symptoms, causes and treatment of hypoglycemia. Mild hypoglycemia is common, especially if tight glucose control is the goal. Treatment with 15 grams of carbohydrate is the first step when hypoglycemia is documented or suspected. Sometimes it is not possible to take time to do a blood glucose test, and treatment action should be taken regardless. Discuss with your patients the need to always carry (or have readily available) a source of carbohydrate and what that might be in a variety of situations. For example, what would they put in the glove compartment of a car, in a gym bag or school backpack. The steps to treat hypoglycemia are listed in Table 4 and can be used as a patient handout.

Meal sizes: half plate

Meal sizes: quarter plate

Half Plate

For people who:

- Are active
- Are younger
- Want to stay at the same weight

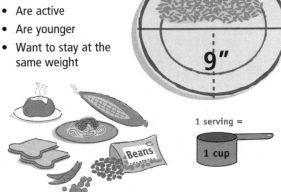

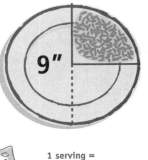

1 serving = **1 cup**

At meals, keep rice, beans, pasta, and starchy vegetables to one half of a plate.

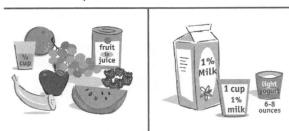

Add 1 serving of fruit   **and/or**   1 serving of milk.

Quarter Plate

For people who:

- Are less active
- Are older
- Need to eat less calories

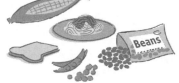

1 serving = **½ cup**

At meals, keep rice, beans, pasta, and starchy vegetables to one fourth of a plate.

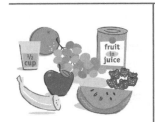
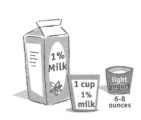

Add 1 serving of fruit   **and/or**   1 serving of milk.

Table 4

Patient Guidelines for Treating Low Blood Sugar

Management of Hypoglycemia

Instructions for Patients

Low blood glucose is a blood glucose test result less than 70 mg/dL.
If you are not able to check your blood glucose, still follow these guidelines if you feel symptoms.

15-15 Guidelines
• When you feel symptoms, do a blood glucose test.
• If your glucose is low, eat or drink 15 grams of carbohydrate (1 carbohydrate choice).

<u>Possible Treatment Options</u> (15 grams carbohydrate)
 • ½ cup fruit juice
 • 1 cup milk
 • ½ cup of regular soft drink (not diet)
 • 3 or 4 glucose tablets
 • 2 or 3 hard candies

• Wait **15 minutes**. Do another test.
• If your glucose is still low, eat or drink another **15 grams** of carbohydrate.
• Wait **15 minutes**. Test again. If necessary, eat or drink another **15 grams** of carbohydrate.
• If your glucose remains low after 4 treatments, call your health care provider or 911.

©2009 International Diabetes Center at Park Nicollet

4. Nutrition Intervention Strategies

Nutrition intervention strategies are carefully selected to provide the guidance that an individual needs at different times during their life. The strategy is selected based on learning needs, and ability and willingness to follow different levels of nutrition recommendations. For example, someone may be able to carefully measure their portion sizes when they are initially diagnosed with diabetes because they want to be as precise as possible. Yet another person may feel so overwhelmed that they need general eating guidelines that include a list of suggested meals and snacks that will keep them safe, until they overcome their initial barriers. Such individualized approaches can facilitate future learning and application, because they are personalized to each individual's immediate needs.

Overwhelming a patient with information is 1 risk of taking a 'shotgun approach' to health education, and can cause patients to become frustrated and embarrassed that they cannot apply all the principles provided to them. A step-by-step approach, based on need-to-know information, is the preferred strategy to behavior change.

The intervention strategy is selected based on a discussion with a patient, usually after a nutrition assessment and diagnosis of nutrition needs. The assessment includes a food history, health and laboratory values review, medications, living situation, daily schedule and other factors that may affect food selection. A discussion of food purchasing, preparation and portioning is warranted, as these factors are key to implementing any food plan. Additionally, learning style and needs are assessed, including health literacy.

Strategies for Translating Nutrition Recommendations

An important strategy in translating nutrition recommendations is to provide the patient with clear expectations that are meaningful to them. For example, a patient may be instructed to "eat less carbs." Such a guideline, however, has various interpretations and may leave a patient confused as to how to implement such a recommendation. Nutrition therapy should provide the individualization of nutrition recommendations so they are translated into practical, understandable, achievable goals for the individual. See Table 5 for an example of how 1 key health message can be translated to clear expectations for an individual, so they have specific implementation guidelines that are appropriate to their eating habits and lifestyle.

Table 5

Example of Translating (Advancing and Individualizing) Nutrition Recommendations

Translation Step	Abbreviated Example
Provide key health message	Eat less fat.
Provide more specific health message	Eat less saturated fat.
Offer education – what to avoid	These foods are high in saturated fat, avoid them.
Offer education – what to replace avoided foods with	These foods are low in saturated fat, use them instead of high saturated fat foods.
Engage patient in individualizing recommendations	Instead of eating _____ what could you eat that is lower in saturated fat _____? Let's discuss options in different situations.
Engage patient in applying recommendations	You could lower your saturated fat intake by a third if you could reduce the amount of _____ you eat each day. Could you prepare your food _____ and /or eat less _____? Let's discuss options.

5. Nutrition Recommendations Throughout the Continuum of Type 2 Diabetes

The principal nutrition recommendations for people with pre-diabetes and newly diagnosed and established type 2 diabetes vary, given the well-described differences in the level of endogenous beta cell function and insulin resistance present. While these core defects play a key role in patients with pre-diabetes and diabetes, nutrition and medication recommendations must change to meet the physiologic demands and progressive nature of diabetes. The concepts for this "natural history" are shown in Figure 5.

A central principle of medical nutrition therapy is to ensure that medication choices are based on an individual's clinical characteristics (such as body weight, duration of diabetes) and a given patient's daily routine, including the pattern of food intake and activity. For glucose-lowering medications to be effective and to be used safely, they must be considered in the setting of this usual pattern of food intake. A careful review of an individual's eating pattern, often with the guidance of a RD. should document these eating behaviors and assist in medication choices or medication adjustments. The goal of the following review is to provide broad-based recommendations for nutrition interventions in patients with type 2 diabetes, and to guide the safe use of medications to match food intake to prevent hypoglycemia, avoid glucose excursions and maximize medication effectiveness.

Figure 5

Natural history of diabetes nutritionia therapy

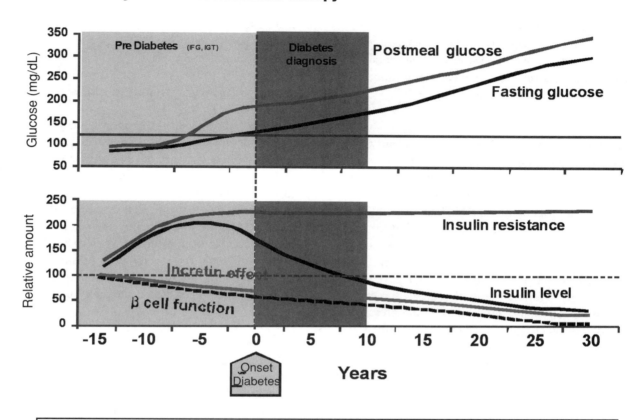

Pre-diabetes	Type 2 Diabetes	Type 2 Diabetes
Insulin resistance *Obesity*	*Insulin resistance*	*Insulin resistance* *Insulin deficiency*
Healthy eating	Consistant carb (portion control)	Insulin-to-carb ratio or or consistant carb
Weight loss	Weight loss	Weight loss or maintenance
Regular activity	Regular activity	Regular activity

6. Pre-diabetes (Preventing Type 2 Diabetes) Through Nutrition Therapy

Pre-diabetes refers to people with either impaired fasting glucose levels or impaired glucose tolerance. With the prevalence of pre-diabetes in 2007, a staggering 57 million people, a number of public health initiatives have focused on preventing and delaying the development of type 2 diabetes. These efforts are based on research that established interventions that effectively prevent/delay the onset of type 2 diabetes.

MNT is a cornerstone of treatment in those with pre-diabetes. The benefit of MNT was clearly established in a series of diabetes prevention studies – including the landmark Diabetes Prevention Program (DPP). In both the Finnish Diabetes Prevention Program and the NIH-sponsored DPP, investigators studied the impact of weight loss and activity (intensive lifestyle intervention) on rates of development of type 2 diabetes. More specifically, DPP compared the impact of intensive lifestyle intervention to drug therapy with metformin in individuals at high risk for progression of pre-diabetes to type 2 diabetes. After only 3.5 years, nutrition therapy/lifestyle intervention significantly reduced the rates of progression. These data showed that overweight persons with either impaired fasting glucose or impaired glucose tolerance, who lost an average of 5%-7% of body weight (typically 10-15 lbs) and increased exercised to 150 minutes a week reduced the risk of developing type 2 diabetes by 58% as compared to placebo. In contrast, those treated with metformin reduced the risk by a lesser amount (31% relative risk reduction vs. placebo).

Of note, intensive lifestyle intervention in DPP was particularly effective in individuals aged 60 years and older, where nutrition therapy reduced risk by more than 70%. Metformin therapy was most effective in people aged 25-44 and in those with a body mass index (BMI) of 35 or higher. Additional analysis of DPP and other studies has found: 1.) weight loss was the most significant predictor of reduced risk for developing diabetes in the lifestyle intervention group; 2.) those in the lifestyle group also experienced reduced blood pressure, while blood pressure increased in those treated with metformin or placebo; 3.) triglyceride and HDL cholesterol levels also improved in the lifestyle intervention group; and 4.) levels of C-reactive protein and fibrinogen—risk factors for heart disease—were lower in both the lifestyle and metformin intervention groups, with a larger reduction in the lifestyle group. Taken as a whole, intensive lifestyle intervention (as evidence by the findings of DPP) should result in a decrease in the yearly incidence of diabetes.

Summary of Interventions: Pre-diabetes

- *Food plan* – Provide healthy eating guidelines that include moderate portion sizes and avoidance of sweetened/sugary beverages. Encourage the use of resources that help each individual translate the guidelines to their eating patterns. For example, help patients plan several breakfast meals that they would enjoy and can have readily available to eat. Registered dietitians can provide individualized recommendations and ongoing support. Additionally, community cooking classes and grocery stores can help support this goal.

- *Weight management* – Discuss the results of the DPP and calculate what a 5%-7% weight loss would be for the individual. Ensure that each patient has the information and structure to achieve weight loss or maintenance. Consistent long-term intervention and follow-up is necessary. Resources include support groups, programs such as WeightWatchers and Overeaters Anonymous and/or RDs, as well as web-based support programs.

- *Activity* – Discuss the value of activity in improving insulin sensitivity and weight management and determine usual activity patterns. Collaboratively set realistic goals to eventually achieve being active 5 days a week for 30 minutes, or refer to community resources that provide activity guidance and support. Consider resources such as community walking programs, YMCAs, community recreation centers, fitness centers and/or physical therapists.

- *Diabetes education* – Provide an overview of the continuum of diabetes and the importance of aggressive attention at this early phase to prevent or delay the progression from pre-diabetes to diabetes. Engage the patient in identifying their treatment needs and setting realistic goals. Teach the patient to do self-blood glucose monitoring so they can observe the effect of the food they eat and their activity on their glucose pattern.

- *Support* – Offer resources that help patients stay motivated to achieve lifestyle goals and address barriers that limit goal achievement, such as local health-related support groups, diabetes education classes, lifestyle support and coaching from a registered dietitian, and/or counseling support with a psychologist or social worker.

7. Recommendations for Medical Nutrition in Recently Diagnosed Type 2 Diabetes

As in pre-diabetes, MNT is a central component of care for all patients who are diagnosed with type 2 diabetes. The use of MNT is recommended both as initial therapy and in the majority of patients, in combination with initial pharmacologic therapy. Additionally, these individuals may have hypertension and dyslipidema that should be treated or co-treated with medical nutrition therapy and medication.

The goal of nutrition therapy early in the course of type 2 diabetes is to optimize glucose control, by appropriately managing carbohydrate intake throughout the day. As noted in Figure 5, the specific focus is to ensure consistent carbohydrate intake, assist with moderate weight loss and encourage regular physical activity. The benefits of weight loss are both well-established and well-known to patients, yet the vast majority of patients struggle with weight management. Further emphasis (or overemphasis) on weight loss as a singular goal of MNT may distract from making other changes that can be of significant benefit.

It is our experience that weight loss can be achieved in many people with type 2 diabetes who receive instruction on carbohydrate counting (food planning) alone. Figure 6 shows data demonstrating the weight loss achieved by patients attending a 4-session diabetes education program that did not emphasize weight loss, but rather focused on carbohydrate counting and modifying intake based on blood glucose test results. This weight loss was achieved for individuals treated with a variety of pharmacologic therapies and supports the central role of carb counting in the initial management of type 2 diabetes.

Many individuals who initially respond to MNT, either alone or in combination with medication, will ultimately require advancing medication therapy, due to the progressive nature of type 2 diabetes. The choices of additional medications should be coordinated with individual patients' food plans and activity patterns. The food plan should be reviewed when medications are added, schedules change, activity patterns change or situations occur that may affect food choices.

Summary of Interventions: Newly Diagnosed Type 2 Diabetes

These interventions build around the recommended interventions in pre-diabetes:

- Food plan – Focus on controlling carbohydrate intake. Initially, eliminate sweetened/sugary beverages and reduce portions of breads, rice, pasta, tortillas, dessert, etc. Provide instruction on sources of carbohydrate and develop a food plan to manage the amount of carbohydrate foods consumed at meals and snacks throughout the day. Engage the patient in identifying food purchasing, preparation and consumption guidelines, based on their typical eating pattern that fits their food plan.

- Weight management – Focus is on weight maintenance, yet a 5%-7% weight loss usually helps improve blood glucose levels. Often, moderating carbohydrate intake leads to reduced caloric intake and supports this focus. Help the patient avoid hypoglycemia, as frequent hypoglycemia can result in excessive caloric intake and result in weight gain.

- Activity – Emphasis is on regular exercise that can be maintained. Discuss and plan activities for different schedules and seasons.

- Diabetes education – Provide instruction on diabetes, its management and goals. Engage patients in setting personal goals and help them track the goals (Appendix B). Initially, have patients monitor their blood glucose at fasting, and before and 2 hours after their largest meal. Review and discuss these values, and engage the patient in determining how their food, activity and medication affects their blood glucose. Ensure that patients are taking their medications appropriately and that medications are advanced as needed.

- Support – Continue to offer resources that help patients stay motivated to achieve lifestyle goals and address barriers that limit goal achievement.

Figure 6

Weight loss as a result of carbohydrate counting

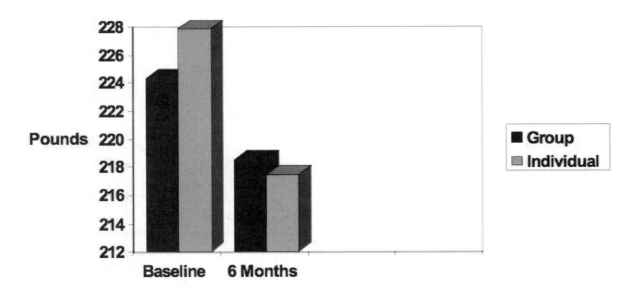

8. Established Type 2 Diabetes

Individuals with longer duration diabetes likely have some experience with MNT. However, the potential need to change medications over time, modify treatment based on individual response and the greater use of insulin therapy with long duration type 2 diabetes warrant additional attention to the patient's nutrition therapy.

Even early in the course of type 2 diabetes, many people will require 1 or more diabetes medications to achieve glycemic targets. After several years, more medications may be necessary. At this point, MNT becomes even more critical, as it is essential to match the specific food intake to the type or types of medications used (eg, meal timing with sulfonylurea or insulin). There is a greater emphasis on consistent carbohydrate intake and the use of insulin-to-carbohydrate ratios.

The following summarizes nutrition-related considerations with non-insulin diabetes medications. Table 6 summarizes nutrition considerations with 3 primary insulin regimens.

Metformin	May cause nausea
Sulfonyureas	May cause hypoglycemia
Incretin-based therapy	May cause nausea, weight loss
TZDs	May cause weight gain, fluid retention, lowering of lipids

Table 6

Meal and Snack Guidelines for 3 Common Insulin Regimens

1 carbohydrate choice - 15 grams carbohydrate

	Meals	Snacks
Background insulin (added to oral agents)	Aim for 3 meals per day: • Women 2–4 carb choices per meal • Men 3–5 carb choices per meal	• Not needed • If desired, should be small: 1–2 carb choices per snack
Premixed insulin	• Eat 3 meals at consistent times with consistent carb intake • Do not skip meals • No more than 10–12 hours between breakfast and dinner	• Rapid-acting: snack not usually needed; if desired should be small, 1–2 carb choices per snack • Regular: may need small snacks
Background & mealtime insulin	• Initially, a consistent carb intake • When patient is ready, advance from carb counting to insulin-to-carb ratio to maximize therapy	• Rapid-acting: not needed; if greater than 1 carb choice may require additional insulin injection • Regular: may need small snacks

Note: A registered dietitian can help assess usual food intake, provide guidance in selecting foods in a variety of situations, and evaluate BG records based on food intake and activity.

Hypoglycemia: All who take insulin should be taught to recognize hypoglycemia and carry a carbohydrate food or beverage to treat it. Usual treatment is 15 grams of carbohydrate.

When insulin is needed

Studies have shown that patients often experience 5-8 years of elevated A1C levels before they start insulin therapy. The delay can be related to a number of factors. To support early and appropriate use of insulin, clinicians can use the insulin gauges in Figure 7 to have a conversation with a patient about the need to start insulin. Also, materials such as an insulin decision aid, in which the gauges are printed, can help engage the patient in the decision about using insulin and address typical concerns about starting insulin, such as those related to fear of injections, hypoglycemia and worsening of diabetes.

The primary goal with insulin therapy is to balance exogenous insulin with food intake and activity using blood glucose testing to monitor and evaluate the treatment. A careful nutrition assessment is necessary when insulin therapy is initiated and adjusted to ensure the insulin regimen corresponds to the typical eating and activity pattern. A focus on MNT will assure both improved effectiveness and safety.

Table 7

Carbohydrate Adjustments for Exercise for People With Diabetes

The recommendations below are guidelines for adding carbohydrates. Testing your own blood glucose levels and evaluating the results is the key to finding the correct adjustments for you.

Duration and Intensity of Exercise	Blood Glucose Level Before Exercise		
	70-120 mg/dL	121-180 mg/dL	181-250 mg/dL
Short Duration Low Intensity Examples: 30 minutes of yoga, walking, or bicycling leisurely	Add 15 grams of carbohydrate	No adjustment needed	No adjustment needed
Moderate Duration Moderate Intensity Examples: 30-60 minutes of vigorous walking, playing tennis swimming, or jogging	Add 15 grams of carbohydrate	No adjustment needed	No adjustment needed
Moderate Duration High Intensity Examples: 30-60 minutes of running, high-impact aerobics or kickboxing	Add 15-30 grams of carbohydrate	Add 15 grams of carbohydrate	No adjustment needed
Long Duration Moderate Intensity Examples: 60 minutes or more of playing team sports, golfing, cycling or swimming. (retest, glucose level to assess, especially if trying a new activity)	Add 15 grams of carbohydrate per hour of activity	Add 15 grams of carbohydrate per hour of activity	After the first hour of activity add 15 grams of carbohydrate

©2009 International Diabetes Center at Park Nicollet

Summary of Interventions: Established Type 2 Diabetes

These interventions build about the recommended interventions in pre-diabetes and newly diagnosed type 2 diabetes:

- *Food plan* – Greater emphasis on consistent carbohydrate intake. Reassess food and activity patterns, and match medication to these patterns to reduce hypoglycemia and improve glycemic outcomes. Ensure the patient's ability to accurately count carbohydrates in a variety of situations.

- *Weight management* – Focus is on weight maintenance, especially if insulin is initiated which has the potential to create weight gain through improved glycemic control, treating hypoglycemia and flexible dosing to accommodate a variety of foods. Consulting with a RD early in the use of insulin can help a patient appropriately address these situations and maximize the use of additional medications.

- *Activity* – If insulin is used, there is greater potential for exercise-induced hypoglycemia. Provide instructions on adjusting insulin doses or food intake; see Table 7.

- *Diabetes education* – Review all areas of diabetes self-care, as advancing diabetes creates renewed interest and attention to self-care behaviors. Specific emphasis should be on problem-solving skills related to blood glucose pattern control.

- *Support* – Openly discuss patients' concerns or fears about diabetes. Emphasize their ability to contribute to goal achievement and refer for additional counseling support as needed.

Figure 7

Visuals that show the change in insulin production during the natural history of diabetes

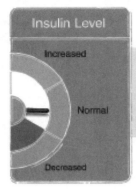

No Diabetes

The pancreas works well and makes enough insulin. Insulin keeps your blood glucose from going too high.

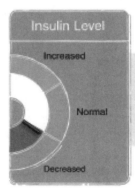

Prediabetes
(10–20 years before diabetes starts)

The pancreas works harder to make more insulin. It's trying to keep up with the body's needs.

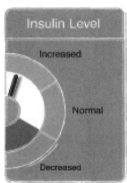

Diabetes

The pancreas starts to wear out. It can't make enough insulin.

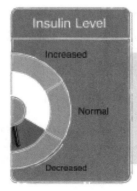

Diabetes Progressing
(5–15 years after diabetes starts)

The pancreas keeps trying to make insulin, but wears out.

9. Monitoring and Evaluating Medical Nutrition Therapy

As with any therapeutic intervention, nutrition therapy requires monitoring and evaluation. Additionally, because nutrition therapy requires behavior change, frequent, ongoing nutrition counseling and support is typically required. Follow-up visits are initially utilized to provide basic education about the food and activity plan and its integration into diabetes management. During these sessions, the appropriateness of the plan is evaluated: is it the correct intervention strategy, is it understood, can it be applied comfortably and confidently in a variety of situations, and does it achieve the desired outcomes? Once the plan is understood, nutrition counseling focuses on the assimilation of the food plan into the patient's life, addressing barriers and facilitators, problem-solving and providing support. Research shows that to maintain changes, counseling support is needed every 3-6 months.

10. Appendices A, B and C

Appendix A. Resources for Diabetes Education and Medical Nutrition Therapy

The following websites can help you locate an accredited "recognized" diabetes education program, certified diabetes educator and registered dietitian in your area.

- www.diabeteseducator.org Click on the box *Find a diabetes educator and/or accredited programs*

- www.diabetes.org Click on *health professionals/recognition programs/education recognition programs*

- www.eatright.org Click on *find a nutrition professional*

Appendix B.
Sample Forms for Diabetes Self Management Training and Medical Nutrition Therapy

Referral Form

Today's Date:	☐ Non-urgent, first available appointment
	☐ Semi-urgent, within 2 weeks
	☐ Medically urgent, within 2 days

Reason for diabetes education

☐ Non-insulin patients newly diagnosed or limited previous diabetes education.

☐ **Insulin Start**

☐ **Insulin Adjust:** education needs, please specify _____

Insulin Pump

    ☐ RN/RD Assessment and Education

    ☐ Training on a new model

       • Date patient expects to receive new pump _____

☐ **Pregnancy (known diabetes) Type 1   Type 2**

☐ **Continuous Glucose Monitoring**

☐ **Health Psychology Consult** (new diagnosis, adherence issues, mood disorder/burnout)

☐ **RD only-Medical Nutrition Therapy: check all that apply**

☐ Diabetes	☐ Eating Disorder	☐ Retinopathy
☐ Hypertension	☐ Nephropathy	☐ Pregnancy
☐ Renal Disease	☐ Non-healing wound	☐ Mental/affective disorder
☐ CHD	☐ Obesity	☐ Stroke
☐ Dyslipidemia	☐ Other:	

Current Diabetes Medications

Diabetes oral medications _____

Insulin (type and dose) _____

I certify that I am managing this patient's condition and the education described in my dictation. The Plan of Care is needed to provide this patient with the skills and knowledge to help manage their diabetes.

Provider signature: _____

Success Plan

This form helps to engage patients in setting realistic goals and tracking their success. The planning tool is used in diabetes education to identify an area of behavior change, the meaningfulness of the goal and areas that will help or hinder goal achievement.

Diabetes Success Plan

Name _____

Date _____

Step 1 – Select **one** lifestyle area to change, then choose a personal goal or write your own.

Food Plan and Nutrition	❑ Count carbohydrates at most of my meals and snacks
	❑ Reduce fat in my diet by eating less _____ at two or more meals a day
	❑ _____
Physical Activity	❑ Increase my activity (for example, take the stairs) at least _____ days a week
	❑ Be active _____ minutes or more _____ times a week
	❑ _____
Medication	❑ Take my diabetes medications as scheduled
	❑ _____
Risk Reduction	❑ Stop smoking by _____ (date)
	❑ _____
Problem-solving	❑ Look for patterns in my record book at least _____ days a month
	❑ _____
Living and Coping	❑ To help manage my stress, I will do _____ at least _____ times a week
	❑ _____
Blood Glucose Testing	❑ Test my glucose at least _____ times a day, _____ days a week
	❑ _____

Step 2 – Is this goal meaningful to **me**? Circle a number after each question.

How <u>important</u> is it to me to do this?

0 1 2 3 4 5 6 7 8 9 10
Not at all   Very

How <u>confident</u> am I that I can do this?

0 1 2 3 4 5 6 7 8 9 10
Not at all   Very

Step 3 – How often am I doing this **now**? Mark the bar below.

The day I write my goal

not at all   about half   always

How will this goal help me?_____

What might get in the way?_____

First follow-up visit Date _____

not at all   about half   always

One benefit of this goal was… _____

This got in my way… _____

Second follow-up visit Date _____

not at all   about half   always

One benefit of this goal was… _____

This got in my way… _____

Appendix C. Frequently Asked Patient Questions about Nutrition for Diabetes

This appendix addresses typical questions patients have about specific foods (foods made with sugar, using low or modified carbohydrate foods), alcohol, protein, fat and exercise. A diabetes food plan will integrate these recommendations into an individualized food plan based on an individual's eating pattern, metabolic needs, activity, schedule and learning needs. The questions and responses can be copied and provided to patients.

Do I have to give up foods made with sugar?
People who have diabetes can eat foods that contain sugar. Sugar is a carbohydrate that raises your blood glucose. But it doesn't raise it higher than other types of carbohydrates. To control your blood glucose, you need to watch your total intake of carbohydrates, not just sugar. Carbohydrates are contained in starchy foods, like potatoes, beans, squash, corn, rice, bread and pasta. They're also found in fruits, fruit juices, dairy products, sweets and sugar. Foods that contain little or no carbohydrate include meats, poultry, fish, eggs, nonstarchy vegetables and fats. It is important to recognize which foods contain carbohydrates and which do not. Then, try to consume a consistent, moderate amount of carbohydrates at meals. That will help you keep your blood glucose levels steadier and in your target range. If you want to choose a sweet food, you can substitute it for another carbohydrate. If you are taking mealtime insulin, you can learn to adjust your dose if you change the carbohydrate content of your meals.

Should I use low-carb products?
There is no need to buy special low-carb food products. There are 3 ways that food manufacturers reduce carbohydrate in a product. The first is to substitute artificial sweeteners like aspartame in place of sugar, such as in diet soda. The second is to use less starch and substitute with more fiber, such as in low-carb, high-fiber breads. The third way is to substitute sugar alcohols for sugar. An example is a "sugar-free" candy bar that contains sorbitol instead of sugar. This can be very misleading, because many low-carb products claim to have zero sugar carbohydrates, when they contain sugar alcohols. In general, half of the sugar alcohol amount should be considered carbohydrate. Sugar alcohols are not completely absorbed from the small intestine into the blood. Unabsorbed sugar alcohols are fermented in the large intestine and may produce some abdominal gas and discomfort.

Compared to regular foods, low-carb products often contain similar amounts of calories. If you like a low-carb product, it's okay to use it. But low-carb products are frequently more expensive, higher in fat and may not taste as good. The key point is that people who have diabetes don't need special foods. They just need to monitor or count their intake of carbohydrates in regular foods.

Do I have to eat whole wheat bread?
No, but eating a diet high in fiber and whole grains is recommended. Whole wheat bread is a better choice than white bread, because it has more fiber and natural nutrients, but both contain carbohydrates and have to be counted as part of the meal plan. Fiber helps lower total and LDL cholesterol, by reducing absorption of dietary fat. It also reduces constipation, bowel cancers and diverticulosis. In addition, fiber can make you feel full, so you may eat less. But if you don't like whole wheat bread, look for other ways to increase fiber in your diet. Eating a diet high in fiber has benefits for everyone. The goal is to increase fiber intake to 25-35 grams per day. You can do this by replacing low-fiber foods with higher fiber foods you enjoy.

Lower fiber	Higher fiber
White bread, 1 g	Whole wheat bread, 2 g
Saltine crackers, less than 1 g	Triscuit® crackers, 3 g
Orange juice, 0 g	Orange, 3 g
Chicken noodle soup, 1 g	Bean or pea soup, 10 g
Cornflakes, less than 1 g	High fiber cereal, 8-13 g

Should I follow a low glycemic index diet?

The glycemic index is a measurement of how a food affects blood glucose levels. There are many factors that can impact the glycemic response of a food: how it is prepared, how ripe it is, how long it was cooked and how much it has been processed. It is important to know that the glycemic response of a food varies significantly from person to person.

The glycemic index values found in books and on the internet are calculated based on individual foods. Foods with a low glycemic index (less than 55%) include all milk products, nuts, dried beans and legumes and most fruits. Foods with an average glycemic index include candy, ice cream, white rice and pasta. Foods with a high glycemic index (greater than 70%) tend to be processed cereals, crackers and starches.

Lower glycemic foods tend to provide more nutrition, but they do not always improve your glucose levels. You also may notice similar types of food affect your blood glucose differently. The amount of diabetes medication you take, together with the total amount of carbs you eat, usually determines your glucose level. However, you may notice that your glucose goes higher after eating certain foods. The glycemic index is a guide to the smaller differences between the glucose rise-and-fall of carbohydrate. The best way to use the glycemic index is to understand your body's glucose response; check glucose levels after eating and figure out your own glycemic index.

What effect does protein and fat have on glucose levels?

If consuming healthy portions of protein and fat, they have little effect on blood glucose levels. Meat, poultry, fish and fats (butter, margarine and oil) do not contain carbohydrates and therefore have little effect on your blood glucose level. Still, they are an important part of your food plan, because they provide necessary protein and other nutrients. Choose lean meats and healthy fats to help protect your heart by reducing saturated and trans fat in the diet.

Can I still have a beer or glass of wine?

In some individuals, a relationship has been shown between drinking a small amount of alcohol and an improvement in insulin resistance, a decrease in the development of diabetes and a reduced risk of coronary artery disease.

Keep in mind, though, that the maximum amount to consume is 1-2 drinks per day (defined as a 12-ounce beer, 5 ounces of wine or a 1.5 ounce shot of liquor). If you are drinking beer, choose light beer, as it contains fewer carbohydrates. 12 ounces of regular beer has about 13 grams of carbohydrate, compared to 5-11 grams in light beer (depending on brand). A 5 ounce glass of wine or a shot of liquor has only trace amounts of carbohydrates.

Because alcohol lowers glucose, there is a potential for hypoglycemia for people who are taking medication to lower blood glucose. To prevent low blood glucose, alcohol should be consumed with carbs. Also, drinking more than the recommended amount of alcohol with metformin can lead to serious health problems (lactic acidosis).

Do I have to exercise?

Physical activity is important for good health whether you have diabetes or not. But it doesn't have to be traditional exercise. The *Dietary Guidelines for Americans 2005* recommends 30 minutes of physical activity most days for general fitness. This activity doesn't have to be in one 30-minute segment. It can be three 10-minute walks around the house or office, or 10 3-minute bouts of an activity. Physical activity is defined as any movement of the body that uses energy. So, activities such as housecleaning, mowing the grass and walking up and down stairs count, in addition to riding a bike, walking the golf course or shooting baskets.

Physical activity uses up glucose and lowers blood glucose levels considerably. In 2 large studies, people who were at risk for developing diabetes lowered that risk by 58% if they exercised at least 150 minutes per week. And people who are physically active tend to live longer, on average, independent of their weight. The message is very clear: get moving!

For the person who has had diabetes for many years and has complications related to diabetes, it is advised that they consult a physician before embarking on a physical fitness program. Of special concern is peripheral neuropathy, because of the potential for foot-related injuries. Everyday, the feet should be checked for any sores or redness and changes should be reported to the physician. Wear shoes that are not binding and provide good support. Cardiovascular disease, unstable retinopathy and nephropathy require gentle or modified activity. Consider a visit with a physical therapist for an assessment and exercise prescription or plan.

Chapter 7: Management of Type 2 Diabetes: Non-insulin Therapies and Insulin Treatment

Richard M. Bergenstal, MD
Gregg Simonson, PhD
Robert Cuddihy, MD

Contents

1. Background

2. Progress in Defining and Reaching Treatment Goals

3. Barriers to Reaching Treatment Goals

4. Approaches to Reaching Glycemic Treatment Targets

5. Conclusion

6. References

1. Background

The growing incidence of type 2 diabetes (T2DM) in adults and children is the major contributor to what is now being referred to as a worldwide epidemic of diabetes. A recent report by the Centers for Disease Control (CDC) stated that 1 out of 3 adults may have diabetes by the year 2050 if the current trends in incidence and prevalence continue. This epidemic of diabetes has dramatic personal health and economic consequences. Diabetes remains the leading cause of blindness in working-age adults, and the leading cause of renal failure and non-traumatic amputations. In addition, individuals with diabetes have 2-4 times the incidence of cardiovascular disease as those without diabetes, and this has earned diabetes the classification as a cardiovascular risk equivalent in most cases. The cost of caring for diabetes is staggering. In the United States alone, 1 in every 10 health care dollars is spent on caring for diabetes-related problems and 1 in every 5 health care dollars are spent on the health care of individuals with diabetes. This translates to an annual cost of approximately 174 billion dollars spent on the direct and indirect expenses of caring for people with diabetes (Figure 1). Worldwide chronic disease is now clearly established as the leading cause of death, led by cardiovascular disease and including diabetes in the top 4 deadly chronic disease categories.

While more effective approaches to preventing diabetes are being developed and tested, it is clear they will be essential to substantially reduce the clinical and economic burden of T2DM. Moreover, employing effective management strategies for diabetes is critical to the well being of the 24 million individuals with diabetes in the U.S., as well as their families, friends and the productivity of companies that employ them.

Figure 1

Diabetes Health Care Expenditures

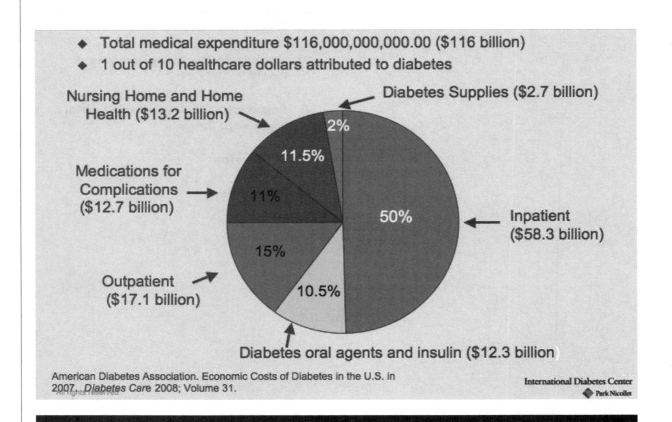

- Total medical expenditure $116,000,000,000.00 ($116 billion)
- 1 out of 10 healthcare dollars attributed to diabetes

Nursing Home and Home Health ($13.2 billion)

Diabetes Supplies ($2.7 billion)

2%

11.5%

Medications for Complications ($12.7 billion)

11%

50%

Inpatient ($58.3 billion)

15%

Outpatient ($17.1 billion)

10.5%

Diabetes oral agents and insulin ($12.3 billion)

American Diabetes Association. Economic Costs of Diabetes in the U.S. in 2007. *Diabetes Care* 2008; Volume 31.

International Diabetes Center
◆ Park Nicollet

2. Progress in Defining and Reaching Treatment Goals

The goal in treating any chronic disease, including diabetes, is to optimize the known metabolic and physiologic abnormalities, prevent or delay the development or progression of complications related to the disease and monitor and treat the common comorbidities found with the disease. In addition, one wants to help the individual lead an active, fulfilling life (good functional status and quality of life) avoiding excessive stress or side effects associated with the necessary treatment of the condition.

Effective management of T2DM starts with a timely diagnosis, followed by self-management education (team-based is ideal) and then a focus on optimizing (treating to target) the various metabolic and physiologic risk factors or abnormalities commonly present in T2DM (as outlined in Figure 2 depicting the priorities of care for adults with T2DM). The goal is to prevent or delay the pro-gression of both cardiovascular (macrovascular) and microvascular complications. In the not-so-distant past, the focus of treating T2DM was only on optimizing glycemic control. This so-called glucocentric approach to diabetes management has clearly been demonstrated to be insufficient in pre-venting the development or progression of compli-cations. Since CVD is the major cause of mortality in T2DM, much of the focus is on what compo-nent of therapy has the biggest impact on mini-mizing CVD. While hyperglycemia is clearly a risk factor for CVD in epidemiologic studies, cur-rent data seems to indicate that smoking cessation and treating blood pressure and lipids aggressively are the most effective in minimizing macrovascu-lar disease. Treatment of hyperglycemia to achieve at least an A1C <7% soon after the diagnosis of T1DM or T2DM seems to have long term benefi-cial CV benefits. Optimizing glucose control and blood pressure are particularly important in mini-mizing microvascular disease.

Figure 2

Priorities of Care for Adults with Diabetes

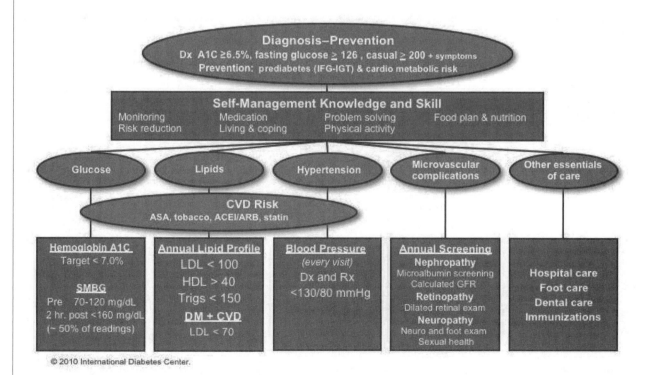

© 2010 International Diabetes Center.

The Steno-2 study tested a multifactorial approach to reducing mortality and CVD in T2DM. In the initial 7.8 year trial, in 160 individuals with T2DM and microalbuminuria (a known CVD risk factor), intensive treatment of the major CVD risk factors (A1C, cholesterol, TG, systolic and diastolic BP) resulted in only a modest improvement in most of the CVD risk factors compared to conventional treatment (see Figure 3). However, this multifactorial approach resulted in approximately a 50% reduction in cardiovascular disease outcomes. The Steno-2 study group then reported an additional 5.5 year follow-up, and the primary outcome was time to death in the intensive vs. conventionally treated group at 13.3 years of total observation. There was a 46% relative reduction in mortality risk (20% absolute reduction in mortality), 57% relative reduction in CV death risk (see Figure 4) and 59% relative reduction in risk of a CV event. The Steno-2 study and follow-up are often referenced regarding the need to address all the major priorities of care for T2DM, if improved morbidity and mortality is the goal. How much improvement would be possible if all the main complication risk factors were treated to optimal levels? This has

recently been addressed by using the Archimedes model. This is one of the most robust and sophisticated modeling programs available, where the user enters all the important characteristics of an individual, or in this circumstance, of a population of individuals, with diabetes. Then the Archimedes model is programmed to calculate the 30-year expected rate of various complications and the mortality rate if current standards of practice are followed vs. if optimal care is delivered (in this case defined as achieving A1C <7%, BP <130/80 mmHg, LDL<100 mg/dL, HDL >40 mg/dL, TG <150 mg/dL, non smoker, +ASA, BMI <25). Figures 5 and 6 show that optimal care for 30 years would indeed dramatically reduce complications, death and save $325 billion dollars.

Figure 3

STENO-2 STUDY

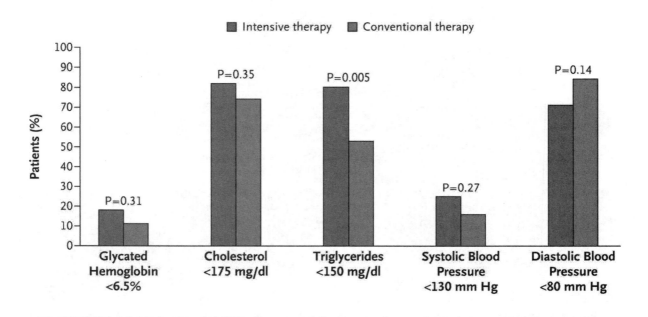

Gaede P et al. *Multifactorial intervention in cardiovascular disease in patients with Type 2 Diabetes.* N Engl J Med. 348(5); 383-393;2003

Figure 4

STENO-2 Study Follow-Up

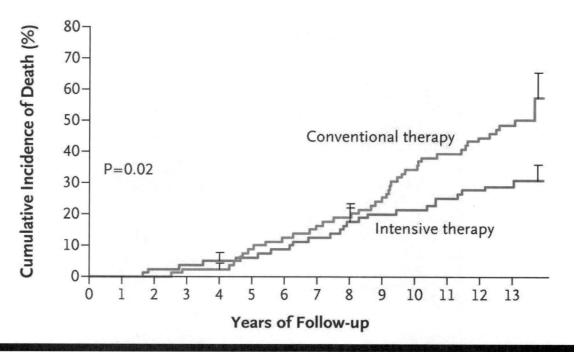

Gaede P et al. Effect of a multifactorial intervention on mortality in Type 2 Diabetes. N Engl J Med. *358; 358-380; 2008.*

Figure 5

Archimedes Model: Reduction in Complications

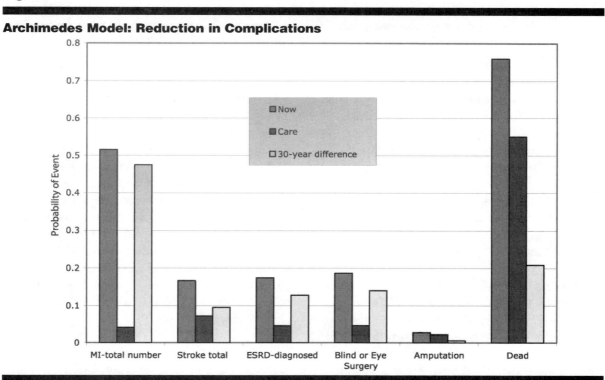

Schlesinger L et al. Archimedes: A new model for simulating healthcare systems - the mathematical formulation. J of Biomedical Informatics. *35; 37-50, 2002.*

Figure 6

Archimedes Model: Cost Savings

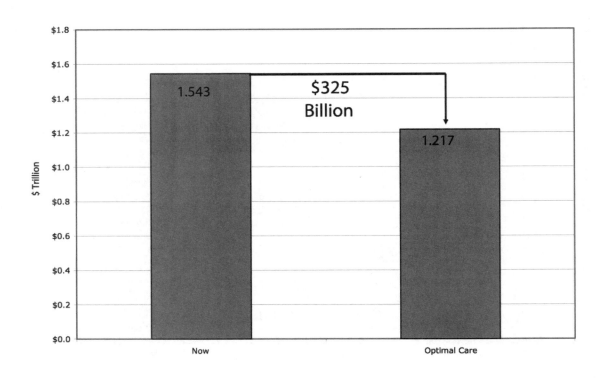

Schlesinger L et al. Archimedes: A new model for simulating healthcare systems - the mathematical formulation. J of Biomedical Informatics. *35; 37-50, 2002.*

Effective treatment starts with a set of target goals that both the provider of care and the patient understand and, ideally, agree upon (see Figure 2). While it is beyond the scope of this section to review all the literature that has resulted in the blood pressure, lipid and glycemic targets outlined in Figure 2, it may be instructive to summarize the recent major clinical trial findings that have informed the dialogue regarding appropriate glycemic targets.

The major trials that have influenced glucose targets include the DCCT and the DCCT follow-up trial (called EDIC), conducted with volunteers with T1DM. These studies established that good glucose control matters and an A1C of 7% dramatically reduced the risk of microvascular complications compared to an A1C of 9%. In addition, this

study was the first to demonstrate and introduce the concept of *metabolic memory*, also referred to as *legacy effect*. Metabolic memory describes the findings that those individuals originally randomized to intensive glycemic control retained their reduced risk for microvascular complications 10-15 years after the trial completion, and even when the glycemic control in the previously intensive and conventionally treated groups was nearly identical for the entire follow-up period. This finding has had lasting implications about the importance of establishing early glycemic control to minimize immediate and future risk of developing complications.

In T2DM, the major trials that have influenced glycemic goals include the original UKPDS trial, studying over 5000 newly-diagnosed T2DM patients, comparing intensive vs. conventional treatment strategies. This study had 2 major subsets: those on sulfonylureas or insulin vs. mainly lifestyle management and those obese T2DM subjects on metformin vs. predominantly lifestyle management. This study demonstrated that an overall A1C of about 7% vs. 7.9% resulted in a significant reduction in microvascular disease and a non-significant (P value 0.052) reduction in macrovascular disease. Again, a 10-year follow-up study of the UKPDS showed a legacy effect of the importance of early good glycemic control. Those randomized to intensive glycemic control in the initial trial maintained a significant reduction in microvascular disease, and also showed a significant reduction in macrovascular disease and all-cause mortality when followed up 10 years after the trial, compared to those who were initially in the conventional treatment arm of the UKPDS.

These findings, other smaller trials and many meta-analyses have shown a good correlation between A1C and cardiovascular outcomes. This led to 3 major randomized controlled trials attempting to answer the following question: does intensive glycemic control reduce cardiovascular events and CV deaths in T2DM? These 3 trials were the ACCORD trial, the ADVANCE trial and the VADT. The papers from these trials summarizing the impact of improving glycemic control on cardiovascular disease and all-cause mortality were each published in the *New England Journal of Medicine* in 2008 and 2009. After an average follow-up of 3.5 years, the ACCORD trial showed an increase (22% relative risk and 1% in absolute risk) in all-cause mortality in the 5000 person treatment arm aiming for an A1C of <6% (achieved median A1C of 6.4%), compared to 5000 individuals aiming for an A1C of between 7% and 7.9% (achieved median A1C 7.5%). There was a non-significant 10% reduction in the ACCORD primary outcome of major cardiovascular events. To date, there is no clear explanation for the unexpected increased mortality finding in the ACCORD intensively treated group. Explanations, such as a very rapid improvement in the A1C, a 3-fold increase in severe hypoglycemia, excessive weight gain, more intensive use of medication (77% on insulin and many individuals with multiple oral agents and insulin thera-

py), and the unknown physiologic and psychosocial effects of aggressive intensive therapy have all been raised as possible explanations. To date, most agree the data available in the ACCORD trial cannot confirm any of these hypotheses. Interestingly, a recent study by Riddle et al. demonstrated that persisting on-treatment elevated A1C was associated with increased mortality in the intensively treated group rather than achieving a low A1C per se. In other words, those in the intensively treated group whose A1C did not respond to regimen intensification were at highest risk of mortality compared to those whose A1C declined significantly from baseline. Two other T2DM trials addressing glycemic control and the risk of CVD were done at the same time as ACCORD. ADVANCE, with over 11,000 participants for 5 years of follow-up (mean endpoint A1Cs of 6.5% and 7.3% in intensive and standard control, respectively), and VADT, with almost 1800 individuals for 5.6 years of follow-up (median endpoint A1C's of 6.9% and 8.4%, intensive and standard control, respectively), did not show an increase in mortality, and also did not show a CVD benefit with intensive vs. conventional glycemic treatment. The ADVANCE trial did show a significant reduction in microvascular outcomes (driven by a reduction in renal disease) with intensive glucose control. The VADT did not show any significant microvascular benefit and the ACCORD trial did not show benefit using a composite microvascular endpoint, but did show benefit in significantly reducing progression of retinopathy as well as delaying the onset of albuminuria. Many health care organizations and clinicians have started to compare, contrast and analyze these major trials to arrive at treatment targets, treatment strategies and the design of studies to address unanswered clinical questions. The American Diabetes Association (ADA), American Heart Association (AHA) and the American College of Cardiology (ACC) summarized the findings of the major T2DM management trials and concluded that individualization of glycemic targets is important. They went on to recommend an A1C target for microvascular disease of 7% or less and a <7% macrovascular disease glycemic target for many individuals, particularly those being treated early in the disease process. These groups also noted that a less stringent (or higher)

Figure 7

Comparison of Recent Glycemia Trials Accord, Advance and VADT

Characteristic	ACCORD	ADVANCE	VADT
N	10,251	11,140	1,791
Mean age	62	66	60.4
Duration of Type 2 DM	10 yr	8 yr	11.5 yr
History of CVD	35%	32%	40%
BMI	32.2	28	31.3
Baseline A1C	8.3%	7.5%	9.4%
Statin	62% → 88%	28% → 47%	58% → 84%
Antiplatelet	55% → 76%	48% → 62%	76% → 93%
Study duration (yrs)	~3.5	5.0	6.0
Target A1C	<6% vs 7-8%	<6.5% vs "Usual"	<6.5% vs 8-9%
Achieved A1C	6.4% and 7.5%	6.5% and 7.3%	6.9% and 8.4%

ACCORD Study Group. *N Engl J Med*. 2008;358:2545-59;
ADVANCE Collaborative Group. N Engl J Med 2008;358:2560-72;
Duckworth W et al. *N Engl J Med* 2009;360

International Diabetes Center
Park Nicollet

A1C target was appropriate for "*patients with a history of severe hypoglycemia, limited life expectancy, advanced microvascular or macrovascular complications, or extensive comorbid conditions or those with long-standing diabetes in whom the general goal is difficult to attain despite diabetes self-management education, appropriate glucose monitoring, and effective doses of multiple glucose lowering agents including insulin.*" The characteristics of patients participating in the 3 major new trials are outlined in Figure 7.

These major trials (and their follow-up studies), evaluating the effect of intensive glycemic therapy on microvascular disease, macrovascular disease and mortality, are summarized in Figure 8.

An A1C target of less than 7% (particularly to minimize microvascular disease or in early T2DM to prevent macrovascular disease) makes sense for many individuals, but not all clinicians and researchers agree at this stage on how to define those individuals in whom a less aggressive goal seems appropriate. Many say the general A1C target should be <7% for T2DM, with a subset which, for safety reasons, should aim for an A1C of <8%; others say the general A1C target should be <8% with a subset in which it is safe to strive for an A1C <7%. The clinician will need to discuss and agree upon an A1C target with each patient he or she cares for, often starting with an A1C <7%, then determining if there is some reason it should be higher (i.e., history of severe hypoglycemia) or lower (i.e., patient is pregnant). Setting the level for a community A1C performance measure is a difficult balance between what is best for each individual, but also with the understanding that it is hard to sort out appropriate exceptions to tight control from audits of electronically submitted clinical data that is often used for

Figure 8

Impact of Intensive Therapy in Diabetes Summary of Major Clinical Trials

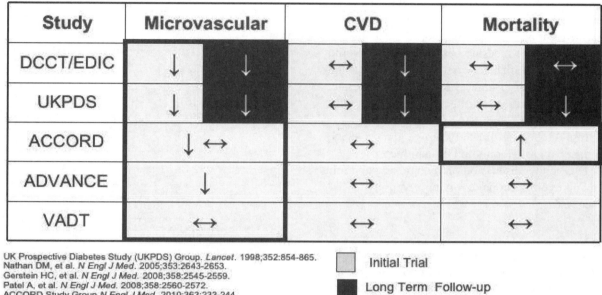

Study	Microvascular		CVD		Mortality	
DCCT/EDIC	↓	↓	↔	↓	↔	↔
UKPDS	↓	↓	↔	↓	↔	↓
ACCORD	↓ ↔		↔		↑	
ADVANCE	↓		↔		↔	
VADT	↔		↔		↔	

UK Prospective Diabetes Study (UKPDS) Group. *Lancet.* 1998;352:854-865.
Nathan DM, et al. *N Engl J Med.* 2005;353:2643-2653.
Gerstein HC, et al. *N Engl J Med.* 2008;358:2545-2559.
Patel A, et al. *N Engl J Med.* 2008;358:2560-2572.
ACCORD Study Group *N Engl J Med.* 2010;363:233-244.
Ismail-Beigi et al. The Lancet 2010; published online

☐ Initial Trial

■ Long Term Follow-up

performance measurement. Some feel it is more appropriate to set only a poor glycemic control (A1C >9%) performance measure and all should be "graded" on how well they minimize the proportion of their patients in poor control. NCQA, a national performance measurement organization, in their Diabetes Physician Recognition Program (DPRP), has devised a way to incorporate the concept of credit for reducing the risk of a population of patients, by moving most people down to an A1C <8% but also including credit and the expectation that many individuals can be safely managed to an A1C <7%. The most commonly followed targets for blood pressure (BP <130/80 mmHg, with much more emphasis today on the systolic BP) and lipid control (LDL <100 mg/dL for most or <70 mg/dL if there is known heart disease) are described in further detail later in this manual.

A much-quoted study in 2003 indicated that Medicare recipients were not receiving optimal care in general, and one specific example given was that individuals with diabetes were only receiving 55% of what was considered optimal care.

Analyzing the last 3 consecutive waves of A1C measurement as part of the US NHANES survey shows that the percentage of adults with diabetes who have an A1C <7% has been improving. Those with A1C <7% went from 37% to 49.7% to between 55.7-56.8% in 1999-2000, 2001-2002 and 2003-2004. While some feel these survey data may not be completely representative of diabetes across the U.S., the trend toward improvement is clear. Whether this improvement represents the introduction of new medications or new technologies, new systems of care and education, the introduction of diabetes registries, transparency in outcomes or pay for performance is not clear.

Before launching into the barriers and facilitators to optimizing glycemic control, it is worthwhile to have a broader discussion of how to define and monitor glycemic control. A1C is the gold standard for measuring glycemic control, because this is a measure of long-term control (2-3 months) and has been the measure best correlated with the development of diabetes complications (particularly microvascular disease). For effective glycemic management, patients will benefit if they are educated about A1C (and new additional ways to express A1C call estimated average glucose eAG), guidance on self-monitored blood glucose (SMBG) and a discussion on recognizing and minimizing hypoglycemia (avoiding severe hypoglycemia).

• **A1C**

  The most widely accepted general A1C goal today is <7%, in order to minimize microvascular complications, but needs to be individualized if circumstances exist that indicate the A1C target should be more lenient or strict.

• **Estimated average glucose (eAG)**

  eAG is another way to express and better understand the A1C, since it presents the A1C in mg/dL, which patients are used to seeing on their glucose meters (A1C of 7% = eAG of 154 mg/dL). An international study showed a good correlation between A1C and average glucose, and a conversion calculator and formula can be located in Table 1.

• **SMBG**

  There is not a broad consensus on SMBG targets (ADA- FPG 70-130 mg/dL, ppg peak <180 mg/dL, IDC- FPG 70-120 mg/dL, 2hr ppg <160 mg/dL or less than 40 mg/dL) rise pre-meal to 2 hours post-meal.

An important clinical variable to be aware of is that if approximately 50% of the patients' SMBG values are within the designated target ranges (assuming fairly commonly used ranges) the A1C will usually be on target or close to target. There is widespread acceptance of the value of performing SMBG in patients with T1DM and T2DM who are

Table 1

Glucose Conversion Calculator

AIC (%)	Mean Plasma Glucose	
	mg/dl	mmol/l
6	126	7.0
7	157	8.6
8	183	10.2
9	212	11.8
10	240	13.4
11	269	14.9
12	298	16.5

Estimates based on ADAG data of ~2,700 glucose measurements over 3 months per AIC measurement in 507 adults with type 1, type 2 and no diabetes. Correlation between AIC and average glucose: 0.92 (42). A calculator fo converting AIC results into cAG, in either mg/dl or mmol/l, is available at http://professional.diabetes.org/eAG.

using insulin. Tests may be fasting and pre-meal (particularly in T2DM) or post-meal when using rapid-acting insulin analogues before meals, or in all patients who are pregnant. There is less agreement on the value of SMBG in patients not on insulin.

Most agree everyone should be taught SMBG as part of an education program, to help them understand their diabetes and the impact of food, exercise and daily stress on their blood glucose levels. Yet, there is not much published data to show overall glucose control or a reduction in complications results from utilizing SMBG in non-insulin-using T2DM patients. The overall recommendation is to perform SMBG in a manner that allows

Figure 9

Adjust SMBG to Therapy

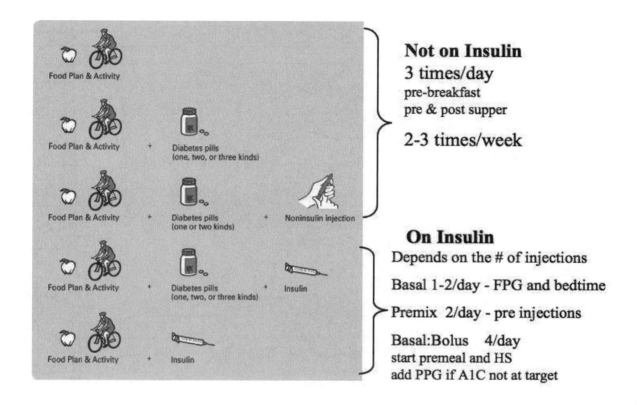

Not on Insulin

3 times/day
pre-breakfast
pre & post supper

2-3 times/week

On Insulin

Depends on the # of injections

Basal 1-2/day - FPG and bedtime

Premix 2/day - pre injections

Basal:Bolus 4/day
start premeal and HS
add PPG if A1C not at target

the patient or health care professional to use the data to make appropriate adjustments in a treatment plan.

Patients will look to the health care provider to suggest how much SMBG testing to do and when to do it. Figure 9 shows one general approach to SMBG testing that suggests testing in a manner that collects enough data to act on, in order to adjust lifestyle or medications to reach glycemic goals.

Downloading the data from a glucose meter is very helpful, but not often done in clinical practice. It reinforces that the provider is interested in the glucose data and ensures the data is verified

(fabricated or inaccurate entered glucose readings can be a problem). Some like to know the average glucose and standard deviation over the last 2-4 weeks, while others like to know the percentage of reading below target, in target and above target. Again, when about 50% of SMBG readings are in target, the patient usually will also reach A1C target. A particularly helpful visual printout of SMBG data is the *modal day*. At a glance the clinician and patient can see how much testing is being done and when. In addition, they can see if there are many high or low readings and visualize glucose patterns (where glucose readings are the highest and where they are the lowest). It is important to minimize the low reading first, then address the highest readings next. Figure 10 is an

Figure 10

Modal Day (Standard Day) Plot

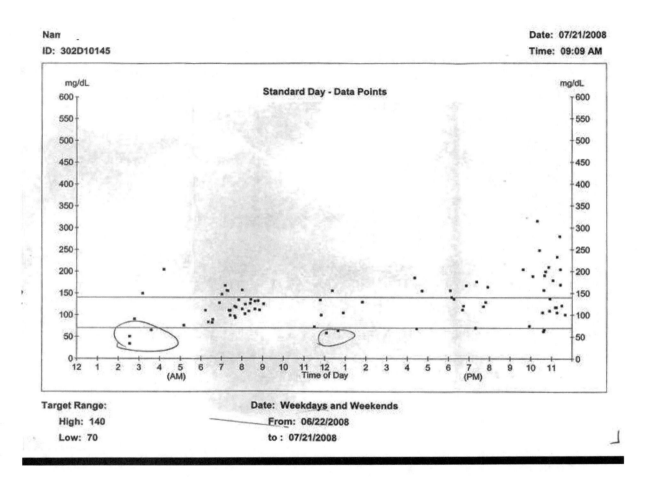

example of a simple but valuable *modal day* or *standard day plot*. You can see the patient test mainly at breakfast and bedtime. There is a problem with low glucoses overnight and high glucoses at bedtime. This is a patient on insulin who continually tries to correct high readings at night, only to get low overnight. Note a long time between lunch and supper which requires good background (basal) insulin coverage, assuming a background and mealtime insulin regimen. It seems that attention to better coverage from supper to bed, and then reducing overnight long-acting insulin or moving the long-acting insulin to the morning, would be a good start in this case. Beyond A1C and eAG, there are considerable data that demonstrate a correlation between postprandi-

al hyperglycemia, glucose excursions or glycemic variability, and oxidative stress or cardiovascular disease. To date, there is no good study (except in treating pregnancy and diabetes) that shows that a targeted intervention to prevent excessive ppg readings or glucose excursions results in a reduction in cardiovascular disease. A recent study specifically designed to target PPG, called Heart 2 D study, concluded that treating diabetic survivors of AMI with prandial vs. basal strategies achieved differences in fasting blood glucose, less-than-expected differences in postprandial blood glucose, similar levels of A1C and no difference in risk for future cardiovascular event rates.

- **Hypoglycemia**

  Severe hypoglycemia is the main safety barrier to achieving glycemic control in both type 1 and type 2 diabetes, and it is important to discuss (detection, treatment and prevention) and consider the possibility of causing hypoglycemia when selecting, adjusting or combining therapeutic agents and types of insulin. There are now good data from the ACCORD Study that those who suffer from an episode of severe hypoglycemia (defined as needing the assistance of another individual to recover) have a higher likelihood of early mortality.

In summary, when setting a glycemic target for a given individual with diabetes, discuss all 3 main

components of glucose control, A1C target (and corresponding eAG target), SMBG testing schedule and targets to fit the individual's stage of therapy, and discuss how to recognize, avoid and treat hypoglycemia.

- **The role of Continuous Glucose Monitoring (CGM) in understanding the full spectrum of glucose control and assisting in achieving glucose targets.**

CGM has become much more accurate and reliable recently, and is now being incorporated more and more into clinical practice. The major use is in T1DM and particularly linked to use of an insulin pump. A recent, very important trial in T1DM demonstrated that if individuals with T1DM wore the CGM sensory regularly, they saw a significant improvement in their A1C with no increase in hypoglycemia. Efforts are now underway to enhance patients' ability to utilize CGM more consistently (particularly adolescents and young children). These devices are very helpful to watch trends in blood glucose values. Watching trends and utilizing glucose alarms (predictive alarms and actual low value alarms) should allow better control with less hypoglycemia, since all agree that hypoglycemia is, in most cases, the major barrier to optimal control (particularly in T1DM, but important in T2DM as well). At the present time, the role of CGM in T2DM is intermittent use

to evaluate glucose profiles in patients that are having a hard time achieving target A1Cs, particularly if on insulin or if having hypoglycemic unawareness. It seems logical that CGM may someday help predict which medication would best match a patient's 24-hour glucose profile. Both individuals with T1DM and T2DM learn a lot about what affects their blood sugars, including stress, food, exercise and medications, when wearing a CGM device. One major problem is that every CGM device has a different read-out, making it hard for clinicians to learn a consistent approach to analysis and lifestyle and medication adjustment.

The IDC has proposed easy-to-visualize graphic display of CGM data that allows both patient and provider to understand where and why an adjustment in therapy is necessary (this display and the associated glucometrics is called the ambulatory glucose profile - AGP™)

3. Barriers to Achieving Glycemic Control

Understanding the Pathophysiology and Natural History of T2DM

Before attempting to achieve optimal glycemic control in individuals with T2DM, it helps to understand both the natural history of T2DM and pathophysiology of the defects that lead to hyperglycemia. This topic is covered in detail in the introduction to this manual. In it, Dr Kendall concludes by stating, *"Specifically targeting the known pathophysiologic defects of insulin resistance and insulin deficiency, while also addressing other potentially important factors, such as the incretin defect, and yet to be discovered pathophysiologic contributors, is critical if good glycemic control is to be both achieved and sustained."*

Clinical Inertia

Patient and provider education, and the availability of effective and safe medications, are just the first steps in optimizing care. Studies have defined clinical inertia as a failure of providers to alter or intensify therapy when there are clear indications for changes.

One problem is that physicians are overburdened by diabetes, and it can be challenging to tackle each component of the disease appropriately and effectively.

Clinical inertia is a common problem in the management of patients with asymptomatic chronic illness. Causes of clinical inertia may include:

• Overestimation of care provided.
• Use of "soft" reasons to avoid intensification of therapy.
• Lack of education.
• Lack of training.
• Lack of practice and organizational focus on achieving therapeutic goals.

Being confident a given treatment target is appropriate and safe for a patient is critical for the provider to take action, be that adjusting medication doses or adding a new medication. Having a team (CDE educator, dietitian and psychologist or social worker) is often critical to engage the patient enough to foster a change in behavior. Having a system in place where patients with diabetes are managed by a multidisciplinary team of providers has been an effective approach to optimizing outcomes. Many practices either do not have their own teams or have not set up an easy referral process to a collaborating diabetes nurse educator, registered dietitian or psychologist. These team members not only provide key clinical information to help make a timely and appropriate clinical decision, but they can also help follow-up with patients and continue to make or assist with therapy adjustments. A good dietitian will often inform a physician when there is not likely to be much more benefit from pursing further changes in meal plans alone and it may be time to consider additional pharmacologic therapy for glucose, blood pressure or lipid control.

Use of algorithms (roadmaps) that guide drug treatment decisions is another important aspect in clinical inertia that will be discussed in detail below. Point-of-care testing is an important consideration, because some studies have shown that physicians are twice as likely to alter medications or make treatment changes when they have access to key lab results (like an A1C) at the time of the office visit. An A1C drawn as the patient leaves the office requires a significant follow-up effort on the part of the physician or an office staff member in order make a change in therapy. Very often, the doctor will wait until the next visit to change therapy, but since that next visit may be 6 months away, often it is felt that a new A1C, that better reflects the patient's current level of glycemic control, must be drawn. Thus, the cycle of delaying a needed change in therapy (clinical inertia) continues.

Involving the patient in the decision-making progress, by letting him or her express their concerns or ask questions and then tailoring the choice in therapy based on the patient's characteristics, is important.

Clinicians should consider the impact of patient factors in clinical inertia. It is important to think about whether or not patients have insurance as you prescribe a new medication. Patients could be on as many as a dozen medications at any point in their course of care, so considering combination pills to reduce the number of copayments for medicines, or exploring other ways to help the patient obtain coverage for their needed medications will help ensure successful outcomes. In addition, a significant number of patients with diabetes will be struggling with depression or anxiety, and addressing these conditions appropriately will allow more effective initiation and adjustment of needed diabetes-specific therapies. Failure to address these types of issues can add to the problem of clinical inertia.

There are many treatment targets that need to be addressed when optimizing care for an individual with T2DM, as outlined in the priorities of care graphic above. This section will focus on reaching the glycemic targets, as the other targets are dealt with elsewhere in this manual. One cornerstone of managing diabetes is to see that patients are well educated in the principles of diabetes self-management (diabetes self-management training: DSMT), including formulating an individual meal plan in consultation with a registered dietitian (medical nutrition therapy: MNT). Ideally, this education and support will be delivered, in part, by a skilled team of certified diabetes educators (CDEs) supporting a provider's practice. If a diabetes education program is recognized by the ADA or American Association of Diabetes Educators (AADE), they may bill an education code for DSMT. In addition, there are separate allowable billing codes for MNT by registered dietitians. It has been clearly demonstrated that this education may be effectively delivered in a group or individual setting. Medicare, for favorable financial reasons, and individuals with diabetes for reasons of enhanced interaction and support, tend to favor education in a group setting.

In addition to diabetes self-management training, the second critical component to optimizing diabetes outcomes is assisting providers in making timely and appropriate clinical decisions. Figure 11 shows the International Diabetes Center at Park Nicollet's depiction of the important interplay of the patient, the educator and the provider that enhances the likelihood of improved outcomes.

One tool to assist in appropriate clinical decision making is the use of a treatment algorithm, sometimes called a *roadmap for care* or a *decision pathway*.

A number of consensus treatment algorithms for the management of type 2 diabetes have been developed, including those from a Consensus Group organized by the ADA and the European Association for the Study of Diabetes (EASD), the American Association of Clinical Endocrinology (AACE) and the Canadian Diabetes Association (see Figures 12-14).

Figure 11

Diabetes Patient Centered Team Care

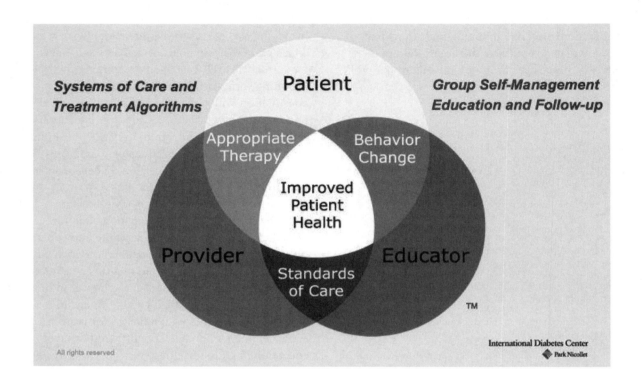

Systems of Care and Treatment Algorithms

Patient

Group Self-Management Education and Follow-up

Appropriate Therapy

Behavior Change

Improved Patient Health

Provider

Educator

Standards of Care

TM

International Diabetes Center
Park Nicollet

The ADA/EASD Consensus Group algorithm added some important concepts to discussion around optimal management of T2DM. This algorithm was the first to suggest all patients with T2DM start metformin at the time of diagnosis of diabetes, along with lifestyle changes. In addition, this algorithm introduced the consideration of adding background (basal) insulin to metformin as a second-line therapy choice. After a series of revisions, this algorithm has two tiers of therapy to consider, when selecting the therapy to follow metformin and lifestyle if patients are not at goal (generally defined as A1C < 7%). Another important concept is that patients not responding to therapy are steadily moved toward the use of metformin and intensive insulin therapy (usually defined as or background-mealtime or basal-bolus insulin therapy).

The AACE roadmap provides a comprehensive set of medication choices based on the A1C and the glucose profiles from the patient's SMBG records. The Canadian Diabetes Association guideline spells out first-line therapy choices based on the A1C, and second-line choices based on the main action of each second-line drug option.

The increased number of drug choices available to practitioners and patients may heighten uncertainty regarding regimen design. There are few published studies with metabolic outcomes associated with specifically implementing any of these association consensus guidelines. The International Diabetes Center (IDC) has perhaps the longest history of algorithm development for glycemic control in diabetes, particularly focused on the needs of primary care providers who see over 90% of

Figure 12

ADA/EASD Consensus Guidelines Treatment Algorithm for Type 2 Diabetes

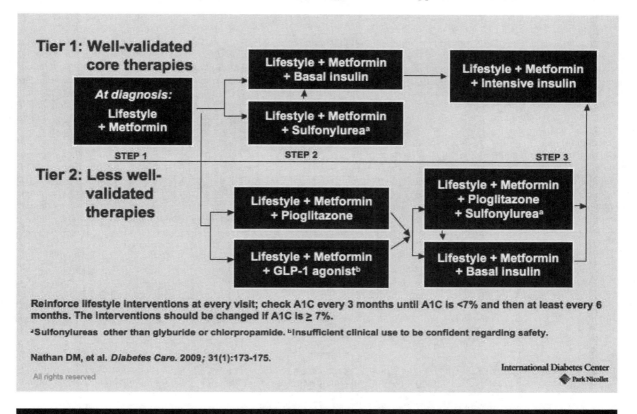

Tier 1: Well-validated core therapies

At diagnosis:
Lifestyle + Metformin

Lifestyle + Metformin + Basal insulin → Lifestyle + Metformin + Intensive insulin

Lifestyle + Metformin + Sulfonylurea[a]

STEP 1 — STEP 2 — STEP 3

Tier 2: Less well-validated therapies

Lifestyle + Metformin + Pioglitazone

Lifestyle + Metformin + GLP-1 agonist[b]

Lifestyle + Metformin + Pioglitazone + Sulfonylurea[a]

Lifestyle + Metformin + Basal insulin

Reinforce lifestyle interventions at every visit; check A1C every 3 months until A1C is <7% and then at least every 6 months. The interventions should be changed if A1C is ≥ 7%.

[a]Sulfonylureas other than glyburide or chlorpropamide. [b]Insufficient clinical use to be confident regarding safety.

Nathan DM, et al. *Diabetes Care.* 2009; 31(1):173-175.

International Diabetes Center
Park Nicollet

the patients with type 2 diabetes. There are published outcomes describing the training, implementation and outcomes achieved by multiple medical group practices implementing their own customized version of the IDC glycemic algorithm or decision path, referred to as Staged Diabetes Management.

ADA/EASD Consensus Guidelines Treatment Algorithm for Type 2 Diabetes

Since the IDC glycemic algorithm (Figure 15) has associated outcome data, is based on addressing glycemic targets (A1C and SMBG) and the pathophysiologic defects of type 2 diabetes, has been updated multiple times since 1994 to include new therapies where appropriate, and has been implemented in multiple U.S. and international clinical settings, the authors will refer to this algorithm in a brief discussion on selecting appropriate thera-

pies, from lifestyle to oral agents and non-insulin injectable agents to the use of insulin therapy.

The IDC algorithm starts with the glycemic targets which can be modified as needed for a given patient. Next is the lifestyle, or nutrition and activity, stage of therapy. It is our contention that the most effective approach to management involves patient-centered team care. Therefore, this algorithm lists key clinical disciplines that might contribute to team care, and a brief highlight of the role each team member might play. All patients with T2DM will ideally receive DSMT and MNT early in the course of their disease. These concepts are greatly expanded on in the MNT chapter of this manual (Chapter 6). This algorithm has patients adding metformin if their A1C is over 7% (which will be the majority of patients unless screening and early detection of diabetes becomes more widespread).

Figure 13

Road Map to Achieve Glycemic Goals: Naïve to Therapy (Type 2)

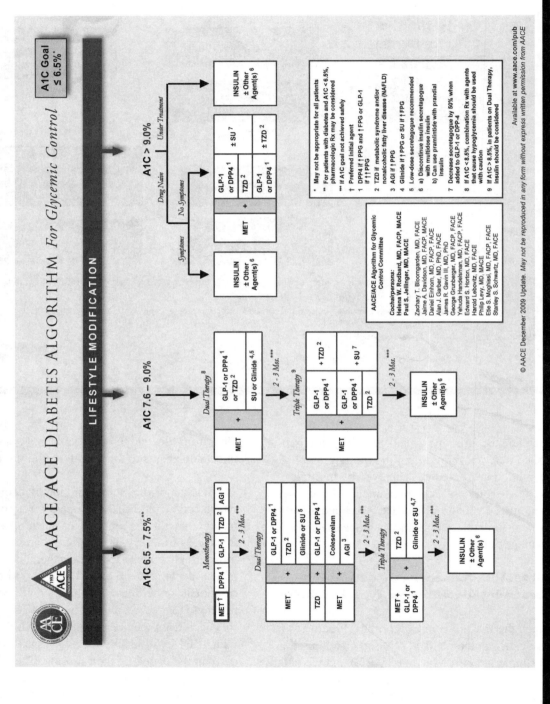

Reprinted with permission of AACE.

Figure 14

Canadian Diabetes Association: Management of Hyperglycemia in Type 2 Diabetes

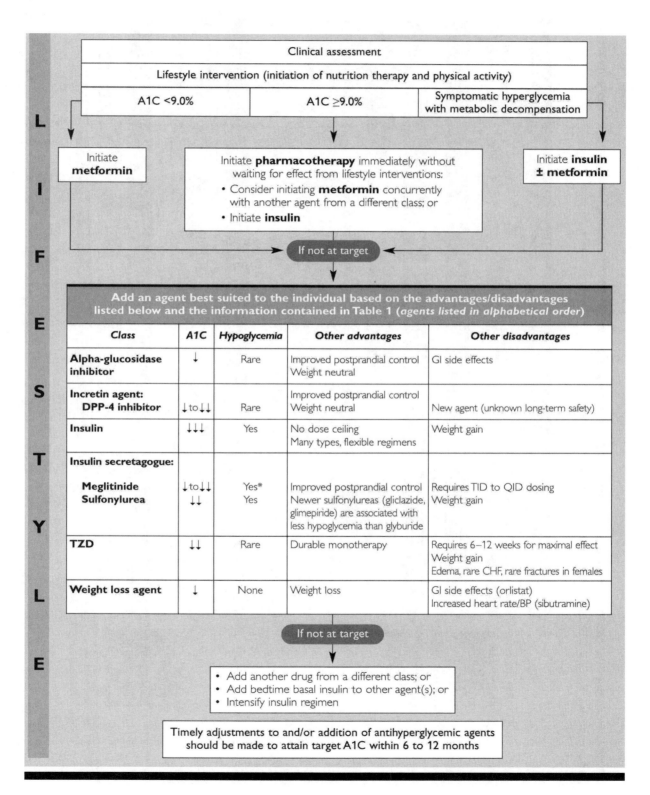

L I F E S T Y L E

Clinical assessment				
Lifestyle intervention (initiation of nutrition therapy and physical activity)				
A1C <9.0%	A1C ≥9.0%	Symptomatic hyperglycemia with metabolic decompensation		

Initiate **metformin**

Initiate **pharmacotherapy** immediately without waiting for effect from lifestyle interventions:
- Consider initiating **metformin** concurrently with another agent from a different class; or
- Initiate **insulin**

Initiate **insulin** ± **metformin**

If not at target

Add an agent best suited to the individual based on the advantages/disadvantages listed below and the information contained in Table 1 (*agents listed in alphabetical order*)

Class	A1C	Hypoglycemia	Other advantages	Other disadvantages
Alpha-glucosidase inhibitor	↓	Rare	Improved postprandial control Weight neutral	GI side effects
Incretin agent: DPP-4 inhibitor	↓ to ↓↓	Rare	Improved postprandial control Weight neutral	New agent (unknown long-term safety)
Insulin	↓↓↓	Yes	No dose ceiling Many types, flexible regimens	Weight gain
Insulin secretagogue:				
Meglitinide	↓ to ↓↓	Yes*	Improved postprandial control Newer sulfonylureas (gliclazide, glimepiride) are associated with less hypoglycemia than glyburide	Requires TID to QID dosing Weight gain
Sulfonylurea	↓↓	Yes		
TZD	↓↓	Rare	Durable monotherapy	Requires 6–12 weeks for maximal effect Weight gain Edema, rare CHF, rare fractures in females
Weight loss agent	↓	None	Weight loss	GI side effects (orlistat) Increased heart rate/BP (sibutramine)

If not at target

- Add another drug from a different class; or
- Add bedtime basal insulin to other agent(s); or
- Intensify insulin regimen

Timely adjustments to and/or addition of antihyperglycemic agents should be made to attain target A1C within 6 to 12 months

Treatment of Type 2 Diabetes: Glycemic Control

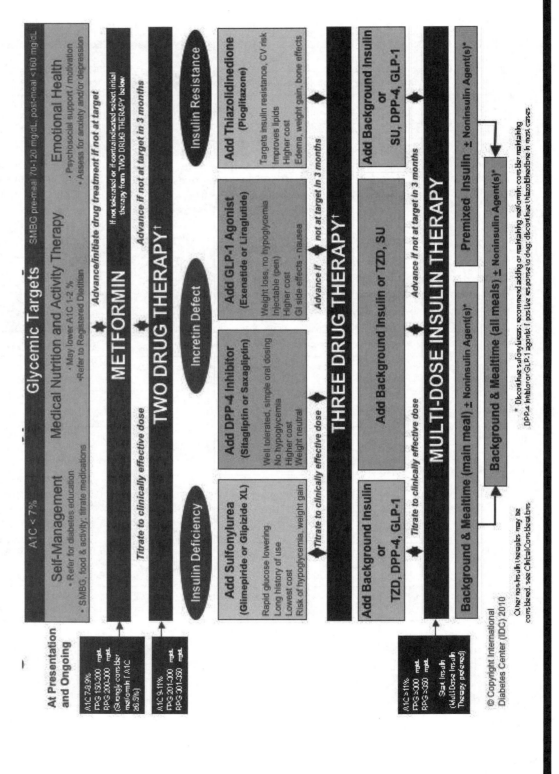

Figure 15b

Clinical Considerations and Abbreviations

Clinical Considerations

1. Check kidney and liver function prior to initiation of non-insulin therapies
2. Pioglitazone recommended over rosiglitazone due to concerns of increased CV risk with rosiglitazone
3. Long-acting background (basal) insulins detemir and glargine reduce risk of nocturnal hypoglycemia compared to intermediate-acting NPH; some patients may benefit from bid dosing of long-acting insulin
4. If a clinically stable patient with A1C >11% and consuming excessive sweetened beverages, consider starting non-insulin agents and re-evaluate need for insulin in 1-2 weeks
5. Pramlintide may be added to mealtime insulin
6. Background & Mealtime Insulin regimen is the most physiological and flexible regimen
7. Focus on modest weight loss of 5-7% total body weight
8. Basic nutrition recommendations include elimination of sweetened beverages, eat minimum 3 meals/day each containing ~3 carbohydrate choices (45 gm/meal)
9. Recommend 150 minutes/week of physical activity
10. Consider referral to Psychologist or Social Worker if persistently elevated A1C
11. If patient treated with metformin and FPG significantly elevated, consider adding background insulin
12. Other non-insulin therapies to consider:
    a) Alpha-glucosidase inhibitor if A1C close to target and post meal glucose elevated due to excessive carb. intake
    b) Nateglinide or repaglinide if post-meal hyperglycemia and need for flexible mealtime dosing schedule
    c) Colesevelam if A1C close to target and LDL remains above target with current statin therapy
    d) Bromocriptine QR if A1C close to target; works though CNS mediated improvement in insulin sensitivity

Abbreviations: **A1C**: glycosylated hemoglobin A$_{1C}$; **CV**: cardiovascular; **DPP-4**: dipeptidyl peptidase-4 inhibitor (sitagliptin and saxagliptin); **FPG**: fasting plasma glucose; **GI**: gastrointestinal; **GLP-1**: glucagon like peptide-1 receptor agonist (exenatide and liraglutide); **RPG**: random plasma glucose; **SMBG**: self-monitored blood glucose; **SU**: sulfonylurea; **TZD**: thiazolidinedione.

A few other general principles of how this algorithm can support care include the notation that if the patient presents with significant hyperglycemia, it is appropriate to consider starting with more advanced therapy, such as a combination of oral agents or insulin. Once the significant hyperglycemia is reduced (reduced glucose toxicity) following additional lifestyle changes, new medications or a procedure like a gastric bypass, it is possible to make the therapy less intense, as noted by the dual flow of the arrows on the algorithm. In addition, each time a new medication is introduced, the algorithm will prompt the provider to titrate the medication in a timely manner and to re-evaluate glycemic control (A1C and SMBG) on a regular basis, and advance therapy if not at target.

Metformin. Metformin should be considered first line pharmacologic therapy in patients with type 2 diabetes, unless contraindicated or poorly tolerated. The Type 2 Diabetes: Glycemic Control algorithm is consistent with the ADA Tier 1 strategy in recommending the biguanide metformin as first line pharmacologic therapy (see Figures 12, 13). Metformin has been in clinical use for more than 3 decades, and has earned first-line status because of its clinical efficacy in lowering A1C 1-2 percentage points, flexibility in combination with other anti-hyperglycemic agents, low risk of hypoglycemia, weight neutrality and lower cost (since it has become available in generic form). Moreover, in the United Kingdom Prospective Diabetes Study (UKPDS), it was the only therapy to show significant benefits in reducing cardiovascular events. Metformin has been shown to be effective in patients throughout the entire spectrum of body mass index. Even with a black box warning for lactic acidosis, metformin has been shown to be a very safe medication, as long as precaution and contraindications for use are followed closely. The primary concern for developing lactic acidosis is in patients with impaired renal function, defined as serum creatinine >1.4 mg/dL in women and >1.5 mg/dL in men. More recent studies have shown that patients with estimated glomerular filtration rate (eGFR) >30 ml/min can safely use metformin.

The Treatment of Type 2 Diabetes: Glycemic Control algorithm recommends metformin as monotherapy when the A1C at presentation is 7%-8.9%, or in combination with other therapies when A1C is >9%. While metformin is a very common therapeutic option for type 2 diabetes, it is often used incorrectly. Chart audits reveal two common themes: providers that fail to titrate metformin to the clinically effective dose of 2000 mg/day and those that initiate too high a dose of the medication and/or advance therapy too quickly. Initiation of 500 mg with an evening meal, coupled with titration (adding 500 mg) every 1-2 weeks is recommended to minimize gastrointestinal side effects. Metformin is being used to prevent diabetes, and was shown to reduce the development of diabetes in patients with prediabetes. Analysis of the data from the Diabetes Prevention Study (DPP) revealed that metformin was most effective in people with body mass index (BMI) >35 and was ineffective at preventing diabetes in leaner patients (BMI <25). Note that lifestyle modifications and 5%-7% weight loss should be recommended before initiating metformin to prevent diabetes. Lifestyle intervention is effective at all BMIs to prevent diabetes, and has shown to be effective prevention strategy for all people at risk of diabetes. The ADA has recently suggested providers consider pharmacologic therapy (preferably metformin) for the prevention of diabetes, in addition to lifestyle therapy, when the individual demonstrates both impaired fasting glucose (IFG) and impaired glucose tolerance (IGT), since this combination doubles one's risk of progressing to diabetes.

Two Drug Therapy
The Treatment of Type 2 Diabetes: Glycemic Control algorithm indicates that *two drug therapy* is indicated when A1C is 9%-11% at presentation, or if metformin therapy coupled with medical nutrition therapy is insufficient to achieve glycemic targets. The first step to consider when selecting two drug therapy is which pathophysiological features you are attempting to address. As described above, the three primary areas to address are relative insulin deficiency, incretin defect or insulin resistance. The addition of sul-

fonylurea to metformin therapy addresses insulin deficiency, and is often considered in patients when cost of therapy is the overriding factor. The combination of metformin and sulfonylurea has a long history of frequent use, and is generally effective at lowering the blood glucose quickly. The addition of sulfonylurea brings with it the increased risk of hypoglycemia and modest weight gain, in the range of 2-3 kg. This algorithm specifically recommends Glimepiride or Glipizide XL, as these SUs in clinical practice are longer-acting and cause less hypoglycemia than glyburide. In addition, with Glimepiride, the very low dosing options and ability to gradually titrate is particularly appealing when used in the elderly or those prone to hypoglycemia, but unable to afford another oral agent.

Other options include the addition of repaglinide or nateglinide to metformin therapy. Similar to sulfonylureas, these two oral agents induce the beta cell to secrete insulin, thus increasing the risk of hypoglycemia and causing modest weight gain. Additional drawbacks are high cost and dosing with meals, leading to the potential for decreased adherence to regimen. These agents have been effectively used with metformin or background (basal) insulin to mimic a basal-bolus type regimen. They can be titrated to cover a given meal, as long as there is adequate beta cell reserve to respond to the medication.

The addition of an incretin-based therapy to metformin is another option that is considered a more "physiological" approach, since neither hypoglycemia nor weight gain are problems to contend with when combined with metformin. The dipeptidyl peptidase-4 (DPP-4) inhibitor class of medications work by inhibiting the ubiquitous DPP-4 enzyme that is responsible for degrading glucagon, like 13 peptide -1 (GLP-1) and glucose-dependent insulinotropic peptide (GIP). Inhibition of DPP-4 allows the level of GLP-1 and GIP to increase 2- to 3-fold in the blood stream, resulting in a modest glucosedependent rise in insulin secretion coupled with suppression of post-meal hyperglucagonemia. Sitagliptin and saxagliptin are the first DPP-4 inhibitors approved by the FDA, with several others (linagliptin and alogliptin) in the pipeline. The addition of DPP-4 inhibitor to metformin main-

tains weight neutrality, low risk of hypoglycemia and is generally very well tolerated. A1C reduction in the range of 0.6-1.0 percentage points is associated with adding a DPP-4 inhibitor to metformin. This is very similar to what is seen clinically upon addition of sulfonylurea to metformin therapy, yet without weight gain or increased hypoglycemia. Combination preparations of sitagliptin/metformin and saxagliptin/metformin XR are available approved as initial therapy, making it consistent with IDC recommendation to consider this combination therapy as initial therapy when A1C is between 9%-11% (see Treatment of Type 2 Diabetes: Glycemic Control algorithm). When used as initial combination therapy, the A1C-lowering potential of DPP-4 Inhibitor and metformin appears to be additive, with A1C reduction >2 percentage points when starting A1C was only modestly elevated (see Figure 16). Although there is concern about the potential for developing a hypersensitivity skin reaction with this class of agents, to date this seems exceedingly rare. Other immunologically-mediated reactions to this class, such as nasopharyngitis or urinary tract infections, have been reported in metaanalysis, but to date have not deterred the clinical usefulness of this class.

Exenatide is a glucagon-like peptide 1 receptor agonist isolated from the salivary secretion of the venomous Gila monster. It mimics the action of naturally-occurring GLP-1, yet has a half-life of approximately 4.5 hours vs. 60-90 seconds for GLP-1. Exenatide is injected subcutaneously before the morning and evening meals. The initial dose is 5mcg BID and is titrated to 10 mcg BID after 1 month, based on the level of glycemic control and tolerability. Approximately 40% of patients will experience transient gastrointestinal side effects when initiating exenatide therapy, but the vast majority of patients will tolerate therapy. The primary action of exenatide is to flatten postprandial glucose excursions. Exenatide should be administered within 1 hour of eating and never after the meal. Data from Linnebjerg et al demonstrated improved flattening of postprandial glucose excursions when exenatide was administered 30 or 60 minutes prior to a fixed meal (see Figure 17).

Figure 16

Combination Therapy: DPP4 Inhibitor and Metaformin

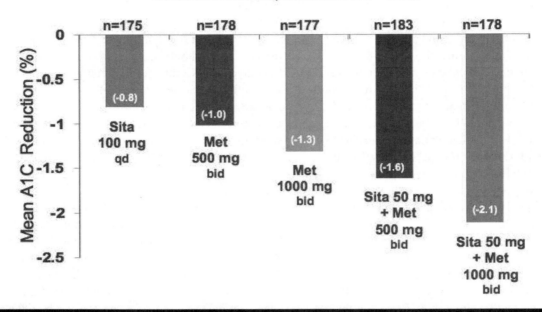

Duration 24 weeks; Baseline A1C = 8.8%

Goldstein et al. Diab Care *2007; 30: 1979-1987*

Figure 17

Exenatide: Effect of Injection Time on Postprandial Glucose

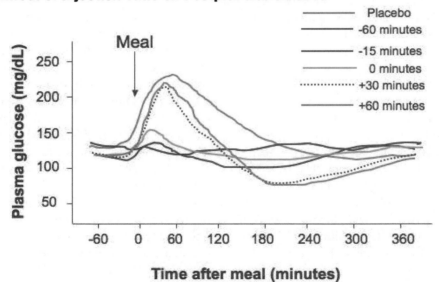

N=18, randomized, six way crossover study, with fixed breakfast

Linnebjerg et al., *Diab Med* 2006; 23:240–245.

Figure 18

Responses in HbA1c and Bodyweight in Individuals Treated with Exenatide Once a Week (x) and Twice a Day (o).

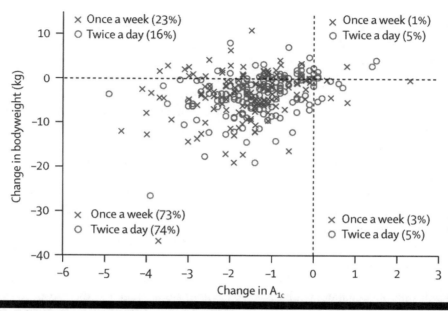

Drucker DJ, Buse JB, Taylor K, Kendall DM, Trautmann M, Zhuang D, Porter L; DURATION-1 Study Group. Exenatide once weekly versus twice daily for the treatment of type 2 diabetes: a randomised, open-label, non-inferiority study. Lancet. 2008 Oct 4; 372:1240-50

Figure 19

PROActive Trial: Reduction in All-Cause Mortality, Non-fatal MI and Stroke-main Secondary Endpoint

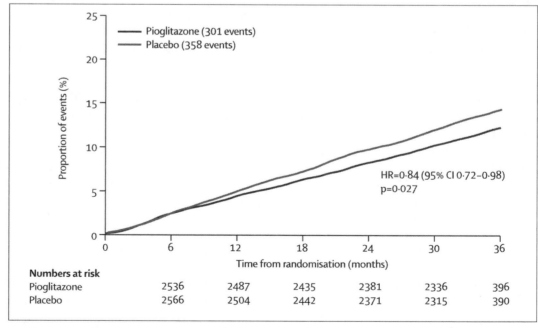

Dormandy JA et al. Lancet 2005; 366: 1279-1289.

Exenatide lowers A1C approximately 1 percentage point and, analogous to other anti-hyperglycemic medications, tends to have a greater A1C lowering effect in patients with higher baseline A1C. When exenatide is added to metformin, there is low risk of hypoglycemia and, more importantly, >85% of patients will lose weight. While the range of weight loss is quite dramatic, most patients lose a modest amount of weight, approaching 3-5 kg after 1 year of therapy. As expected with weight loss, modest improvement in lipid parameters and blood pressure occurs with the addition of exenatide. A long-acting, once-weekly formulation of exenatide has been developed and studied. This formulation is injected 1 time per week and a steady state exenatide concentration is achieved within 6-7 weeks. Preliminary studies demonstrate that long-acting exenatide maintains similar (if not slightly greater) A1C-lowering and weight loss, compared to BID dosing of exenatide, with the convenience of fewer injections. The long-acting exenatide appears to reduce fasting blood glucose more effectively than BID exenatide and does not reduce postprandial excursions as effectively. Drucker et al, in 2008, demonstrated that over 70% of individuals treated with either exenatide BID or once-weekly exenatide both lost weight and improved their A1C (Figure 18). Recently, the FDA held up approval of onceweekly exenatide due to a request for additional QT interval data at higher than normal doses.

More recently, a second GLP-1 agonist has been approved by the FDA. . Liraglutide is a GLP-1 receptor agonist that has a half-life of 13 hours, making it a 1 injection/day medication. Preliminary data show that liraglutide lowers A1C approximately 1 percentage point and causes modest weight loss. In a head-to-head study with BID exenatide, liraglutide therapy resulted in slightly better A1C control, better fasting blood glucose control and similar weight reduction. Liraglutide has a black-box warning for risk of thyroid c-cell tumors that were found in rodent models, making it contraindicated in patients with history of medullary thyroid carcinoma (MTC) and/or Multiple Endocrine Neoplasia Syndrome (MEN 2). Whether there will be an increased risk of this rare cancer in humans is still undetermined. Because of the potential of the incretin-based ther-apies, many other GLP-1 receptor agonists are being developed.

The addition of thiazolidinedione (TZD) to metformin therapy is yet another option. This approach should be considered in patients with significant insulin resistance, because TZDs improve insulin sensitivity throughout the body by activation of the nuclear peroxisome proliferator-activated receptorgamma pathway. This results in improved fasting blood glucose control and A1C reduction of approximately 1.0-1.5 percentage points. The TZD class improves lipid levels by increasing high density lipoprotein levels and lowering triglycerides. They have also been shown to lower blood pressure and reduce c-reactive protein levels. Given this overall profile, it was thought that TZDs should be considered first-line or expectant therapy. However, prospective CV outcomes studies, such as the Prospective Pioglitazone Clinical Trial in Macrovascular Events (PROactive) have shown the TZD pioglitazone only modestly reduced risk of all-cause mortality, non-fatal myocardial infarction (MI) and stroke in high-risk individuals with diabetes (Figure 19). The modest risk reduction did not occur without significant increase in weight and an increased number of cases of heart failure requiring admission to hospital. More recently, rosiglitazone has received significant attention because a metaanalysis of rosiglitazone studies revealed a 43% increased risk of MI.

It is very well established that TZD therapy may cause increased fluid retention in a dose-dependent manner, and it is especially a concern in patients treated with insulin. This has led to black box warnings to not use TZDs in patients with heart failure. Recently, more data showing that TZD therapy may increase bone fracture rates has been published. For example, in the A Diabetes Outcome Progression Trial (ADOPT), patients taking a TZD (rosiglitazone) were at nearly twice the risk of fracture compared to those taking metformin or sulfonylurea. Other epidemiological cohort studies have shown increased fracture risk for both TZDs and in both men and women. Duration of therapy appears to be critical with significantly increased fracture rates occurring after 2 or more years of TZD therapy. Bone studies in animals have shown that TZDs suppress osteoblast differentiation, promote adipogenesis, and increase osteoclast differentiation, ultimately reducing done density. If a TZD is to be initiated, the Treatment of Type 2 Diabetes: Glycemic Control algorithm recommends starting pioglitazone vs. rosiglitazone, because the current data support this decision. In support of this is the FDA's decision in September 2010 to dramatically reduce access to rosiglitazone through a Risk Evaluation and Mitigation Strategy (REMS). Patients and providers would need to verify they are aware of increased CV risk associated with rosiglitazone and that they were unable to achieve glycemic control on other glucose-lowering medications.

Three Drug Therapy

If glycemic control is not established or maintained on a two drug regimen of metformin + SU, or DPP4 I, or GLP-1 agonist or TZD, the next step is usually to proceed to three drug therapy. The option here is to add a third non-insulin drug, or to add insulin and, according to this algorithm usually a basal or background long-acting insulin. was always considered the therapy of last resort. In the ADA/EASD algorithm basal (background) insulin is one of the second drug choices, whereas in the IDC algorithm, it is a third drug choice.Three non-insulin agents used together is also widely utilized. In practice today, this is often metformin + SU to which either a DPP4 inhibitor, GLP-1 agonist or TZD is added. As many providers and patients are considering therapy that is less likely to cause weight gain or hypoglycemia, that will guide them in the direction of metformin plus either a DPP4 inhibitor or a GLP-1 analogue. If one is determined to avoid hypoglycemia, the third drug would be a TZD. Adding a basal or background insulin to metformin and either a DPP-4 inhibitor or GLP-1 agonist can be a very effective therapy, although to date there are limited published data on the combination of insulin- and incretin-based therapy.

Emerging, recently-approved non-insulin therapies

Bromocriptine has been recently approved for the treatment of type 2 diabetes. Bromocriptine is an ergot alkaloid dopamine D (2) receptor agonist that has been used to treat hyperprolactinemia and galactorrhea. While the exact mechanism of glucose-lowering is not clearly delineated, it is thought to work by lowering insulin resistance by resetting circadian rhythm, inducing improvement in insulin sensitivity. A quick release formulation has been developed (bromocriptine QR) that is taken within 2 hours of waking that results in A1C lowering of up to 0.5 percentage points from baseline with no increase in hypoglycemia and no weight gain. The most common adverse effects associated with bromocriptine QR are transient nausea, rhinitis and headache. Preliminary evidence of cardiac safety, and potential benefit, have been shown recently in an article by Gaziano et al. with significantly fewer patients experiencing CVD end-point versus placebo group (hazard ratio 0.60 [0.35-0.96]). Where bromocriptine QR fits for the management of type 2 diabetes is still evolving, and its place in the treatment paradigm will emerge more clearly as more information on this new class of medication becomes available through research and clinical use.

Colesevelam is a bile-acid sequestrant used to treat primary hypercholesterolemia and has a new indication as an adjunct therapy to treat T2DM. While the mechanism of action for lowering glucose is still not completely understood, evidence suggests it may work through suppression of hepatic gluconeogenesis coupled with stimulation of glucagon like peptide 1 (GLP-1) release. When added as an adjunct to metformin, sulfonylurea or insulin it promotes an additional ~0.5 percentage point reduction in A1C along with LDL lowering of 12-17%. The most common side effects are constipation and dyspepsia.

In clinical trials

Sodium-glucose cotransport inhibitors are a new class of oral medication being developed that use the kidney to remove excess glucose. Dapagliflozin and canagliflozin are currently undergoing clinical study and have been shown to lower blood glucose by reducing renal glucose reabsorption via inhibition of the sodium-glucose cotransporter 2 (SGLT2) found in the proximal tubule. Preliminary phase 3 data show reduction in A1C in the range of 0.6 to 0.9 percentage points at 24 weeks along with modest weight loss due to loss of excess glucose (calories) in the urine. The risk of urinary tract infections and genital infection was higher compared with placebo and may be a limiting factor in the acceptance of this class of medications.

Insulin Therap

How many patients with T2DM really need insulin and why?

Estimates of T2DM patients that will require insulin within 10 years of diagnosis, or over the course of their diabetes to achieve an A1C target of <7%, run from 40%-80%. Experience would say it is on the higher side of this estimate if the A1C target is ≤6.5%.

The natural history of the progression of T2DM reveals a steady decline in beta cell function, starting before diabetes is even diagnosed. If one could alter the natural history of beta cell deterioration (likely needing to start an insulin sensitizer and or GLP-1 agonist soon after the onset of T2DM, or even in the pre-diabetes stage) it may be possible that the need for insulin to achieve glycemic control could be delayed. This has not been demonstrated to date.

It is possible that the use of insulin soon after the onset of diabetes (or pre-diabetes) may be beneficial, even if not necessary, to achieve glycemic targets. This hypothesis is being tested in the ongoing ORIGIN trial, in which basal insulin (glargine) is \ being given to individuals with pre-diabetes or T2DM to see if CV events and mortality (as well as glycemic control) are improved, compared to usual care without insulin. This and other outcome studies using insulin early in the course of treating T2DM are important to show if some of the recent findings, such as an anti-inflammatory effect (reduced CRP and interleukin [IL-6]) of insulin vs. metformin (separate from the glucose-lowering effect) translates into reduced clinical outcomes.

Currently Available Insulin Preparations

There are data indicating that when pushing for fairly tight glycemic goals, like A1C <7%, the use of insulin analogues results in less hypoglycemia (particularly overnight) and less postprandial hyperglycemia (for rapid-acting analogues). Some reviews, and most clinicians, comparing analogue insulin to human insulin are positive regarding the benefits of analogues on reducing hypoglycemia and postprandial hyperglycemia, and some feel these promote less weight gain (long-acting analogues). Other comparisons show only modest benefits of the analogue insulins and a recent metaanalysis reviewing the benefits of insulin analogues fails to show any significant benefit of insulin analogues in the trials felt to be appropriate for this analysis. This article does conclude that more, good quality studies are needed to evaluate if insulin analogue might reduce complications compared to non-analogue insulins. A recent review of pharmacoeconomic modeling studies and database retrospective analyses concluded that the insulin analogues were cost-effective compared to other alternatives. If the cost of insulin is a major barrier to its use, the human insulin preparations should be prescribed with careful attention to avoiding hypoglycemia. Regular human insulin preparations premeal are sometimes preferred, if individuals snack often after meals without covering with an additional bolus, or if they steadily eat or "graze" after meals.

While slight differences have been demonstrated in the PK and PD characteristics of the three Rapid Acting (bolus or mealtime insulins – Lispro, Aspart, Glulisine) and the two Long Acting (basal or background – Glargine, Detemir) insulin analogues, for clinical purposes in the management of most patients with type 2 diabetes these preparations are often used interchangeably. The choice depends mostly on provider experience and preference, formulary/cost issues and familiarity with the pen delivery devices.

Table 2

Summary of Insulin Types and Insulin Action (in hours, unless noted)

Brand Names	Onset	Working Hardest	Stops Working Effectively
Background (Basal) Insulin			
Humulin® N Novolin® N	2-4	Intermediate 4–8	Intermediate 10–16
Lantus® Levemir®	2	Long-acting Up to 24 hours[a]	Long-acting Up to 24 hours[a]
Premixed Insulin			
Premix with rapid-acting insulin analogue			
Humalog® Mix	5–15 min	1–2[b]	10–16
NovoLog® Mix	5–15 min	1–2[b]	10–16
Premix with Regular Insulin			
Humulin® Novolin®	30–45 min	4–8/2–3	10–16
Humulin®	30–45 min	4–8/2–3	10–16
Mealtime (Bolus) Insulin			
Humalog® NovoLog® Apidra®	5–15 min	1–2	3–4
Humulin® R Novolin® R	30–45 min	2–3	4–8

[a] Some patients will benefit from BID dosing of long-acting insulin
[b] Insulin activity gradually decreases over next 8–14 hours

Figure 20

Insulin Time Action Curves

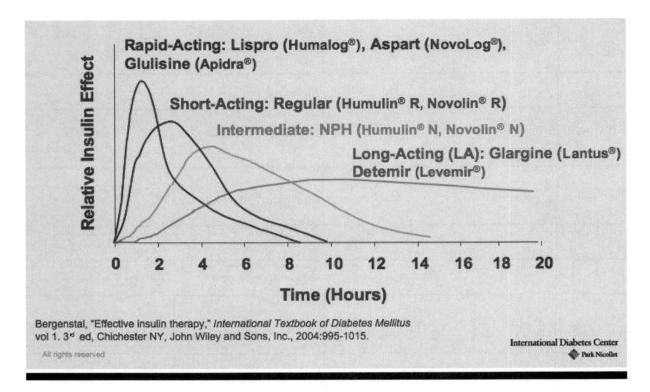

Rapid-Acting: Lispro (Humalog®), Aspart (NovoLog®), Glulisine (Apidra®)

Short-Acting: Regular (Humulin® R, Novolin® R)

Intermediate: NPH (Humulin® N, Novolin® N)

Long-Acting (LA): Glargine (Lantus®) Detemir (Levemir®)

Relative Insulin Effect (y-axis)

Time (Hours) (x-axis): 0 2 4 6 8 10 12 14 16 18 20

Bergenstal, "Effective insulin therapy," *International Textbook of Diabetes Mellitus* vol 1. 3ʳᵈ ed, Chichester NY, John Wiley and Sons, Inc., 2004:995-1015.

International Diabetes Center
Park Nicollet

How to Start Insulin in T2DM

Three main approaches to starting insulin will meet the needs of most patients and providers.

- Consider which insulin regimen fits each patient's:

    * Glycemic data (SMBG in particular and A1C) and current meds
    * Lifestyle and psychosocial factors

- Determine starting dose of insulin (weight-based [units/kg] and glycemic control-based [<9% or ≥9%]). By using a weight-based and A1C-based approach, the starting dose is more likely to have some clinically meaningful impact on glucose-lowering, but still will be relativity low and will need several upward adjustments to achieve optimal control.

- Give patient a SMBG monitoring schedule and SMBG targets (>50% of values at a given time above target range, or 1 or more below target on a weekly basis).

- Teach patient to review glucose data (patterns) each week if out of target and make an insulin adjustment (or call/email for assistance if out of target).

- If all values are high, consider increasing total insulin dose by 10% and spreading it out evenly among the insulins, if there is more than one insulin). We suggest one consider 3 insulin regimens and chose the one that best matches the patient's needs, based on their lifestyle and glycemic factors.

Background (basal) insulin added to oral agent(s):

• Lifestyle factors: patient overwhelmed, fearful of injections.

• Glycemic factors: elevated fasting BG main problem, post-meal BG targets achieved.

   * Glucose at bedtime not significantly higher than fasting BG (e.g. bedtime glucose not more than 50 mg/dL >fasting BG)
   * Most effective if A1C <8.5%

Premixed (analogue) insulin ± oral agent(s):

• Lifestyle factors—opposed to >2 injections, consistent meals times.

• Glycemic factors – elevated fasting and post-meal BG, high A1C's, symptomatic.

Background and mealtime (basal-bolus) insulin ± oral agent(s):

• Lifestyle factors: desires flexible schedule and tight glycemic control.

• Glycemic factors: elevated fasting and post-meal BG.

When starting insulin, you may select an insulin regimen that is not considered the most physiologic, but if it matches the patient's needs at that point in time, it is likely more important to just get the insulin started and you can change regimens later if indicated.

Selecting a Starting Dose Based on Weight and A1C
A few simple guiding principles make selecting a starting insulin dose relatively easy, safe and effective. We use 0.1 units per kg of insulin if the A1C is <9%, and 0.2 units per kg if the A1C is >9% when starting a once-daily background (basal) insulin. Background insulin is always paired with at least one oral agent and background insulin covers half the general insulin needs. When starting BID premixed insulin or QID back-

ground and mealtime insulin, since the insulin is covering the entire day's needs, you give 0.1 or 0.2 units per kg BID for premixed insulin or split into 0.1 or 0.2 units/kg as background and 0.1 or 0.2 units/kg split among the mealtime doses. See Table 3.

It is very helpful and important to give nutritional advice that matches the insulin regimen prescribed, as outlined in Tables 4 and 5. While all clinicians can deliver and reinforce these basic nutrition messages, it is also very valuable for a dietitian to review food records and come up with a more detailed food plan for each patient early in the course of their disease, and again later as needed.

How to adjust insulin in T2DM

See Table 5 and 6 for monitoring and adjusting initial insulin regimen.

Additional Insulin Adjustment Tips:

Background (basal) insulin (plus orals)—making the transition to background and mealtime insulin regimen

• Start hs or AM (occasionally at dinner).

• Usually require about 40-50 units (0.40-0.50 units/kg) to achieve A1C<7%.

• Some patients benefit from BID dosing of background (basal) insulins.

   * Hypoglycemia 4-8 hours after dose, yet hyperglycemia 12 hours after dose

   * Hyperglycemia 20-23 hours after dose with adequate control at 10-12 hours

• Once at 50 units (or ~0.5 units/kg).

   * Often need to add mealtime (bolus) insulin: rapid-acting analogue

   * Be sure you are check post-meal glucose (begin with pre- and post-dinner)

Table 3

Select a Starting Insulin Dose

	A1C <9%	A1C ≥9%
Background insulin (added to oral agents) • **Start with 1 dose; take at same time each day**	0.1 units/kg	0.2 units/kg
Premixed insulin[a] • Start with 2 doses: before breakfast and before evening meal	0.1 units/kg (2 times/day) (Total = 0.2 units/kg)	0.2 units/kg (2 times/day) (Total = 0.4 units/kg)
Background and mealtime insulin[a] • Calculate background and mealtime doses • Initially, mealtime insulin dose is divided evenly between meals	Background 0.1 units/kg (once daily) + Mealtime 0.1 units/kg (divide evenly between meals) (Total = 0.2 units/kg)	Background 0.2 units/kg (once daily) + Mealtime 0.2 units/kg (divide evenly between meals) (Total = 0.4 units/kg)

Note: A referral to diabetes educators (dietitian and nurse) can be helpful for carbohydrate meal planning, instruction on insulin administration and BG monitoring, and guidance on insulin selection and adjustment.

[a] *Discontinue sulfonylureas; consider adding or maintaining Metformin and/or Actos or Avandia*

• When adding rapid-acting (RA) analogue before meal:

  * Consider starting one RA before largest meal (most CHOs or largest post-meal glucose excursion)

  * Start 0.1 units/kg (10 units) RA and reduce LA background insulin by same amount

* Adjust RA to cover the meal, if continues to increase RA also monitor fasting BG, as you may need to reduce LA insulin more

* If one meal is stabilized but A1C still elevated, add second dose RA before next largest meal (add 0.1units/kg) again usually reducing same amount from background (basal) insulin.

* Repeat if needed (A1C still high) to cover third meal with RA insulin.

• When adding RA insulin (before one meal at a time: "basal plus therapy") to LA insulin, most often can monitor SMBG before next meal or bedtime to make an adjustment (if this is in target but still high A1C then do 2-hour PPG readings and adjust bolus insulin to reach PPG target). In type 1 diabetes, we use PPG readings routinely to adjust bolus insulin.

• Starting with background (basal) insulin and then adding concept of mealtime (bolus) insulin makes the transition to background and mealtime insulin very straightforward and logical.

Premixed insulin (±orals)

• Start premixed insulin in individuals with significant hyperglycemia all day and often with symptoms of hyperglycemia. Simple pen use BID makes this very simple.

• There are studies which show you can start premixed once daily at dinner, then if not at goal progress to BID and even to TID premixed insulin. It is a fairly straightforward progression, and results in many patients getting to goal. It is less physiologic and less clear how to titrate a TID premixed regimen compared to a background and mealtime (basal-bolus) regimen, but it can be done.

• Some start with 70/30 or 75/25 analogue premixed BID and then, depending on the SMBG patterns, consider substituting 50/50 premixed analogue (Lispro protamine/lispro) at either breakfast of dinner, or add 50/50 at lunchtime.

• 70/30 premixed come as human insulin as well, and can be used where cost is an issue. While you sacrifice some post-meal coverage and may increase rates of overnight hypoglycemia, one must be sure patients can afford their insulin.

• Systematic approach to transition from premixed bid to background and mealtime (basal-bolus) insulin (if BID premixed is not effective after a period of time (patient needs more flexibility, has postlunch hyperglycemia or has excess hypoglycemia]). Take total daily insulin dose of premixed insulin.

* If A1C <9% subtract 10% for modified TDD. A1C >9 the modified TDD is same as original TDD

* Give half of modified TDD as long-acting background (basal) insulin

* Give half of modified TDD as rapid-acting bolus insulin split between meals (usually over 3 meals and split either evenly to start [or my preference of 30%/30%/40%]; or ideally work with a dietitian to match the proportion of CHO at each meal compared to total CHOs in a day)

* Then adjust ba and bolus insulin according to glucose patterns

Background and Mealtime (Basal-Bolus) Insulin (± orals)

• One may start background and mealtime insulin initially, but usually one arrives at this regimen as a transition from background only or premixed (both transitions described above).

• Once on background and mealtime insulin, pattern control on a weekly basis initially (less often when stable) is used to continue to fine-tune background insulin and mealtime doses.

• Mealtime (bolus) insulin can be given and adjusted in one of two ways to meet a patient's (and provider's) needs.

* Determine and adjust mealtime insulin, based on unit of insulin per carbohydrate (units/CHO choice or units/gram of CHO) as is usually done in T1DM

* Give a usual or set dose of bolus insulin at meals and try to eat a relatively consistent amount of carbohydrate at meals

* Both approaches have recently been shown to effectively lower A1C's in T2DM, and depend on weekly evaluation of glucose patterns leading to insulin adjustments

* Each of these approaches to mealtime insulin can also include a simple insulin correction factor with meals, if desired

Titrate Insulin for High and Low Blood Glucose

Titrate 1–2 times per week using fasting or pre-meal BG as guide.

<70 mg/dL Decrease by 1-3 units

70–120 mg/dL No change

121–200 mg/dL Increase by 1-3 units

>200 mg/dL Increase by 3-5 units or 10%

Should oral agents be used with insulin in T2DM?

• Background (basal) insulin regimen

  * When using background insulin alone, oral agents should be added (since there are few trials on patients without orals on background insulin)

  * Metformin (if tolerated should be continued)

  * Often SU is continued to help maintain glucose control when starting on a low dose of background insulin, as is usually done. In the long run, as one increases the background insulin to close to 0.5 units/kg, it is not clear if keeping the SU is helpful or leads to more hypoglycemia, so background insulin cannot be fully titrated

  * If on background and metformin and SU, and making transition to background and mealtime insulin, most would agree if on full background and mealtime (bolus at each meal) one should stop the SU agent. But for adding bolus 1 meal at a time, there is currently no definitive study. One suggestion is to reduce SU dose in half as you add the first bolus (usually at supper) and then when second bolus is added, stop SU

• Premixed and background and mealtime insulin regimens.

  * Most studies show using metformin with more advanced insulin regimens reduces insulin doses 20%-30%, may allow slightly less complex regimen, and may help get more patients to A1C target while minimizing hypoglycemia and weight gain

  * TZDs with insulin may lead to significant fluid retention and weight gain, thus are discontinued in most cases; if TZDs is to be used, usually mid-dose level (e.g. 30 mg pioglitazone) is recommended

  * Insulin plus incretins, while not approved, have been used in clinical practice with some anecdotal success. Background insulin and an incretin makes a lot of sense from the standpoint of background insulin controlling glucose overnight and between meals, and the incretin helping with post-meal glucose control. If longer-acting preparations of GLP-1 analogs become available (which also lower FPG) one would need to be careful of the evening background (basal) insulin dose, or consider dosing background insulin in the AM.

  * If insulin is titrated effectively and aggressively one does not need to have an oral agent with insulin, but the practice of including metformin is very common today

Table 4

Nutrition Guidelines to Match an Insulin Regimen
1 carbohydrate choice = 15 grams carbohydrate

	Meals	Snacks
Background insulin (added to oral agents)	Aim for 3 meals per day: • Women 2–4 carb choices per meal • Men 3–5 carb choices per meal	• Not needed • If desired, should be small; 1–2 carb choices per snack
Premixed insulin	• Eat 3 meals at consistent times with consistent carb intake • Do not skip meals • No more than 10–12 hours between breakfast and dinner	• Rapid-acting: snack not usually needed; if desired should be small; 1–2 carb choices per snack • Regular: may need small snacks
Background and mealtime insulin	• Initially, a consistent carb intake • When patient is ready, advance from carb counting to insulin-to-carb ratio to maximize therapy	• Rapid-acting: not needed; if greater than 1 carb choice may require additional insulin injection • Regular: may need small snacks

---

Note: A registered dietitian can help assess usual food intake, provide guidance in selecting foods in a variety of situations, and evaluate BG records based on food intake and activity.

Hypoglycemia: All who take insulin should be taught to recognize hypoglycemia and carry a carbohydrate food or beverage to treat it. Usual treatment is 15 grams of carbohydrate.

Table 5

Monitor BG Level and Adjust Insulin[a]

Background insulin	Check morning fasting BG level every day (minimum). • **If most AM fasting >120 mg/dL** use titration guide (Table 6) until fasting target blood glucose reached; if dose reaches 0.5 units insulin/kg body weight consider adding mealtime insulin. • **If most AM fasting <120 mg/dL** and A1C remains above target, consider 2-hour post-meal testing and consider need for mealtime insulin.

Premixed insulin[b]	Check fasting and pre-dinner BG every day (minimum).
	
	 • **If most BG >200 mg/dL,** increase total insulin by 0.1 units/kg, then distribute equally between doses.
	
	 • **If most BG <200 mg/dL,** use titration guide to adjust out-of-target BG values 1 insulin at a time:
	
	      * *AM fasting BG*: adjust pre-dinner insulin dose
	
	      * *Predinner BG*: adjust pre-breakfast insulin dose

Background and mealtime insulin[b]	Check BG before all meals and 2 hours after evening meal (minimum).
	
	 • **If most BG >200 mg/dL,** increase total insulin by 0.1 units/kg, then add half to background and distribute remaining half equally between meals.
	
	 • **If most BG <200 mg/dL,** use titration guide to adjust out of target BG values:
	
	      * *AM fasting BG*: adjust background insulin
	
	      * *Prelunch or predinner BG*: adjust previous mealtime insulin
	
	      * If on rapid-acting and more than a 40 mg/dL pre- to post-meal rise, increase that meal's insulin by 1–3 units. If there is a pre- to post-meal drop, decrease insulin by 1–3 units.

[a] *Ensure that BG data is accurate—checking BG correctly, no food intake 2 hours prior to BG check.*
[b] *Discontinue sulfonylureas; consider adding or maintaining Metformin and/or Actos or Avandia.*

Table 6

Titrate Insulin for High and Low Blood Glucose

Titrate 1–2 times per week using fasting or pre-meal BG as guide.	
<70 mg/dL	Decrease by 1-3 units
70–120 mg/dL	No change
121–200 mg/dL	Increase by 1-3 units
>200 mg/dL	Increase by 3-5 units or 10%

Other Insulin Issues in T2DM

• For patients requiring large doses of insulin >2 units/kg, consider using U500 insulin. This is 5 times the concentration and needs to be used carefully, but in very insulin-resistant patients is often the most effective approach to reducing hyperglycemia.

• Insulin pumps are not commonly used in T2DM, in part because they are not covered by Medicare or most insurance companies (unless a low C-peptide is documented). In addition, to date there are no studies showing a clear benefit of pump therapy in T2DM over background and mealtime (basal-bolus) therapy.

• Patch pumps that deliver bolus only, basal only or fixed basal and bolus on demand are being developed. The use of CGM in T2DM is being studied to sort out its best application. Clinical experience indicates one use of CGM in T2DM be intermittent, and use blinded CGM to establish a reliable glucose pattern (usually takes 10-14 days) for adjusting meds and knowing which time of day needs focused SMBG testing to correct highs or lows. Then repeat CGM in another quarter and continue guide SMBG testing, medication selection and adjustment (oral agents or insulin).

• One marker of effective insulin use to consider is the A1C level at which insulin is typically initiated. One should not wait until A1C is 9%-10 %, which is a typical A1C when insulin is initiated in T2DM today.

In summary, insulin is very often needed in type 2 diabetes to achieve glucose control targets (A1C and SMBG). The benefits of insulin should be discussed early in the course of diabetes management and instituted in a timely manner when A1C cannot be maintained less than 7% (not waiting to start when A1C is 9% or 10%, as is common practice today). It is acceptable and effective to start with a "simplified" insulin regimen, and then, if unable to reach or maintain glycemic targets (or accommodate variable lifestyles and schedules), make a transition to the more physiologic background and mealtime (basal-bolus) insulin regimen. While being comfortable with starting insulin is important, equally critical to reaching and maintaining glycemic targets is making systematic insulin adjustments. Weekly observation of glucose patterns and insulin adjustment is effective and acceptable to patients and providers after insulin initiation. Most providers find it helpful to continue metformin if tolerated along with insulin therapy. Effective use of insulin in combination with newer antidiabetic medications (such as incretins) appear promising but awaits further trial data. New insulin analogs with ultra-long action times and new preparations of insulin with ultra-rapid action times are under development. Degludec is an ultra-long, peak-less background (basal) insulin that is currently being studied that may be injected daily or three times per week in order to provide for background insulin needs.

5. Conclusion

Our understanding of the pathophysiology of T2DM has progressed from the "triumvirate" (insulin resistance in the liver and muscle and Beta cell deficiency) to what Dr. DeFronzo has described as the "Ominous Octet" (adding to the known defects in the muscle, liver and Beta cell, abnormalities in the fat cell [accelerated lipolysis], gastrointestinal tract [incretin deficiency/resistance], alpha-cell [hyperglucagonemia], kidney [increased glucose reabsorption], and brain [insulin resistance]). Likewise, our approach to the effective management of T2DM changed. No longer is our management focused only on glucose control. We now strive to make an earlier diagnosis, start treatment early, teach patients self-management skills, utilize team care and work to control blood pressure, lipids and glucose (without weight gain and hypoglycemia). In addition, we push to stop tobacco use, start aspirin in appropriate patients, check feet, eyes and kidneys, and be sure an annual flu shot is delivered.

The management of glucose control is also evolving. NHANES data shows we are making some progress toward improving A1C control. But in light of data demonstrating a lasting harmful effect of early hyperglycemia (metabolic memory or legacy effect), we need to establish effective glucose control much sooner after the diagnosis of diabetes. We have an ever-growing list of agents to reduce hyperglycemia; we now need to match the most appropriate agents to a given patient's needs.

If diabetes care is to continue improving, it will not only take continued advances in science and medicine but advances in health care reform as well. Donald Berwick, MD, in an article entitled *The Triple Aim: Care, Health, and Cost* states "…the remaining barriers to integrated care are not technical, they are political." Mayer Davidson summarizes the diabetes care improvement literature in his recent editorial, entitled *How Our Current Medical Care System Fails People with Diabetes: Lack of timely, appropriate clinical decisions*. He concludes that the only effective diabetes disease management intervention is to use a specialty-trained nurse or pharmacist under appropriate supervision, with authority to make medication changes that fall within an approved algorithm. So, it is clear we must understand the steps needed to improve diabetes care, many of which are described in this chapter, and have a health care system that supports the implementation of these measures.

6. References

ACCORD Study Group and ACCORD Eye Study Group. Effects of Medical Therapies on Retinopathy Progression in Type 2 Diabetes. *N Engl J Med*. 2010:363:233-244.

Amori RE, Lau J, Pittas AG. Efficacy and safety of incretin therapy in type 2 diabetes: systematic review and meta-analysis. *JAMA*.2007;298(2): 194-206.

Benjamin EM, Bradley R. Systematic implementation of customized guidelines: the staged diabetes management approach. *J Clin Outcomes Manag*. 2002;9:81-86.

Bergenstal RM. Treatment models from the International Diabetes Center: Advancing from oral agents to insulin therapy in type 2 diabetes. *Endocr Pract*. 2006;12(suppl 1):98-104.

Bergenstal RM, Johnson ML, Powers MA, et al. Adjust to target in type 2 diabetes: comparison of a simple algorithm with carbohydrate counting for adjustment of mealtime insulin Glulisine. *Diabetes Care*. 2008;31(7):1305-1310.

Berwick DM, Nolan TW, Whittington J. The Triple aim: care, health and cost. *Health Affairs*. 2008;27:759-769.

Bonds DE, Miller ME, Bergenstal RM et al. The association between symptomatic, severe hypoglycaemia and mortality in type 2 diabetes: retrospective epidemiological analysis of the ACCORD study. BMJ. 2010;340:b4909.

Brixner D, McAdam-Marx C. Cost-effectiveness of insulin analogs. *Am J Manag Care*. 2008;14(11):766-775.

Buse JB, Rosenstock J, Sesti G, et al. Liraglutide once a day versus exenatide twice a day for type 2 diabetes: a 26-week randomised, parallel-group multinational, open -label trial (LEAD-6). *The Lancet*. 2009; 374:39-47.

Cochran E, Musso C, Gorden P. The use of U-500 in patients with extreme insulin resistance. *Diabetes Care*. 2005;28:1240-1244.

Crasto W, Jarvis A, Hackett V, Nayyar P, Davies M. Insulin U-500 in severe insulin resistance in type 2 diabetes mellitus. *Postgrad Med J*. 2009;85:219-222.

Cryer P. Hypoglycaemia: the limiting factor in the glycaemic management of Type I and Type II Diabetes. *Diabetologia*. 2002;45:937-948.

Davidson MB. How our current medical care system fails people with diabetes: lack of timely, appropriate clinical decisions. *Diabetes Care*. 2009;32:370.

DeFronzo RA. From the triumvirate to the ominous octet: a new paradigm for the treatment of type 2 diabetes mellitus. *Diabetes*. 2009;58:773-795.

Diabetes Prevention Program Research Group. Reduction in the incidence of type 2 diabetes with lifestyle intervention or metformin. *N Engl J Med*. 2002;346:393-403.

Dormandy JA, Charbonnel B Eckland DJA, et al. Secondary prevention of macrovascular events with patines with type 2 diabetes in the PROactive study (PRospective PioglitAzone Clinical Trial in MacroVascular Events): a randomized controlled trial. *Lancet*. 2005; 366:1279-1289.

Drucker DJ, Buse JB, Taylor K, et al for the DURATION-1 Study Group. Exenatide once weekly versus twice daily for the treatment of type 2 diabetes: a randomised, open-label, non-inferiority study. *Lancet*. 2008;372:1240-1250.

Etzwiler DD, Mazze R S, Bergenstal RM. Diabetes translation: a blueprint for the future. *Diabetes Care*. 1994;17(suppl 1):1-4.

Ferrannini E, Ramos SJ, Salsali A, et al. Dapagliflozin monotherapy in type 2 diabetic patients with inadequate glycemic control by diet and exercise: a randomized, double-blind, placebo-controlled, phase 3 trial. *Diabetes Care*. 2010; 33:2217-24.

Fonseca VA, Handelsman Y and Staels B. Colesevelam lowers glucose and lipid levels in type 2 diabetes: the clinical evidence. *Diabetes, Obesity and Metab*. 2010; 12:384-392.

Freeman J. Insulin analog therapy: improving the match with physiologic insulin secretion. *J Am Osteopath Assoc*. 2009;109:26-36.

Gæde P, Vedel P, Larsen N, et al. Multifactorial intervention and cardiovascular disease in patients with type 2 diabetes. *N Engl J Med*. 2003;348:383-393.

Gæde P, Lund-Andersen H, Parving H-H, Pedersen O. Effect of a multifactorial intervention on mortality in type 2 diabetes. *N Engl J Med*. 2008;358:580-591.

Gaziano JM, Cincotta AH, O'Connor CM, et al. Randomized Clinical Trial of Quick-Release Bromocriptine Among Patients with Type 2 Diabetes on Overall Safety and Cardiovascular Outcomes. *Diabetes Care*. 2010; 33:1503-1508.

Gerstein HC. Dysglycemia and cardiovascular risk in the general population. *Circulation* 2009; 119:773–75.

Goldstein BJ, Feinglos MN, Lunceford JK, et al. Effect of initial combination therapy with sitagliptin, a dipeptidyl peptidase-4 inhibitor, and metformin on glycemic control in patients with type 2 diabetes. *Diabetes Care*. 2007;30:1979-1987.

Grant RW, Buse JB, Meigs JB. Quality of diabetes care in U.S. academic medical centers: low rates of medical regimen change. *Diabetes Care*. 2005;28:337-342.

Green BD., Flatt PR, Bailey CJ. Dipeptidyl peptidase IV (DPP IV) inhibitors: a newly emerging drug class for the treatment of type 2 diabetes. *Diab Vasc Dis Res*. 2006;3(3):159-165.

Heisler M, Vijan S, Anderson R, et al. When Do Patients and Their Physicians Agree on Diabetes Treatment Goals and Strategies, and What Difference Does It Make? *J Gen Intern Med*. 2003;18:893-902.

Herman WH, Ilag LL, Johnson SL, et al. A clinical trial of continuous subcutaneous insulin infusion versus multiple daily injections in older adults with type 2 diabetes. *Diabetes Care*. 2005;28:1568-1573.

Hirsch IB, Bergenstal RM, Parkin CG, Wright E Jr, Buse J. A real-world approach to insulin therapy in primary care practice. *Clinical Diabetes*. 2005;23(2):78-87.

Hoerger TJ, Segel JE, Gregg EW, Saaddine JB. Is glycemic control improving in U.S. adults? *Diab Care*. 2008;31:81-86.

Holt RI, Barnett AH, Bailey CJ. Bromocriptine: old drug, new formulation and new indication. *Diabetes Obes Metab*. 2010; 12:1048-1057.

Horvath K, Jeitler K, Berghold A, et al. Longacting insulin analogues versus NPH insulin (human isophane insulin) for type 2 diabetes mellitus. *Cochrane Database of Systematic Reviews*. 2007;2.

Ismail-Beigi F, Craven T, Banerji MA , et al. Effect of intensive treatment of hyperglycemia on microvascular outcomes in types 2 diabetes: an analysis of the ACCORD randomised trial. *The Lancet*. 2020:376:419-430.

Jabbour S. Primary care physicians and insulin initiation: multiple barriers, lack of knowledge or both. *Int J Clin Pract*. 2008;62(6):845-847.

Kahn SE, Zinman B, Lachin JM et al. Rosiglitazone-associated fractures in type 2 diabetes: an Analysis for A Diabetes Outcome Progression Trial (ADOPT). *Diabetes Care*. 2008; 31:845-851.

Lane WS, Cochran EK, Jackson JA, et al. High-dose insulin therapy: is it time for U-500 insulin? *Endocr Pract*. 2009;15(1):71-79.

Linnebjerg H, Kothare PA, Skrivanek Z, et al. Exenatide: effect of injection time on postprandial glucose in patients with Type 2 diabetes. *Diab Med*. 2006;23:240-245.

Loke YK, Singh S, Furberg CD. Long-term use of thiazolidinediones and fractures in type 2 diabetes: a meta-analysis. *CMAJ*. 2009;180(1):32-39.

Mao XM, Liu H, Tao XJ, Yin GP, Li Q, Wang SK. Independent anti-inflammatory effect of insulin in newly diagnosed type 2 diabetes; *Diabetes Metab Research Rev*. Online ahead of print April 2009. DOI 10.1002/dmrr.968

Marshall SM, Flyvbjerg A. Prevention and early detection of vascular complications of diabetes. *BMJ*. 2006; 333:475-480.

Mazze RS, Etzwiler DD, Strock E, et al. Staged diabetes management: toward an integrated model of diabetes care. *Diabetes Care*. 1994;17(suppl 1):S56-S66.

Mazze RS, Strock E, Simonson GD, Bergenstal RM. Staged diabetes management, *a systematic approach*. 2nd ed rev. St. Louis Park, MN: John Wiley & Sons, Ltd, ;2006.

Mazze R, Strock E, Wesley D, et al. Characterizing glucose exposure for individuals with normal glucose tolerance using continuous glucose monitoring and ambulatory glucose profile analysis. *Diabetes Technol Ther*. 2008;10:149-159.

Mazze RS, Powers MA, Wetzler HP, Ofstead CL. Partners in advancing care and education solutions study: impact on processes and outcomes of diabetes care. *Population Health Management*. 2008;11:297-305.

McGlynn EA, Asch SM, Adams J, et al. The quality of health care delivered to adults in the United States. N Engl J Med. 2003;348:2635-2645. Montori VM, Fernández-Balsells M. Glycemic control in type 2 diabetes: time for an evidence based about-face? *Ann Intern Med*. 2009;150(11).

Nathan D, Davidson M, DeFronzo R, et al. Impaired Fasting Glucose and Impaired Glucose Tolerance: Implications for care. *Diab Care*. 2007; 30:753-759.

Nathan DM, Kuenen J, Borg R, et al. for the A1c-Derived Average Glucose (ADAG) Study Group. Translating the A1C assay into estimated average glucose values. *Diab Care*. 2008;31:1473-1478.

Nissen SE, Wolski K. Effect of rosiglitazone on the risk of myocardial infarction and death from cardiovascular causes. *N Engl J Med*. 2007;356(24):2457-2471.

Ong CR, Molyneaux LM, Constantino MI, et al. Long-term efficacy of metformin therapy in nonobese individuals with type 2 diabetes. *Diab Care*. 2006;29:2361-2364.

Perlin JB, Pogach LM. Improving the outcomes of metabolic conditions: managing momentum to overcome clinical inertia. *Ann Intern Med*. 2006;144(7):525-527.

Philis-Tsimikas A, Walker C, Rivard L, et al. Improvement in diabetes care of underinsured patients enrolled in Project Dulce. *Diabetes Care*. 2004;27:110-115.

Phillips LS, Branch WT Jr, Cook CB, et al. Clinical inertia. *Ann Intern Med*. 2001;135:825-834.

Raskin P, Bode BW, Marks JB, et al. Continuous subcutaneous insulin infusion and multiple daily injection therapy are equally effective in type 2 diabetes: a randomized, parallel-group, 24-week study. *Diabetes Care*. 2003;26:2598-2603.

Raz I, Wilson PW, Strojek K, et al. Effects of prandial versus fasting glycemia on cardiovascular outcomes in type 2 diabetes: the HEART2D trial. *Diab Care*. 2009;32:381-386.

Riddle MC, Ambrosius WT, Brillon DJ, et al. Epidemiologic Relationships Between A1C and All-Cause Mortality During a Median 3.4-Year Follow-up of Glycemic Treatment in the ACCORD Trial. *Diabetes Care* 2010; 33:983-990.

Rith-Najarian S, Branchaud C. Beaulieu O, et al. Reducing lower extremity amputation due to diabetes. Application of staged diabetes management approach in a primary care setting. *J Fam Pract*. 1998;47:127-132.

Rizza R, Eddy D, Kahn R. Cure, care, and commitment: what can we look forward to? *Diab Care*. 2008 31(5):1051-1059.

Schwartz AV, Sellmeyer, DE. Thiazolidinedione Therapy Gets Complicated Is bone loss the price of improved insulin resistance? *Diab Care*. 2007; 30:1670-1671.

Siebenhofer A, Plank J, Berghold A, et al. Short acting insulin analogues versus regular human insulin in patients with diabetes mellitus. *Cochrane Database of Systematic Reviews*. 2006;2.

Skyler JS, Bergenstal RM, Bonow RO, et al. Intensive Glycemic Control and the Prevention of Cardiovascular Events: Implications of the ACCORD, ADVANCE, and VA Diabetes Trial. *Diab Care*. 2009;32(1).

Shah BR, Hux JE, Laupacis A, Zinman B, van Walraven C. Clinical inertia in response to inadequate glycemic control: Do specialists differ from primary care physicians? *Diab Care*. 2005;28:600-606.

Shaw JS, Wilmot RL, Kilpatrick ES, et al. Establishing pragmatic estimated GFR thresholds to guide metformin prescribing. *Diab Med*. 2007; 24:1160-1163.

Sidorov J, Shull R, Tomcavage J, et al. Does diabetes disease management save money and improve outcomes? *Diabetes Care*. 2002;25:684-689.

Simonson GD, Kendall DM. Different actions of peroxisome proliferator-activated receptors: molecular mechanisms and clinical importance. *Curr Opin Endocrinol Diabetes*. 2006;13;162-170.

Singh SR, Ahmad F, Lal A, et al. Efficacy and safety of insulin analogues for the management of diabetes mellitus: a meta-analysis. *CMAJ*. 2009;180(4):385-397.

Solomon DH, Cadaretter SM, Choudhry NK, et al. A cohort study of thiazolidinediones and fractures in older adults with diabetes. *J Clin Endocrinol Metab* 2009;94:2792-2798.

The Emerging Risk Factors Collaboration. Diabetes mellitus, fasting blood glucose concentration, and risk of vascular disease: a collaborative meta-analysis of 102 prospective studies. *Lancet* 2010;375:2215–22.

UKPDS Study Group. Effect of intensive blood glucose control with metformin on complications in overweight patients with type 2 diabetes (UKPDS 34). *Lancet*. 1998;352:854-865.

Yach D, Hawkes C, Gould CL, Hofman KJ. The global burden of chronic diseases overcoming impediments to prevention and control. *JAMA*. 2004;291:2616-2622.

Ziemer DC, Miller CD, Rhee MK, et al. Clinical inertia contributes to poor diabetes control in a primary care setting. *Diabetes Educ*. 2005;31:564-571.

Chapter 8: Diabetes and Cardiovascular Disease –The Impact of Glycemic Control

David M. Kendall, MD
John B. Buse, MD, PhD

Contents

1. Introduction

Type 1 and type 2 diabetes are associated with a significant increase in the risk for major cardiovascular disease including CVD death, fatal and non-fatal myocardial infarction (MI) and stroke.[1] Regardless of the type of diabetes, there is also data supporting an increase in CVD risk with increasing hyperglycemia. Over the past decade, a number of clinical trials have shed further light on the potential impact of glucose lowering on CVD risk in both type 1 diabetes[2] and type 2 diabetes.[3] Most recently, the ACCORD, ADVANCE and VADT trials[4-6] specifically addressed the impact of unique approaches to intensive diabetes control on CVD risk. The epidemiology of hyperglycemia and CVD risk in diabetes, as well as the key features of these landmark trials, will be reviewed: seeking to identify both common and distinct features of each that may help clinicians better understand the impact on clinical decision-making. In addition, this review will serve to focus on the role of individualized treatment glycemia goals for patients—highlighting data that allow both patients and providers to identify the proper approach to care—while achieving the best control of diabetes, as early as possible, as safely as possible and for as long a period as possible. Ultimately, clinical care for diabetes must be driven by choices that provide maximal protection from CVD while assuring that glycemic targets provide for low risk of microvascular disease.

2. Glucose Control and Complications Risk

Intensive glycemic control significantly reduces the risk of microvascular complications of diabetes.[2,3] However, the impact of intensive glucose lowering on CVD risk remains less clear. Epidemiologic data support the assumption that lower blood glucose values may be associated with lower rates of CVD events and mortality.[7] Which specific combinations of glucose-lowering therapies may be of greatest benefit is also not known, although short-term data from uncontrolled observations support the use of metformin[8] and insulin-sensitizing medications like the thiazolidinediones.[9]

Data from epidemiologic studies and post hoc analyses of randomized, controlled intervention trials suggest a significant relationship between blood glucose lowering and a reduction in the risk of macrovascular disease in diabetes.[2,3,8,10] Both DCCT and UKPDS demonstrated unequivocally that intensive treatment of both type 1 and type 2 diabetes significantly reduces the risk of retinopathy, nephropathy and peripheral neuropathy. In general, a 1% reduction in A1C resulted in a 20%-40% reduction in the risk of microvascular disease, and this effect has now been shown to be sustained many years following the interval of intensive therapy.[10,11]

Even with the well-established relationship between glucose lowering and microvascular risk, the association between glucose lowering and the risk of CV disease remains poorly understood. Prospective trials of glucose lowering and its impact on macrovascular disease risk were needed to address the question as to the potential impact of more intensive glucose control on CVD risk.

In the following section, we provide detail on both the epidemiologic studies connecting hyperglycemia and CVD risk, and discuss the implications of recent large-scale, randomized clinical trials which assessed the impact of intensive glycemic control on the rate of cardiovascular events in high-risk individuals with diabetes.

3. Hyperglycemia and Cardiovascular Disease Risk

There are compelling data from numerous studies that provide strong evidence of the epidemiologic association between hyperglycemia (and diabetes) and cardiovascular risk. Data from the Framingham Heart Study,[12] the Honolulu Heart Study[13] and other large population analyses, including Epic-Norfolk,[14] ARIC,[15] and UKPDS,[8] have identified the association between increasing levels of glucose and an increased CVD risk. This was most clearly demonstrated in populations with type 2 diabetes. Cardiovascular risk is increased 2- to 4-fold in patients with diabetes; and most analyses described above estimated that for every 1% increase in A1C, there is an associated 10%-15% increase in the risk of CVD (Figure 1).

Perhaps the most widely accepted epidemiologic analysis of glycemia and CVD risk is derived from data from UKPDS.[8] In this analysis, Stratton et al identified a linear increase in risk of fatal or nonfatal MI and fatal and nonfatal stroke with increasing A1C. There was a 12%-14% higher risk of these selected CVD events for every 1% increase in mean updated A1C during the trial. This observation was also supported by data from UKPDS, where patients randomized to early intensive pharmacologic therapy with either sulfonylurea or insulin therapy (as compared to patients treated conventionally with initial medical nutri-

tion therapy [MNT]) exhibited a non-significant trend towards a reduction in rates of MI (16% risk reduction in the rate of first fatal or nonfatal MI, $P=0.052$).[3] Notably, both the epidemiologic analysis and the observation from the UKPDS were derived from a population of patients with a recent diagnosis of type 2 diabetes, rather than those with many years of poor glycemic control. Whether this feature—or others—plays an important role in the risk/benefit of glycemic control and CVD risk will be discussed later in this chapter.

The DCCT was a landmark trial establishing the impact of intensive glycemic control on microvascular risk in type 1 diabetes. This study was not designed to assess the impact of glycemic control on CVD risk. Overall, the rate of CVD was quite low in this young, healthy population with shorter-duration type 1 diabetes. However, the initial study did report fewer major cardiovascular events in the subject randomized to intensive insulin therapy.[2]

The observations from both UKPDS and DCCT provided support for the hypothesis that intensive glycemic control may favorably affect subsequent cardiovascular risk in patients with diabetes. In both trials, post-study follow-up was initiated to evaluate the impact of the initial period of inter-

Figure 1

Hazard ratios of myocardial infarctions and strokes

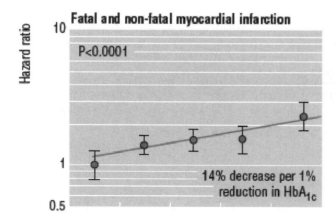
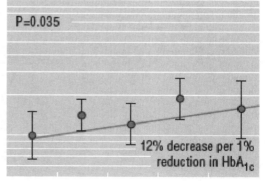

Hazard ratios, with 95% confidence intervals (as absolute risks), as estimate of association between category of updated mean hemoglobin A1C concentration and the risk of myocardial infarction or stroke.[8]

vention on subsequent risk of complications. The Epidemiology of Diabetes Interventions and Complications (EDIC) trial was an observational period that began following completion of DCCT. Since 1993, this cohort has been evaluated for rates of both micro- and macrovascular disease. Despite similar levels of glycemic control in both the intensive and conventional treatment groups after the randomized treatment was stopped, a significantly lower rate of microvascular disease has been noted in the 3-10 years following completion of the initial 6.5 years of intervention. Subsequent follow-up of this cohort also demonstrated a significantly lower rate of CVD events in the intensive treatment cohort. After an average of ~17 years of follow-up, there was a 42% reduction in the risk of CVD events (Figure 2).[16]

Whether this same effect might be present in patients with type 2 diabetes was addressed by Holman and colleagues, with data detailing a 10-year, post-trial follow-up of subjects from UKPDS. In this analysis, the initial trend suggesting a reduction in rates of first MI was maintained and intensive treatment resulted in a significant 15% risk reduction at 10 years post-study (Figure 3). Again, this finding was observed despite similar levels of glycemic control in the UKPDS cohort, regardless of the initial treatment assignment.[11] In both studies, the findings were consistent, namely, that early initiation of intensive therapy in both type 1 and type 2 diabetes resulted in a significant reduction in later cardiovascular risk.

Figure 2

Incidence of cardiovascular outcomes

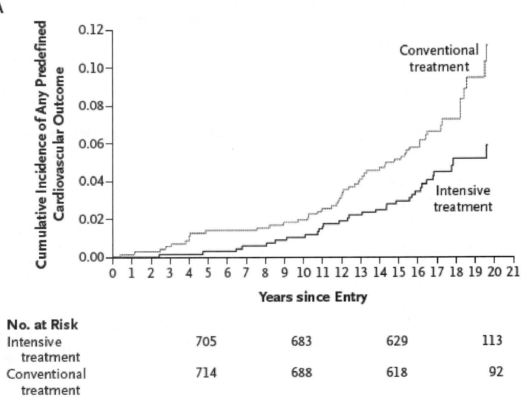

Cumulative incidence of the first major CVD event in the EDIC study. A 42% reduction in risk was observed in the cohort of patients with initial intensive therapy during the first 5 years of DCCT/EDIC.[16]

Again, both studies support the hypothesis that early intensive therapy can reduce the subsequent risk of cardiovascular disease. However, neither study was originally designed, nor adequately powered, to specifically address this question. In addition, the significant reduction in CVD risk was observed only after many years of post-trial follow-up. Despite this, however, these findings continued to raise questions as to the potential impact of glycemic control on later cardiovascular risk.

Despite the demonstrated benefit on microvascular disease risk, and the suggestion of a later impact on CVD risk in both the UKPDS and DCCT trials, many clinicians and investigators have remained skeptical of the potential for glycemic control alone to further reduce risk in higher risk patients with type 2 diabetes. A number of key, unanswered questions remained, even with the completion of DCCT/EDIC and UKPDS and its 10-year follow-up.

- What is the impact of more intensive control (targeting near normal glucose levels) on CVD risk?

- Can intensive glycemic control reduce both micro- and macrovascular risk in higher risk individuals with longer duration diabetes?

- What interval of intensive glycemic control (and what level of glycemia) must be achieved to adequately assess the impact of glucose control on CVD risk?

- What are the potential risks of more intensive glycemic control in high-risk patients with type 2 diabetes?

Figure 3

Hazard ratio of myocardial infarction

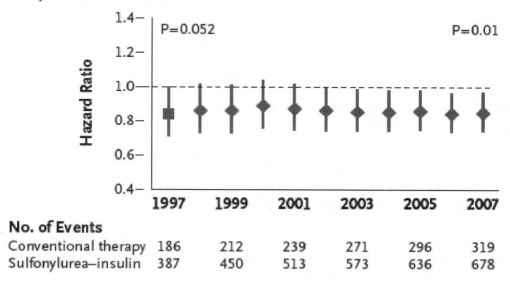

C Myocardial Infarction

No. of Events	1997	1999	2001	2003	2005	2007
Conventional therapy	186	212	239	271	296	319
Sulfonylurea–insulin	387	450	513	573	636	678

Kaplan–Meier Curves for Myocardial Infarction in UKPDS reflecting the proportions of patients in the study who myocardial infarction at the time of initial study completion and at each annual time point for out to 10 years of post-study follow-up. Overall, those treated with early intensive therapy had a significant 15% reduction in the risk of MI over 10 additional years of follow-up.[11]

4. Recent Clinical Trials: ACCORD, ADVANCE and the VADT

Even with the results of UKPDS and DCCT in hand, substantial questions regarding the impact of intensive glucose control on CVD risk remained unanswered. While these studies demonstrated conclusively that the risk of microvascular complications is reduced by intensive glycemic control, long-term, randomized and controlled clinical trials of intensive control and CVD risk were necessary. It is on this background that 2 large-scale clinical trials were performed. The recently completed Action to Control Cardiovascular Risk in Diabetes (ACCORD) trial, the Action in Diabetes and Vascular Disease: Preterax and Diamicron Modified Release Controlled Evaluation (ADVANCE) trial and the Veterans Affairs Diabetes Trial (VADT) have significantly added to our understanding of intensive glycemic control in type 2 diabetes. In addition, a number of new questions regarding the benefits and risks of intensive therapy were raised. A clear understanding of the unique study designs, patient populations and approach to care in ACCORD, ADVANCE and VADT are necessary to enable clinicians to understand both the benefit and potential risk of intensive glycemic control in patients at risk for CVD.

These trials were specifically designed to compare the effects of intensive vs. standard glycemic control on CVD outcomes in relatively high-risk individuals with established type 2 diabetes. Each of the studies enrolled individuals at significant risk for CVD, including patients with pre-existing CVD, multiple CVD risk factors or both. While similar in many respects, these trials differed in important ways; enrolling patients with varying severity and duration of antecedent hyperglycemia, varying control of concomitant CVD risk factors, and varying duration and intensity of the glycemia intervention. These studies have been well summarized in the recent position statement of the American Diabetes Association (ADA), the American Heart Association (AHA) and the American College of Cardiology (ACC),[18] and the key patient characteristics of these studies are outlined in Table 1.

A1C values achieved with either intensive or standard treatment approaches, and the hazard ratio (with 95% CI) of major CVD events and mortality in the ACCORD, ADVANCE and VADT Trials.[4-6]

Middle-aged and older subjects with varying degrees of antecedent glycemic control at higher risk for CVD were included in all 3 trials. While a trend towards lower rates of CVD events was seen in all 3 trials (Relative Risk [RR] CVD Events) when comparing intensive vs. standard glycemia treatment, no significant effect was observed in any these trials. Only ACCORD demonstrated a statistically significant increase ($P=0.04$) in the RR of mortality at a hazard ratio of 1.22.

ACCORD

The ACCORD study randomized 10,251 participants with either history of a CVD event (aged 40-79) or significant CVD risk (aged 55-79 years). ACCORD employed a glycemia treatment strategy using multiple medications in either intensive or less intensive approaches to glycemic control. Investigators used a therapeutic strategy targeting A1C levels less than 6% (intensively treated) vs. 7.0%-7.9% (standard treatment) to determine if such an approach could significantly reduce the risk of CVD events. Other CVD risk factors, including blood pressure and lipids, were treated aggressively and similarly between groups. ACCORD trial participants were middle-aged, with average diabetes duration of approximately 10 years. Median baseline A1C values for ACCORD subjects were ~8.3% within 4 months of intensive treatment and patients achieved a significantly greater reduction in median A1C: 6.4% as compared to 7.5% in the standard treatment group, in the 3.5 years of follow-up.[4]

ACCORD Glycemia

The intensive glycemic control group was more commonly treated with insulin and utilized multiple combinations of oral agents. This group also experienced significantly more weight gain and episodes of severe hypoglycemia than the standard group. While the primary outcome measure for ACCORD was the first occurrence of major CVD events (including fatal or nonfatal MI, fatal or nonfatal stroke or cardiovascular death), the glycemia intervention was discontinued in February 2008 at the recommendation of the data safety monitoring committee, due to the finding of increased all-cause mortality in intensively treated

Table 1

Selected Demographic Features from the ACCORD, ADVANCE and VADT Trials

Characteristic	ACCORD[4]	ADVANCE[5]	VADT[6]
N	10,251	11,140	1791
Mean age (years)	62	66	60
Duration of T2DM	10	8	11.5
Prior history of CVD	35%	32%	40%
BMI (kg/m^2)	32	28	31
A1C at baseline	8.3%	7.5%	9.4%
A1C (intensive vs. standard)	6.4% vs. 7.5%	6.5% vs. 7.3%	6.9% vs. 8.4%
RR CVD events	0.9 (0.78-1.04)	0.94 (0.84-1.06)	0.88 (0.74-1.06)
RR mortality	1.22 (1.01-1.46)	0.93 (0.83-1.06)	1.07 (0.80-1.42)

subjects. With the discontinuation of the intensive treatment strategy, all patients continued in the trial and all were converted to the standard glycemia treatment strategy.[4]

During the 3.5 years of average follow-up, there was no significant reduction in the rate of major CVD events or CVD death (hazard ratio 0.90 [95% CI 0.78-1.04], P=0.16). At that same time, all-cause mortality was increased by 22% (HR 1.22 [95% CI 1.01-1.46], P=0.04) in intensively treated subjects, resulting in the discontinuation of the intensive treatment strategy before the planned 5.5 years of average follow-up was completed.

Despite the trend toward modestly lower rates of major CVD events observed with intensive therapy in ACCORD, the apparent increase in mortality raised substantial questions about the potential risk of very intensive treatment strategies in such high-risk individuals. In the first 3.5 years of ACCORD, rates of nonfatal MI were significantly lower in the intensively treated cohort (HR 0.76 [95% CI 0.62-0.92], P=0.004) while there was no significant difference in the rate of either nonfatal stroke or congestive heart failure between the 2 treatment groups. The intensive treatment strategy was associated with an increase in the rates of fatal cardiovascular events. The potential mechanisms for the higher mortality, despite a reduction in total CVD events, are not known.

A number of hypotheses have been suggested to explain the higher mortality observed early in ACCORD. The intensively treated cohort in ACCORD differed in a number of important ways. Evaluation of specific baseline characteristics, diabetes treatments, rates of severe hypoglycemia, weight gain and other factors have yet to reveal specific features that may have predicted risk. In addition, ongoing analyses will assess the impact of antecedent cardiovascular disease, glycemic control and other factors. Initial analysis of the ACCORD trial cohort suggests that those individ-

Figure 4

Incidence of cardiovascular outcomes

A Primary Outcome

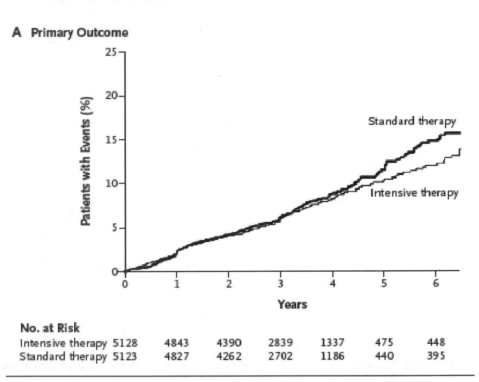

No. at Risk							
Intensive therapy	5128	4843	4390	2839	1337	475	448
Standard therapy	5123	4827	4262	2702	1186	440	395

B Death from Any Cause

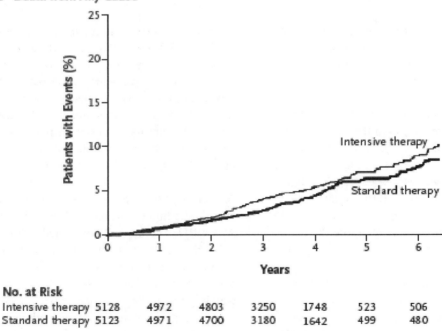

No. at Risk							
Intensive therapy	5128	4972	4803	3250	1748	523	506
Standard therapy	5123	4971	4700	3180	1642	499	480

Kaplan Meier curves for the rates of major CVD endpoint and total mortality during the 3.5 years of follow-up from the ACCORD Trial.[4]

uals with lower baseline A1C values may have been at lesser risk of early mortality. However, further post hoc analysis of this data set—along with analysis of data from ADVANCE, VADT and other trials—will be needed to further clarify the potential risks associated with such an intensive treatment approach.

The data from the initial evaluation of ACCORD suggest that, as compared to standard therapy targeting A1C values in the 7% range, an intensive treatment strategy targeting A1C levels <6% results in an unanticipated increase in all-cause mortality, with no significant impact on rates of major CVD events. While these findings identified potential and previously unidentified risk with a very intensive treatment strategy in high-risk subjects, extensive additional analysis—and prolonged follow-up—will be required to better understand the clinical implications of these findings. *To date, ACCORD is the only intensive treatment trial in patients with T2DM where more intensive glucose lowering was associated with an increase in early mortality*. Further exploration of this population, baseline characteristics and the specific treatment approach used in ACCORD will be needed to provide clinicians with a better understanding of how to appropriately target glycemia to maximize benefit for micro- and macrovascular disease risk, while limiting the possible risks of more intensive therapy.

It is critical to note that intensive treatment in ACCORD targeted blood glucose and A1C values substantially lower than those currently recommended. Whether this very intensive treatment approach, or other factors, contributed to the increase in early mortality is not known. The 2 treatment groups differed in a number of important ways (eg, A1C, hypoglycemia, weight gain, medication combinations) and these differences must all be carefully analyzed. Undoubtedly, subsequent studies will be needed.

ADVANCE Trial

The ADVANCE study randomized 11,140 participants at centers in Europe, Asia, Canada, Australia and New Zealand. Treatment assignment was a strategy of intensive glycemic control (with initial

sulfonylurea/gliclazide therapy followed by additional medications as needed to achieve an A1C = 6.5) vs. a strategy of standard therapy (use of any medication except gliclazide, with glycemic target set according to local guidelines).[20] In contrast to ACCORD, ADVANCE participants were modestly older (required to be at least 55 years) with either known vascular disease or at least 1 other vascular risk factor. However, ADVANCE study participants had an average duration of diabetes of only 8 years (2 years shorter than ACCORD subjects), with lower baseline A1C values (median 7.2%) and almost no use of insulin.[5]

Over 5 years of treatment, significantly lower HgbA1C values were achieved in the intensive treatment group (6.5%) vs. the standard treatment group (7.3%). As in ACCORD, outcomes from the ADVANCE trial demonstrated no significant effect on rates of major CVD events from intensive treatment.[5] However, ADVANCE also included microvascular disease in its primary composite endpoint, and the investigators did report a significant reduction in the primary endpoint of combined CVD events, nephropathy and retinopathy. Overall, this risk was reduced approximately 10%, with much of the overall risk reduction seen as a consequence of lower rates of new onset or progressive renal disease. ADVANCE demonstrated no significant difference in the risk of all-cause mortality. These data supported evidence that further reductions in A1C can significantly reduce the risk of microvascular complications, but may provide no significant benefit on the risk of major CVD events as compared to usual treatment approaches targeting A1C values near 7%.

Veterans Affairs Diabetes Trial (VADT)

The VADT randomized nearly 1800 individuals with type 2 diabetes and uncontrolled diabetes on either insulin or maximal-dose oral agents (median entry A1C 9.4%). Investigators utilized a strategy of intensive glycemic control (goal A1C=6.0%) or standard glycemic control. Medication treatment algorithms were employed to achieve glycemic goals.[6] Median A1C levels of 6.9% and 8.5% were achieved in the intensive and standard arms, respectively, and were maintained thru the 5+ years of follow-up. Other CVD risk factors were treated aggressively and effectively in both groups. The primary clinical question addressed by VADT investigators was whether older males with poor glycemic control, and established type 2 diabetes with significant risk for cardiovascular disease might benefit from more intensive glycemic control. Importantly, the VADT population had poorly controlled diabetes at baseline, a longer duration of diabetes, and the cohort was of older age and higher BMI as compared to the populations of ACCORD and ADVANCE. In addition, the VADT population had substantial number of patients with established (or pre-existing) macro- and microvascular disease.

The primary outcome of VADT was a composite of CVD events, including: fatal and non-fatal MI, stroke, cardiovascular death, revascularization, hospitalization for heart failure and amputation for ischemia. Over 5.5 years of treatment, the cumulative risk of CVD events was similar in the intensive vs. standard treatment arms (HR 0.88 [95% CI 0.74 –1.05], $P = 0.12$). While there was a numerically greater number of CVD deaths in the intensive treatment group as compared to standard care (38 vs. 29), as well as an excess of sudden death (11 vs. 4), neither of these differences were statistically significant. Additional analyses suggested that duration of diabetes may have impacted outcomes, as a duration of diabetes less than ~12 years appeared to be associated with a CVD benefit with intensive control, while those with longer disease duration at entry had a neutral or possibly adverse effect.[6]

Assessment of rates of hypoglycemia in VADT suggested that severe hypoglycemia within 90 days was a strong predictor of both CVD events and CVD mortality. One additional, embedded study within VADT suggested that higher baseline coronary or aortic calcium scores predicted future CVD events. The intensive therapy approach significantly reduced CVD events in those with lower baseline coronary artery calcium score, but not those with high scores, suggesting a modest benefit from intensive control in those with lower disease burden. These findings are consistent with the observations in both ACCORD and ADVANCE, where both trials demonstrated reductions in CVD event (but not in mortality) in those without preexisting CVD.

5. Clinical Implications and Conclusions

The results of the ACCORD, ADVANCE and VADT trials, as well as the follow-up of the UKPDS study, were all published in the summer and fall of 2008. These results have engendered a great deal of confusion and concern regarding the appropriate glycemic targets and treatment approaches in patients with diabetes. Though each of these trials individually failed to demonstrate clear benefits with more intensive glycemic interventions on CVD event rates, meta-analysis of these trials suggests that there is modest benefit of A1C reduction on CVD endpoints and no adverse effect on mortality.[17,18] The summary of results of these trials, with a summary of the baseline features of the subjects treated, is shown below.

The following conclusions seem reasonable, based on the totality of evidence:[17]

1. Based on the findings of the DCCT and UKPDS studies, as well as epidemiological analysis, the glycemic goal of therapy for the prevention of microvascular complications (eye, kidney, nerve disease) should, in general, be <7%. Microvascular disease is a major cause of morbidity in type 1 and type 2 diabetes, and prevention of these complications is an important clinical goal of diabetes care.

2. Though the ACCORD, ADVANCE and VADT trials did not provide evidence for CVD reduction, the long-term follow-up of the DCCT and UKPDS cohorts suggests that treatment to A1C targets below or around 7%, particularly soon after the diagnosis of diabetes, is associated with reduction in CVD risk with long-term follow-up (10-20 years).

3. Based on the ADVANCE trial and subgroup analysis of the UKPDS and DCCT trials, lower A1C targets may be associated with a small but incremental benefit in microvascular outcomes. In selected patients, such as those with recent onset disease, long life-expectancy and no significant CVD, A1C targets of <6.0%-6.5% may be reasonable, if they can be achieved without significant hypoglycemia or other adverse effects.

4. Based on the ACCORD trial, A1C targets of 7.0%-7.9% may be appropriate for patients with advanced CVD or other complications, multiple risk factors, limited life expectancy, and those with longstanding diabetes whose care is complicated by severe hypoglycemia despite diabetes self-management education, appropriate glucose monitoring and effective doses of multiple glucose-lowering agents, including insulin.

1 remaining question is whether the lack of benefit of more intensive control on CVD endpoints in the ACCORD, ADVANCE and VADT trials is the result of the specific treatment strategies employed. In the overweight subgroup of the UKPDS, metformin was associated with a significant benefit on MI. Likewise, the PROactive study suggested CVD benefit from pioglitazone therapy in patients with clinical cardiovascular disease. Could novel agents with benefits on CVD risk factors and lesser risk of hypoglycemia provide for CVD benefits? Would more intensive lifestyle efforts provide for CVD risk reduction? These issues are being examined in trials that have yet to be completed. However, the long-term benefits of intensive early treatment on microvascular and CVD complications in the UKPDS and DCCT suggest that early aggressive treatment, when the general A1C target of <7% can be safely achieved with rational treatment approaches, is arguably the most evidence-based strategy for glycemic control. Early screening for type 2 diabetes and treating those individuals with combined therapy with lifestyle and metformin at diagnosis is now widely recommended.

It is certain that prevention of complications is best accomplished by targeting the multiple co-morbidities of diabetes – glycemia as well as blood pressure and lipids. The STENO-2 trial[19] demonstrated a substantial benefit of combined approaches to lower glucose, blood pressure and lipids. Thus, the overarching principle of diabetes care should not be to solely focus on glycemic control, but to target equally the ABCs of diabetes:

- A1C <7%

- Blood pressure <130/80 mm Hg

6. References

- Cholesterol (LDL <100 mg/dl in general and <70 mg/dl in those at highest risk)

Additionally, those people with diabetes and CVD or over the age of 40 with additional CVD risk factors should use antiplatelet agents, and people with diabetes should not use tobacco. With a comprehensive, proactive approach, the risk of major complications of diabetes can be prevented or delayed, and most people should be able to achieve a long life without disabling complications.

1. Haffner SM, Lehto S, Ronnemaa T, et al. Mortality from coronary heart disease in subjects with type 2 diabetes and in nondiabetic subjects with and without prior myocardial infarction. *N Engl J Med*. 1998;339:229-234.

2. The Diabetes Control and Complications Trial Research Group (DCCT). The effect of intensive treatment of diabetes on the development ond progression of long term complications in insulin dependent diabetes mellitus. *N Engl J Med*. 1993;329:977-986.

3. UK Prospective Diabetes Study (UKPDS) Group. Intensive blood-glucose control with sulphonylureas or insulin compared with conventional treatment and risk of complications in patients with type 2 diabetes (UKPDS 33). *Lancet*. 1998;352:837-853.

4. Action to Control Cardiovascular Risk in Diabetes Study Group (ACCORD). Effects of intensive glucose lowering in type 2 diabetes. *N Engl J Med*. 2008;358(24):2545-2559.

5. The ADVANCE Collaborative Group. Intensive blood glucose control and vascular outcomes in patients with type 2 diabetes. *N Engl J Med*. 2008;358(24):2560-2572.

6. Duckworth WC, Abraira C, Moritz T, et al. Glucose control and vascular complications in veterans with type 2 diabetes. *N Engl J Med*. 2009;360(2):129-139.

7. Selvin E, Marinopoulos S, Berkenblit G, et al. Meta-analysis: Glycosylated hemoglobin and cardiovascular disease in diabetes mellitus. *Ann Intern Med*. 2004;141(6):421-431.

8. Stratton IM, Adler AI, Neil HA, et al. Association of glycaemia with macrovascular and microvascular complications of type 2 diabetes (UKPDS 35): prospective observational study. *BMJ*. 2000;321(7258):405-412.

9. Dormandy JA, Charbonnel B, Eckland DJ, et al for the PROactive investigators. Secondary prevention of macrovascular events in patients with type 2 diabetes in the PROactive Study (PROspective pioglitAzone Clinical Trial In macroVascular Events): a randomized controlled trial. *Lancet*. 2005;366(9493):1279-1289.

10. Writing Group for the Diabetes Control and Complications Trial/Epidemiology of Diabetes Intervention and Complications (DCCT/EDIC) Research Group. Sustained effect of intensive treatment of type 1 diabetes mellitus on development and progression of diabetic nephropathy. *JAMA*. 2003;290:2159-2167.

11. Holman RR, Paul SK, Bethal MA, et al. 10-year follow-up of intensive control of type 2 diabetes. *N Engl J Med*. 359:1577-1589.

12. Fox CS, Pencina MJ, Wilson PW, Paynter NP, Vasan RS, D'Agostino RB Sr. Lifetime risk of cardiovascular disease among individuals with and without diabetes stratified by obesity status in the Framingham Heart Study. *Diabetes Care*. 2008;31(8):1582-1584.

13. Donahue RP, Abbott RD, Reed DM, Yano K. Postchallenge glucose concentration and coronary heart disease in men of Japanese ancestry. Honolulu Heart Program. *Diabetes*. 1987;36(6):689-692.

14. Khaw KT, Wareham N, Luben R, et al. Glycated haemoglobin, diabetes, and mortality in men in Norfolk cohort of european prospective investigation of cancer and nutrition (EPIC-Norfolk). *BMJ*. 2001;322(7277):15-18.

15. Selvin E, Coresh J, Golden SH, Brancati FL, Folsom AR, Steffes MW. Glycemic control and coronary heart disease risk in persons with and without diabetes: the atherosclerosis risk in communities study. *Arch Intern Med*. 2005;165(16):1910-1916.

16. Nathan DM, Cleary PA, Backlund JY, et al for the Diabetes Control and Complications Trial/Epidemiology of Diabetes Interventions and Complications (DCCT/EDIC) Study Research Group. Intensive diabetes treatment and cardiovascular disease in patients with type 1 diabetes. *N Engl J Med*. 2005;353(25):2643-2653.

17. Skyler JS, Bergenstal R, Bonow R, et al. Intensive glycemic control and the prevention of cardiovascular events: implications of the ACCORD, ADVANCE, and VA diabetes trials. *Diabetes Care*. 2009;32(1):187-192.

18. Gaede P, Vedel P, Larsen N, et al. Multifactorial intervention and cardiovascular disease in patients with type 2 diabetes. *N Engl J Med*. 2003;348:383-393.

Chapter 9:
Managing CV Risk - Hypertension

David C. Goff Jr, MD, PhD
William C. Cushman, MD

Contents

Overview

High blood pressure is a common coexisting condition in patients with type 2 diabetes mellitus, affecting over a third of adults with diabetes. The presence of high blood pressure increases the risk of numerous macro- and microvascular complications of diabetes, including cardiovascular disease, nephropathy, retinopathy and, possibly, neuropathy. The association of blood pressure with complications extends into the blood pressure range usually considered normal in persons without diabetes. The relative increase in risk attributable to high blood pressure is comparable in persons with and without diabetes, but the combination of high baseline risk of complications in patients with diabetes and this relative risk generate a much larger absolute excess risk of high-blood-pressure-related complications in persons with diabetes, than in those without. Clinical trial data have proven the benefits of blood pressure-lowering therapy in patients with diabetes; however, the most appropriate goal for the treated blood pressure level is unknown. The clinical trial evidence clearly supports systolic blood pressure levels less than 140 mm Hg, and diastolic blood pressure levels less than 80 mm Hg. Lower systolic blood pressure goals are supported by observational data. The relative benefits of various blood pressure-lowering medications has received much attention and generated much controversy. Since most patients with diabetes will require triple-drug therapy with a diuretic, ACE inhibitor (or angiotensin receptor blocker) and calcium channel blocker to achieve blood pressure control, this debate is largely academic. In patients with high blood pressure but not diabetes, the risk of developing diabetes may be reduced by ACE inhibitors, angiotensin receptor blockers and calcium channel blockers relative to diuretics and beta-blockers. Prevention of diabetes and high blood pressure remain important long-term public health goals; however, given the frequency and complications of high blood pressure in patients with diabetes, and the proven benefits of blood pressure control, attention to improving the quality of care for high blood pressure in patients with diabetes is of major importance.

1. Risks of High Blood Pressure in Type 2 Diabetes

High blood pressure is a common medical problem in patients with type 2 diabetes. According to results from the National Health and Nutrition Examination Survey (NHANES) 1999-2000, 31% of men and 43% of women with diabetes in the United States had high blood pressure.[1] These high prevalence figures contrast with 28.3% of all men and 28.7% of all women in the U.S.[.] In addition, diabetes has been shown to increase the incidence of high blood pressure by approximately 50%.[3] This increased risk may be due to mechanisms related to insulin resistance[4] and hyperinsulinemia,[5-7] including effects on salt sensitivity, the nocturnal fall in blood pressure,[8] the response of blood pressure to exercise,[9] and left ventricular mass and structure.[10]

High blood pressure is an important risk factor for the major forms of cardiovascular disease (CVD), including coronary heart disease, heart failure, stroke and peripheral arterial disease.[11] CVD is the leading cause of death and a major cause of morbidity in the U.S., regardless of diabetes status.[11] The adverse effect of high blood pressure on risk of coronary heart disease and stroke has been recognized for several decades,[12-14] and for over a decade in persons with diabetes.[15] The risk of major CVD events increases, in a continuous manner, across the distribution of blood pressure.[16] In patients with type 2 diabetes, there is also a graded increase in risk for CVD and microvascular complications, across the entire range of blood pressure levels, including blood pressure levels below current treatment thresholds.[15,17,18] Among 347,978 middle-aged men screened for participation in the Multiple Risk Factor Intervention Trial (MRFIT), the absolute risk of CVD mortality increased more steeply across progressively higher systolic blood pressure (SBP) categories among men with diabetes than among men without diabetes.[15] Consequently, as shown in Table 1, the absolute excess risk of CVD mortality attributable to higher blood pressure was much greater in men with diabetes than in men without diabetes, regardless of serum total cholesterol concentration or cigarette smoking status.[15] In the observational component of the United Kingdom Prospective Diabetes Study (UKPDS), higher baseline and subsequent SBP levels were associated with greater relative and absolute risk of total mortality, deaths and complications related to diabetes, including CVD events and microvascular complications (Table 2).[17]

Stroke is the third leading cause of death and a major cause of morbidity in the U.S., in persons with and without diabetes.[11] At the population level, high blood pressure is probably the most important risk factor for stroke, whether ischemic or hemorrhagic;[14,19] nevertheless, diabetes and high blood pressure each independently increase the risk of stroke.[19-23] Little evidence exists regarding the precise nature of the association between blood pressure and the risk of stroke in patients with diabetes; however, Hu et al reported that the effect of high blood pressure on risk of stroke was similar among persons with and without diabetes.[24] It seems prudent to presume that the continuous

relationship observed between blood pressure and risk of stroke in persons without diabetes[16] exists in persons with diabetes. Consequently, given the greater absolute risk of stroke in patients with diabetes vs. those without, the excess risk of stroke related to high blood pressure is likely to be much greater in people with diabetes than in those without diabetes.

Heart failure is a major public health problem in people with diabetes. Bertoni et al reported a prevalence of heart failure of 22% of Medicare beneficiaries with diabetes; in addition, the incidence of heart failure was 12.6 per 100 person-years.[25] In the general population of people ≥65 years old, the prevalence of heart failure is less than 10%;[11] a difference that underscores the effect of diabetes on heart failure risk. The independent

Table 1

Relative and Absolute Risks for Cardiovascular Disease (CVD) Mortality Associated With Systolic Blood Pressure (SBP) Below or at Least 120 mm Hg in Men With and Without Diabetes According to Serum Total Cholesterol Concentration and Cigarette Smoking Status at Initial Screening for the Multiple Risk Factor Intervention Trial.[15]

Diabetes	Serum Cholesterol (mg/dL	Cigarette Smoking	Age-adjusted CVD Mortality (per 10,000 person-years)		Relative Risk (≥120/<120 mm Hg)	Excess Risk (≥120 mm Hg-<120 mm Hg [per 10,000])
			SBP <120 mm Hg	SBP ≥120 mm Hg		
No	<200	No	6.02	12.96	2.15	6.94
Yes	<200	No	30.68	60.33	1.97	29.65
No	<200	Yes	14.33	28.50	1.99	14.17
Yes	<200	Yes	57.12	102.71	1.80	45.59
No	200+	No	9.99	20.59	2.06	10.6
Yes	200+	No	52.17	87.03	1.67	34.86
No	200+	Yes	23.48	47.38	2.02	23.90
Yes	200+	Yes	86.01	125.23	1.46	39.22

roles of high blood pressure and diabetes in the etiology of heart failure have been recognized for at least 2 decades;[26] however, early research on heart failure etiology and prevention focused primarily on high blood pressure, perhaps because the relative risk for heart failure was greater for high blood pressure than for diabetes, and because high blood pressure was much more common than diabetes. Recent research has documented a continuous relationship between blood pressure and heart failure risk. For example, in the Framingham Heart Study, a 20 mm Hg greater SBP was associated with a 56% greater risk for heart failure.[27] As is the case with stroke, limited evidence exists regarding the precise nature of the association between blood pressure and risk of heart failure in people with diabetes; however, Iribarren et al showed no interaction between blood pressure and hemoglobin A1C on risk of heart failure.[28] It seems likely that the continuous relationship exists in patients with diabetes as well as in those without.

The excess risk for heart failure due to higher blood pressure levels is likely to be much greater in persons with diabetes, given their greater absolute risk of heart failure, even at optimal blood pressure levels, when compared with persons without diabetes.

Diabetes and high blood pressure are the top 2 causes of end-stage renal disease (ESRD) in the U.S.[29] The incidence of chronic renal failure in diabetes has been estimated to range between 133 per 100,000 person-years in Rochester, Minnesota[30] to 200 per 100,000 person-years among MRFIT screenees,[31] to 1570 per 100,000 person-years among Oklahoma Indians.[32] Diabetes increased the risk of ESRD by a factor of almost 10 (RR, 9.0 [95% CI, 7.4-11.0]) among MRFIT screenees.[31] The clinical diagnosis of high blood pressure is reported to double the risk of nephropathy in patients with diabetes;[32] however, the relationship is probably continuous in nature.

Table 2

Adjusted[a] Relative Risk Increment Associated With a 10 mm Hg Greater Systolic Blood Pressure (SBP), Measured at Baseline and as an Updated Mean, Among 3642 Participants in the Observational Component of the United Kingdom Prospective Diabetes Study.[17]

Endpoint	Number of Events	Baseline SBP		Updated Mean SBP	
		Relative Risk Increment (%)	95% CI (%)	Relative Risk Increment (%)	95% CI (%)
Total mortality	597	13	10, 17	12	9, 16
Diabetes related deaths	346	19	15, 23	17	13, 21
Diabetes complications	1255	9	7, 12	12	9, 14
Microvascular disease	323	10	4, 15	13	9, 26
Myocardial infarction	496	13	9, 16	12	7, 16
Heart failure	104	14	5, 21	15	4, 19
Stroke	162	13	7, 19	19	14, 24
Peripheral arterial disease	41	30	20, 39	16	9, 23

[a]Adjusted for age at diagnosis of diabetes, sex, ethnicity, smoking, microalbuminuria, hemoglobin A1c, high and low density cholesterol, and triglycerides.

Among 332,544 men who were screened for entry into the MRFIT, a strong gradient was observed between baseline blood pressure level and risk of ESRD. As compared with men possessing an optimal level of blood pressure (systolic pressure <120 mm Hg and diastolic pressure <80 mm Hg), the relative risk of ESRD for those with stage 4 hypertension (systolic pressure ≥210 mm Hg or diastolic pressure ≥120 mm Hg) was 22.1 ($P<0.001$).[33] The excess risk of ESRD due to higher blood pressure is certainly greater in patients with diabetes than in those without. Even after adjustment for baseline glomerular filtration rate, which is probably influenced by high blood pressure and diabetes, Fox et al reported elevated odds ratios for the development of new onset kidney disease attributable to diabetes (2.6) and high blood pressure (1.6), based on data from the Framingham Heart Study.[34]

In the U.S., diabetic retinopathy is the fifth most common cause of legal blindness and occurs in about 4.8 people per 100,000 population.[35] Higher blood pressure increases the risk of retinopathy in patients with diabetes.[36-43] In the Barbados Eye Study, the relative risk (RR) for diabetic retinopathy increased by 30% for every 10 mm Hg higher SBP at baseline (RR, 1.3 [95% CI, 1.1–1.4]). This relationship was observed even within the normal range for blood pressure. A 10 mm Hg increase in SBP from baseline to the 4-year follow-up was associated with a similar increase in risk (RR, 1.3 [95% CI, 1.1–1.4]).[36] In a study of Pima Indians, the incidence of exudates in those with SBP of at least 145 mm Hg was more than twice that of those with SBP of <125 mm Hg.[37] In the San Luis Valley Diabetes Study, the RR for retinopathy was 80% greater for a 20 mm Hg higher SBP.[42]

The risk of diabetes-related neuropathy, for autonomic,[44] peripheral sensory neuropathy[45] and composite definitions[46] has been associated with hypertension in patients with type 1 diabetes, but evidence regarding this relationship in type 2 diabetes is sparse and inconsistent. Cohen et al reported an association between high blood pressure and sensory, but not autonomic, neuropathy in patients with type 2 diabetes, based on data from the Appropriate Blood Pressure Control in Diabetes Trial.[47] In contrast, high blood pressure was not associated with risk of sensory neuropathy in patients with type 2 diabetes in the San Luis Valley Diabetes Study.[48] At present, the role of high blood pressure in the etiology and progression of diabetes-related neuropathy is unclear.

In summary, type 2 diabetes is associated with increased risk for numerous macrovascular and microvascular complications. The risk for all of the complications reviewed above, with the possible exception of neuropathy, is increased in the presence of high blood pressure. As a consequence of the multiplicative nature of the interaction between diabetes and high blood pressure, the excess risk attributable to high blood pressure is much higher in patients with diabetes than in patients without diabetes. Therefore, it would seem reasonable to expect that treatment of high blood pressure would be especially effective in reducing the absolute risk of these complications in patients with diabetes.

2. Benefits of Blood Pressure Control in Type 2 Diabetes

As reviewed above, the increase in CVD risk associated with higher blood pressure is independent of the increase in CVD risk associated with diabetes; therefore, diabetes and hypertension combined confer a much higher risk than either alone.[15] In part because of this higher risk, observed even in the prehypertensive range, the Seventh Report of the Joint National Committee on the Prevention, Detection, Evaluation, and Treatment of High Blood Pressure (JNC 7) recommended beginning drug treatment at lower blood pressure levels in patients with diabetes than in patients without diabetes. In patients with diabetes, blood pressure lowering treatment is recommended when the SBP is ≥130 mm Hg or the diastolic blood pressure (DBP) is ≥80 mm Hg, with treatment goals of <130/80 mm Hg.[18] However, there is a paucity of randomized clinical trial evidence to support these recommendations. The 2004 Veterans Affairs-Department of Defense (VA-DoD) hypertension guidelines, relying primarily on available evidence from clinical trials, recommend a goal blood pressure in diabetes mellitus of <140/80 mm Hg.[49] Table 3 provides summary information from randomized clinical trials regarding the effect of blood pressure-lowering treatment on risk of CVD endpoints.

The Systolic Hypertension in the Elderly Program (SHEP) was designed to test the hypothesis that treatment of isolated systolic hypertension would reduce the risk of stroke and CVD in elderly persons.[50] In the overall SHEP population, stroke was reduced by 36% and major CVD by 32% by chlorthalidone-based therapy.[51] In a *post hoc* subgroup analysis of participants with type 2 diabetes in SHEP, major CVD events were reduced by 34%.[52] Whereas the relative risk reduction was similar in participants with and without diabetes, the absolute risk reduction was twice as great in participants with diabetes as in those without. The Systolic Hypertension in Europe (Syst-Eur) Trial, was a similar trial conducted in Europe but using nitrendipine as the initial blood pressure-lowering drug.[53] Stroke was reduced by 42% and CVD by 31%.[54] Patients with diabetes were reported in a *post hoc* subgroup analysis to have significant reductions in total mortality (55%), CVD mortality (76%), all CVD events (69%) and stroke (73%).[55]

The Hypertension Optimal Treatment (HOT) study was designed to test the relative effectiveness of treatment to 3 different DBP goals (≤90, ≤85 and ≤80 mm Hg) on risk of CVD.[56] Participants in the more intensively treated group received ACE inhibitors, beta-blockers and diuretics more often than did the less intensively treated participants; however, there was little difference in use of felodipine (the initial therapy used per protocol). No difference in CVD event rates was observed between the treatment groups in the overall study population.[57] In a *post hoc* analysis of participants with diabetes, major CVD events were reduced by 51% (P=0.005) among those randomized to a DBP goal of ≤80 mm Hg compared to a goal of ≤90 mm Hg.[57] The large size of the observed treatment effect in participants with diabetes was impressive. However, the number of major CVD events observed in participants with diabetes was relatively small (n=101), and the difference between the blood pressure achieved for the more intensively treated participants with diabetes (144/81 mm Hg) compared with the less intensively treated group (148/85 mm Hg) was small (4/4 mm Hg).[58] Furthermore, as indicated above, no difference in CVD event rates was observed between randomized groups in the entire HOT population, despite an identical difference in achieved blood pressures. The authors did not report how many subgroup analyses they examined; hence, the role of chance cannot be completely excluded.

In the UKPDS, hypertensive patients with type 2 diabetes were randomized to more or less intensive blood pressure control (goals <150/85 vs. <180/105 mm Hg). Participants randomized to more intensive control were also randomized to initial therapy with either captopril or atenolol. The suggested sequence for adding medications was furosemide, slow-release nifedipine, methyldopa, and prazosin. Nifedipine was the agent used most often in the less intensively treated group. Average blood pressure over 9 years was 144/82 and 154/87 mm Hg in the more and less intensively treated groups, respectively. In the more intensively treated group, 29% of participants were taking at least 3 drugs, just over 30% were taking 2

Table 3

Clinical Trials of Blood Pressure-lowering in Patients with Diabetes

Trial	N	Duration	Mean BP, less intense	Mean BP, more intense	Initial Therapy	Outcome	Relative Risk Reduction
SHEP[52]	583	5 years	155/72[a]	146/68[a]	Chlorthalidone	Stroke CVD events CHD	22% (ns) 34% 56%
Syst-Eur[55]	492	2 years	162/82	153/78	Nitrendipine	Stroke CV events	69% 62%
HOT[57,58]	1501	3 years	148/85	144/81	Felodipine	CV events MI Stroke CV mortality	51% (ns) 50% 30% 67%
UKPDS[59]	1148	8.4 years	154/87	144/82	Captopril or atenolol	Diabetes-related endpoints Deaths Strokes Microvascular	34% 32% 44% 37%
ABCD[61-63]	470	5.3 years	138/86	132/78	Nisoldipine or enalapril	CCr Albuminuria Retinopathy Neuropathy Mortality MI, Stroke, CHF	nc nc nc nc 49% ns

Continued

Table 3 (continued)

Clinical Trials of Blood Pressure-lowering in Patients with Diabetes

Trial	N	Duration	Mean BP, less intense	Mean BP, more intense	Initial Therapy	Outcome	Relative Risk Reduction
ADVANCE[64,65]	11,140	4.3 years	140/77	135/75	Perindopril and indapamide	Major macrovascular and microvascular events	9%
						Macrovascular	8% (ns)
						Microvascular	9% (ns)
						Renal events	21%
						CV mortality	18%
						Total mortality	14%
SANDS[66]	499	3 years	129/73	117/67	JNC 7 based stepped care	CV events	ns

BP = blood pressure, CCr = Creatine Clearance, CHD = Coronary heart disease, CHF = Congestive heart failure, CV = Cardiovascular, CVD = Cardiovascular Disease, MI = Myocardial infarction, nc = no change, ns = not significant,
[a] Personal communication from Sara Pressel, School of Public Health, University of Texas Health Science Center.

drugs and fewer than 40% were taking 1 or 0 drugs. Diabetes-related endpoints were reduced by 24% (95% CI, 8% to 38%; P=0.005), deaths related to diabetes by 32% (95% CI, 6% to 51%; P=0.019), strokes by 44% (95% CI, 11% to 65%; P=0.013) and microvascular endpoints by 37% (95% CI, 11% to 56%; P=0.009), with intensive therapy to reduce blood pressure. Although not statistically significant, all-cause mortality was lowered by 18% and myocardial infarction (MI) by 21%.[59] In a report based on extended follow-up for a median duration of 14.5 years, these benefits were not sustained; however, it is important to note that the BP differential was also not sustained during post-trial follow-up.[60] It seems reasonable to conclude that the lower BP level must be sustained if the benefits are to be maintained.

The Appropriate Blood Pressure Control in Diabetes (ABCD) trial, a prospective, randomized, blinded trial in hypertensive patients with diabetes, compared the effects of moderate control of blood pressure (target DBP 80-89 mm Hg) with those of intensive control (DBP 75 mm Hg or less) on the incidence and progression of diabetes-related nephropathy, retinopathy, cardiovascular disease and neuropathy.[61-63] Therapy was based on the use of nisoldipine and enalapril. The mean blood pressure achieved in the intensive group was 132/78 mm Hg vs. 138/86 mm Hg in the moderate control group. There were no differences in any microvascular endpoints for the 2 BP goals. The intensive therapy group had a lower mortality rate (5.5% vs. 10.7%, P=0.037), but there were no statistically significant differences in MI, cerebrovascular events or heart failure to account for the mortality difference.

The Action in Diabetes and Vascular disease: preterAx and diamicroN-MR Controlled Evaluation (ADVANCE) trial assessed the effects on vascular disease of an approach using a fixed combination of the ACE inhibitor, perindopril and the diuretic, indapamide, in a diverse population of patients with type 2 diabetes and a broad range of blood pressure values. Although there were no specific BP goals, the study achieved average differences of 5.6 mm Hg and 2.2 mm Hg for SBP and DBP, respectively, and mean values of about 140/77 and 135/75 in the less and more intensive-

ly treated groups, respectively. This treatment led to a 9% reduction in relative risk of the primary endpoint, a composite that combined major macrovascular and microvascular disease endpoints. Mortality from CVD was reduced by 18% (3.8% vs. 4.6%, P=0.027) and total mortality by 14% (7.3% vs. 8.5%, P=0.025).[64] This trial also documented a reduction in risk of renal events by 21% (P<0.0001), driven by reduced risks for developing microalbuminuria and macroalbuminuria (both P<0.003).[65]

The Stop Atherosclerosis in Native Diabetics Study (SANDS) was a randomized trial with an open-label, blinded endpoint assessment design, comparing intensive control of BP and lipids with a standard approach. The intensive (and corresponding standard) treatment goals were SBP ≤115 (130) mm Hg, DBP ≤75 (85) mm Hg, LDL cholesterol ≤70 (100) mg/dL and non-HDL cholesterol ≤100 (130) mg/dL. Achieved intensive (and standard) mean values were as follows: SBP, 117 (129) mm Hg; DBP, 67 (73) mm Hg; LDL cholesterol,[72] (104) mg/dL; and non-HDL cholesterol 102 (138) mg/dL. Carotid artery intimal-medial thickness regressed in the intensive group and progressed in the standard group (P<0.001), and left ventricular mass index decreased more in the intensive group (P=0.03); however, adverse events related to the BP-lowering medications were more common in the intensive group (P=0.005), and there was no difference in clinical cardiovascular events in this small trial (N=499).[66] Given the simultaneous intensive treatment of BP and lipids, it is difficult to attribute the effects on atherosclerosis to a specific therapy; however, it seems reasonable to conclude that the seemingly beneficial effects on left ventricular mass index were likely attributable to the intensive BP intervention.

The UKPDS, HOT and ADVANCE trials provide the most definitive clinical trial evidence to date, and support BP goals of <150/85 mm Hg (UKPDS), DBP <80 mm Hg (HOT) and BP < 140/80 (ADVANCE) in patients with both hypertension and diabetes. These goals and the achieved BP levels in these and other trials are consistent with an SBP goal of less than 140 mm Hg in patients with diabetes. No trials have confirmed CVD benefits of treating to lower BP goals (eg,

3. Relative Efficacy of Various Classes of Blood Pressure-lowering Medications

SBP <130 mm Hg). In particular, no trial has tested whether reduction to *optimal* levels, as defined by JNC 7 (ie, SBP <120 mm Hg), would provide additional CVD benefits. The Action to Control Cardiovascular Risk in Diabetes (ACCORD) trial was designed to provide evidence relevant to this question.[67,68] Of the 10,251 participants in ACCORD, 4733 were randomized in a factorial substudy examining the effects of an intensive blood pressure-lowering strategy, targeting a SBP <120 mm Hg vs. a standard strategy, targeting a SBP <140 mm Hg. The primary outcome measure for the trial is the first occurrence of a major cardiovascular event, specifically nonfatal MI, nonfatal stroke or cardiovascular death. Participants will be followed for 4-8 years (mean 5.6 years), and follow-up is planned to continue through the summer of 2009.[69]

The best choice of pharmacologic therapy for lowering blood pressure has been a much debated topic, both for persons with and without diabetes. Multiple clinical trials have been conducted to compare various antihypertensive agents to placebo or to other active comparators. Metabolic considerations have been discussed to support the use of newer agents (eg, ACE inhibitors, alpha-adrenergic receptor blockers, angiotensin receptor blockers and calcium channel blockers) with potentially fewer detrimental effects than older agents on electrolyte concentrations (thiazide-type diuretics), lipid and lipoprotein concentrations (thiazide-type diuretics and beta-adrenergic receptor blockers), and glucose and insulin metabolism (thiazide-type diuretics and beta-adrenergic receptor blockers). Several recent trials and meta-analyses have contributed important information relevant to this issue.

Psaty et al reported the results of a meta-analysis of 42 clinical trials testing 7 major treatment strategies (placebo, ACE inhibitors, alpha-blockers, angiotensin receptor blockers, beta-blockers, calcium channel blockers and low-dose diuretics) involving 192,748 participants with and without diabetes.[70] None of the alternative agents were superior to low-dose diuretics (the equivalent of 12.5-25 mg per day of chlorthalidone or 25-50 mg per day of hydrochlorothiazide) for any of the outcomes examined (coronary heart disease, heart failure, stroke, CVD events, CVD deaths or total mortality). Low-dose diuretics were superior to ACE inhibitors for heart failure, CVD events and stroke; to alpha-blockers for heart failure and CVD events; to beta-blockers for CVD events; and to calcium channel blockers for heart failure and CVD events. Blood pressure effects were similar between active agents.[70] No results were reported specific to patients with diabetes.

The Blood Pressure Lowering Treatment Trialists' Collaboration reported the results of a prospectively planned meta-analysis of 29 randomized trials involving 162,341 participants, and reported results similar to those of Psaty. Neither of the newer agents examined (ACE inhibitors and calcium channel blockers) were superior to the older agents examined (beta-blockers or diuretics) for any of the outcomes examined (coronary heart disease, heart failure, stroke, CVD events, CVD death or total mortality). The older agents were superior to ACE inhibitors for stroke and to calcium channel blockers for heart failure and CVD events.[71] A subsequent meta-analysis by this collaboration from the same database reported drug comparisons in hypertensive patients with and without diabetes.[72] They concluded that "*the short- to medium-term effects on major cardiovascular events of the BP-lowering regimens studied were broadly comparable for patients with and without diabetes.*" 2 limitations of these meta-analyses are: 1.) there are no separate analyses using diuretics alone as a comparator group (diuretics were superior to beta-blockers in several trials and other meta-analyses); and 2.) many studies were excluded because it was a prospective meta-analysis.

The Antihypertensive and Lipid-Lowering Treatment to Prevent Heart Attack Trial (ALL-HAT) randomized over 42,000 participants to 1 of 4 active anti-hypertensive agents: chlorthalidone (a thiazide-type diuretic), amlodipine (a calcium channel blocker), doxazosin (an alpha blocker) and lisinopril (an ACE inhibitor). The primary outcome measure was the combined occurrence of fatal coronary heart disease (CHD) or nonfatal MI, analyzed by intent to treat (ITT). The doxazosin arm was terminated early, after a mean follow-up of 3.2 years. Although there was no difference in the primary outcome (RR, 1.02 [95% CI, 0.92-1.15]) or all-cause mortality (RR, 1.03 [95% CI, 0.94-1.13]) between these 2 arms, the doxazosin arm had a higher risk of stroke (RR, 1.26 [95% CI, 1.10-1.46]) and combined CVD (RR 1.20 [95% CI, 1.13-1.27]) in all participants.[73] In the subgroup of patients with diabetes, a greater risk of heart failure (RR, 1.85 [95% CI, 1.56-2.19]), stroke (RR, 1.21 [95% CI, 0.97-1.50]) and combined CVD (RR, 1.22 [95% CI, 1.11-1.33]) was observed in those treated with doxazosin, despite lower glucose levels seen on follow-up.[74]

The 3 other arms in ALLHAT continued until the planned termination of the trial, following a mean follow-up of 4.9 years. Overall, there was no difference in the primary endpoint or all-cause mortality between the treatment groups; however, in

comparison to chlorthalidone, amlodipine was associated with greater incidence of heart failure (RR, 1.38 [95% CI, 1.25-1.52]) and lisinopril was associated with greater risk of stroke (RR, 1.15 [95% CI, 1.02-1.30]), combined CVD (RR, 1.10 [95% CI, 1.05-1.16]) and heart failure (RR, 1.19 [95% CI, 1.07-1.31]).[75] Similar results were observed in the subgroup of patients with diabetes. Amlodipine was associated with greater risk of heart failure (RR, 1.42 [95% CI, 1.23-1.64]), and lisinopril was associated with greater risk of combined CVD (RR, 1.08 [95% CI, 1.00-1.17]) and heart failure (RR, 1.22 [95% CI, 1.05-1.42]). These findings in favor of chlorthalidone were seen, despite the expected lesser decreases in total cholesterol, greater increases in fasting glucose and greater decreases in potassium among participants assigned to chlorthalidone. About 8% of the chlorthalidone group were receiving potassium supplementation at 5 years, compared with 4% in the amlodipine group and 2% in the lisinopril group.[75] A more extensive analysis of the ALLHAT data by diabetes status, published by Whelton et al, confirmed these results and showed no evidence of a benefit of therapy with amlodipine or lisinopril vs. chlorthalidone in patients with diabetes.[76] Whereas the estimated glomerular filtration rate (GFR) was preserved more effectively by amlodipine and lisinopril than by chlorthalidone,[75] there was no difference between the treatment groups in the development of ESRD, and this latter finding held true in participants with diabetes as well as in those without diabetes.[77] In comparison to the chlorthalidone-treated group, the relative risk of developing ESRD in participants with diabetes was 1.30 (95% CI, 0.98-1.73) for amlodipine-treated participants and 1.17 (95% CI, 0.87-1.57) for lisinopril-treated participants.[77] Large, beneficial effects of amlodipine or lisinopril relative to chlorthalidone on development of ESRD in patients with diabetes are not consistent with these findings.

In contrast to ALLHAT, the Second Australian National Blood Pressure Study Group reported that an antihypertensive regimen beginning with ACE inhibitors led to better outcomes than treatment with diuretics, despite similar reductions in blood pressure; however, this relatively small trial had few participants with diabetes (7%) and has not reported the results in the subgroup with diabetes.[78] The Anglo-Scandinavian Cardiac Outcomes Trial-Blood Pressure-Lowering Arm (ASCOT-BPLA) tested the relative efficacy of atenolol with bendroflumethiazide (a thiazide-type diuretic [added if needed]) vs. amlodipine with perindopril (added if needed), and the study was stopped early. The investigators reported a significant reduction in fatal and non-fatal stroke (RR, 0.77 [95% CI 0.66-0.89]), total cardiovascular events and procedures (RR, 0.84 [95% CI 0.78-0.90]), and all-cause mortality (RR, 0.89 [95% CI, 0.81-0.99]) in the amlodipine/perindopril group.[79] There was no statistically significant difference between groups in the primary endpoint (non-fatal MI [including silent MI] and fatal CHD). Reductions in total cardiovascular events and procedures were similar for participants with diabetes (RR, 0.87 [95% CI, 0.76-0.99]) and without diabetes (RR, 0.82 [95% CI, 0.75-0.90]), suggesting that the relative superiority of amlodipine over atenolol is similar across both subgroups.[79] However, it is difficult to compare the ASCOT findings to those from previous outcome trials for several reasons: the addition of agents from different antihypertensive classes to the 2 treatment arms makes it impossible to determine whether 1, or the combination of both, might be responsible for beneficial cardiovascular outcomes; and, the thiazide dose used in the trial is one-fourth to one-half the dose used in prior trials.

The effect of different blood pressure-lowering medications on renal function has received great attention in patients with type 2 diabetes.[80-111] Overwhelming evidence supports the effectiveness of ACE inhibitors and angiotensin receptor blockers, in slowing the progression of microalbuminuria and preventing the development of overt nephropathy.[80-111] The relative superiority of these medications over blood pressure-lowering medications from other classes has been less well-studied. 1 small trial (N=21) reported a benefit with enalapril and no benefit with hydrochlorothiazide;[82] however, other reports have shown similar efficacy of indapamide (an indoline diuretic) and ACE inhibitors.[81,90,105] Similarly, some studies have shown relative equivalence of ACE inhibitors and calcium channel blockers;[86,87,91,96,106,108] whereas others have shown superiority of ACE inhibitors over calcium channel blockers.[99,103,107] Irbesartan was superior to amlodipine in the Irbesartan Diabetic Nephropathy Trial.[110] In addition, ramipril was superior to atenolol in 1 trial.[92] Combined use of ACE inhibitors and angiotensin receptor blockers was superior to monotherapy with either alone in some,[95,109] but not all, trials.[98,111] Similarly, whereas a trial of the combination of amlodipine and fosinopril demonstrated superiority of combination therapy over either monotherapy,[103] a trial of the combination of trandolapril and verapamil showed no benefit of adding verapamil to trandolapril or even of verapamil vs. placebo.[107] Based on this evidence, it may be reasonable to prefer ACE inhibitors or angiotensin receptor blockers in the presence of microalbuminuria; however, this evidence should be considered along with the results of ALLHAT, described above, that showed no superiority of lisinopril over chlorthalidone in the development of ESRD in patients with high blood pressure and type 2 diabetes.[77]

4. Diabetes Prevention With Antihypertensive Agents

The potential role of antihypertensive agents to prevent the development of diabetes has also received attention. In the Captopril Prevention Project (CAPPP), the effect of therapy based on the ACE inhibitor captopril was compared with conventional treatment, consisting of beta-blockers and diuretics. Atenolol and metoprolol were the most commonly used β-blockers, and hydrochlorothiazide and bendrofluazide were the most commonly used diuretics. There was no difference in the primary endpoint (a composite of fatal and non-fatal MI, stroke and other cardiovascular deaths); however, the incidence of diabetes was lower in the captopril group than in the conventional group (RR, 0.86; P=0.039).[112,113] In the Heart Outcomes Prevention Evaluation (HOPE) Study, a placebo-controlled trial, use of the ACE inhibitor ramipril was associated with a reduction in the development of diabetes (RR, 0.66 [95% CI, 0.51-0.85]).[114] In the Diabetes Reduction Assessment with Ramipril and Rosiglitazone Medication (DREAM) study of persons with pre-diabetes, use of ramipril was not associated with a reduction in incidence of diabetes, but rather with an increase in reversion to normoglycemia.[115] In the Losartan Intervention For Endpoint reduction in hypertension (LIFE) study, the risk of developing diabetes was 13.0 in 1000 patient-years in the group randomized to begin therapy with the angiotensin receptor blocker losartan and 17.4 in 1000 patient-year in the atenolol-based group (RR, 0.75 [95% CI, 0.63-0.88]).[116] In a substudy to the LIFE trial, losartan was shown to have more favorable effects than atenolol on insulin resistance.[117]

In ALLHAT, the risk of developing diabetes during 4 years of follow-up was also associated with treatment. The group treated with chlorthalidone had the highest 4-year incidence (11.6%) followed by amlodipine (9.8%, P=0.04 vs. chlorthalidone) and lisinopril (8.1%, P<0.001 vs. chlorthalidone).[75] In ASCOT-BPLA, the incidence of developing diabetes was less on the amlodipine-based regimen than on the atenolol-based regimen (RR, 0.70 [95% CI, 0.63-0.78]).[79] In aggregate, these results support the contention that ACE inhibitors, angiotensin receptor blockers and calcium channel blockers may provide some protection against the development of diabetes. The failure of this protection against diabetes to translate into superiority over diuretics in trials of CVD outcomes may relate to the duration of the CVD outcomes trials having been too brief to observe the long-term effects of diabetes prevention on risk of CVD. However, in the 14.3 year follow-up of the SHEP participants, there was no increase in cardiovascular or all-cause mortality for those who had developed incident diabetes during the trial in the chlorthalidone group, whereas those in the placebo group with *incident diabetes* had significantly higher mortality than those who did not develop diabetes or those with incident diabetes in the chlorthalidone group.[118] In addition, the 2-6 mg/dl lower glucose seen in trials with ACE inhibitors or angiotensin receptor blockers compared with other drugs would be predicted to have a rather small effect on CVD outcomes. In the ACCORD trial, for example, a Hgb A1c difference of 1.5%, similar to a fasting glucose difference of approximately 55-60 mg/dl, is estimated to be needed to produce a 15% difference in CVD events in 10,000 participants over 5 years. This is 10 times the glucose difference observed between antihypertensive drugs. Therefore, it is not surprising that, in studies like ALLHAT and SHEP, there were no CVD outcome effects of differences in glucose or diabetes incidence. Furthermore, other differences between the antihypertensive agents in mechanisms of cardiac protection may be operative.

5. Practical Aspects of Blood Pressure Control in Diabetes

A summary of treatment recommendations is provided in Table 4.

The literature reviewed above supports the conclusion that high blood pressure is a major risk factor for macro- and microvascular disease in patients with diabetes. Indeed, as a consequence of the higher baseline risk in patients with diabetes and the manner in which the presence of high blood pressure multiplies that already elevated risk, the absolute excess risk of adverse outcomes related to high blood pressure is much greater in patients with diabetes than in those without diabetes. Due to the aforementioned increased risk for macro-and microvascular disease, treatment of high blood pressure is a high priority in patients with diabetes. As recommended by JNC 7, it may be reasonable to treat patients with diabetes at lower blood pressure levels, and to aim for lower blood pressure goals; however, strong evidence from clinical trials is currently lacking to support this approach.

In the interim, control of SBP to <130 mm Hg and DBP to <80 mm Hg is recommended in JNC 7.[18] This level of control can be challenging to achieve, and usually requires combination antihypertensive therapy. However, identification of an evidence-based approach to combination therapy is difficult, because most of the randomized trials have applied constraints on the regimens that have impaired their subsequent clinical applicability. In ALLHAT, approximately 60% of participants were controlled to SBP <140; however, the ALLHAT protocol prohibited, or at least strongly discouraged, any combined use of diuretics, ACE inhibitors and calcium channel blockers. The second- and third-line agents approved by the protocol included atenolol, clonidine, reserpine and hydralazine.[75] In the subgroup of participants with diabetes, the mean SBP ranged from 135-137 mm Hg across the treatment groups, despite the use of 2 medications on average.[76] In ASCOT, 53% of participants reached both their systolic and diastolic blood-pressure targets, but only 32% of patients with diabetes reached their intensive targets of SBP <130 and DBP <80 mm Hg. ASCOT also limited the use of therapies to amlodipine plus perindopril vs. atenolol plus bendroflumethiazide.[79] In UKPDS, just over 60% of participants

in the more intensively treated group received 2 or more medications, and 29% received 3 or more medications to achieve a mean blood pressure of 144/82 mm Hg; however, the protocol discouraged the combined use of ACE inhibitors and beta-blockers.[59] In ADVANCE, adherence to the intensive (2-drug) treatment was 83%, and 74% of intensively-treated participants were taking at least 1 additional BP-lowering medication in order to achieve the mean BP of ~135/75 mm Hg.[64] In SANDS, the intensive participants were treated with a mean of 2.3 BP-lowering medications (vs. 1.6 on average in standard participants), and 67% of intensively treated participants achieved the SBP target of <117 mm Hg for at least 50% of visits.[66] No study has examined the effectiveness of triple drug therapy with a diuretic, ACE inhibitor (or angiotensin receptor blocker) and calcium channel blocker, either in patients with or without diabetes.

Nevertheless, it is clear from the ALLHAT, ASCOT, UKPDS, ADVANCE and SANDS experiences that the majority of patients with diabetes and high blood pressure will need 3 or more medications to achieve SBP <130 mm Hg.[59,75,79] Since most patients will need multiple drugs to achieve good blood pressure control, it may be reasonable to begin therapy with a combination medication that includes a diuretic and an ACE inhibitor. In those instances in which a single agent may be sufficient to achieve good blood pressure control, cost and efficacy considerations support the use of diuretics. ACE inhibitors may be reasonable alternatives, especially in patients with microalbuminuria or macroproteinuria.

Angiotensin receptor blockers are reasonable substitutes for ACE inhibitors when the latter are not tolerated due to cough; however, angioedema has been reported in patients on angiotensin receptor blockers, so other alternative therapies may be preferable when patients experience angioedema with an ACE inhibitor. When a third medication is needed, a calcium channel blocker may be a reasonable choice. Beta-blockers, reserpine or alpha blockers may be useful when more than 3 medications are needed, or when patients do not tolerate medications from other classes. The choice of BP-lowering medications should

Table 4

Practical Recommendations for the Treatment of High Blood Pressure in Type 2 Diabetes Mellitus

Category	Recommendation	Evidence Grade
Treatment Goals	SBP should be controlled to <140 mm Hg	1A
	SBP should be controlled to <130 mm Hg consistent with JNC 7	2C
	DBP should be controlled to <80 mm Hg consistent with JNC 7	1A
Drug Therapy	Thiazide-type diuretics should be used as first-line therapy for uncomplicated high blood pressure in patients with diabetes.	1A
	ACE inhibitors and calcium channel blockers should be used as second line agents or as alternative first line agents for patients who do not tolerate diuretics.	1A
	Angiotensin receptor blockers (ARB) may be used for patients who do not tolerate ACE inhibitors (except when angioedema is the reason for intolerance).	1A
	Many, if not most, patients with diabetes will need 3 medications to reach goal (especially SBP <130 mm Hg).	1A
	Initial therapy with a combination of a diuretic and an ACE inhibitor (or ARB) would be reasonable for most patients with diabetes and high blood pressure.	Expert opinion
	When 3 medications are needed, combination therapy with a diuretic, ACE inhibitor (or ARB) and calcium channel blocker would be reasonable.	Expert opinion
	Beta adrenergic receptor blockers, alpha blockers, reserpine, hydralazine and centrally acting sympatholytics are reasonable alternatives as third-line agents.	Expert opinion
	Choice of blood pressure lowering medications should be influenced by other indications for use of specific agents.	Varies by agent and indication

also be influenced by other specific indications (eg, beta-blockers in patients with compensated heart failure or known CAD).

In the ACCORD trial, an intensive BP-lowering strategy was developed by 1 of the clinical sites to assist them in pursuing the target SBP <120 mm Hg. That strategy, which was influenced by the formulary available in ACCORD, recommends initiation with benazepril/hydrochlorothiazide as step 1, switch to diuretic plus benazepril/amlodipine for step 2, switch to metoprolol/hydrochlorothiazide plus benazepril/amlodipine for step 3 and addition of reserpine, when needed, for step 4. An alternative strategy was developed for participants who do not tolerate ACE inhibitors. Both candesartan with (and without) hydrochlorothiazide and valsartan with (and without) hydrochlorothiazide are available in the ACCORD formulary, so the use of either of these combination medications with amlodipine and metoprolol would provide presumably similar BP-lowering effectiveness to the step 3 regimen described above. This alternative strategy requires participants to use a larger number of pills per day, possibly decreasing adherence and increasing cost. Strategies that minimize the number of different pills taken per day may help enhance adherence and limit the cost to patients, at least in terms of copays. Another strategy to consider in clinical practice, which is also available in ACCORD, is to change the thiazide-type diuretic from hydrochlorothiazide to chlorthalidone, since chlorthalidone 12.5-25 mg per day appears to have more antihypertensive efficacy than hydrochlorothiazide 25-50 mg per day, especially throughout the 24-hour dosing period.[119]

6. Prevention of High Blood Pressure and Diabetes as Approaches to Control Complications

Prevention of diabetes and high blood pressure may be the most effective long-term approaches to preventing highbloodpressure-related events in patients with diabetes. The Finnish Diabetes Study[120] and the Diabetes Prevention Program[121] provide strong evidence that lifestyle-change approaches to promote healthy diet and increased physical activity can reduce the risk of diabetes by more than 50%. The Dietary Approaches to Stop Hypertension trial provides strong evidence that similar lifestyle changes can reduce blood pressure levels.[122] In the long-term, it may be much more effective to promote lifestyle change approaches than to attempt to medicate the >60 million Americans with hypertension[2] and the >20 million Americans with diabetes.[123] Although there are currently no long-term studies indicating that prevention of diabetes and hypertension is sustainable, or that short-term prevention translates into reduced morbidity or mortality attributable to either disease, trends in blood pressure and diabetes reflect the importance of societal influences on diet, physical activity and adiposity in populations. Greater attention should be placed on understanding and improving these influences on health. Until efforts to prevent high blood pressure and diabetes are more effective, efforts to improve the quality of medical care will remain crucial to the control of diabetes- and high blood pressure-related complications.

7. References

1. Imperatore G, Cadwell BL, Geiss L, et al. Thirty-year trends in cardiovascular risk factor levels among US adults with diabetes: National Health and Nutrition Examination Surveys, 1971-2000. *Am J Epidemiol.* 2004;160:531-539.

2. Fields LE, Burt VL, Cutler JA, Hughes J, Roccella EJ, Sorlie P. The burden of adult hypertension in the United States 1999 to 2000: a rising tide. *Hypertension.* 2004;44:398-404.

3. Wang W, Lee ET, Fabsitz RR, et al. A longitudinal study of hypertension risk factors and their relation to cardiovascular disease: the Strong Heart Study. *Hypertension.* 2006;47:403-409.

4. Goff DC Jr, Zaccaro DJ, Haffner SM, Saad MF. Insulin sensitivity and the risk of incident hypertension: insights from the Insulin Resistance Atherosclerosis Study. *Diabetes Care.* 2003;26:805-809.

5. Liese AD, Mayer-Davis EJ, Chambless LE, et al. Elevated fasting insulin predicts incident hypertension: the ARIC study. Atherosclerosis Risk in Communities Study Investigators. *J Hypertens.* 1999;17:1169-1177.

6. Dyer AR, Liu K, Walsh M, Kiefe C, Jacobs DR Jr, Bild DE. Ten-year incidence of elevated blood pressure and its predictors: the CARDIA study. Coronary Artery Risk Development in (Young) Adults. *J Hum.Hypertens.* 1999;13:13-21.

7. Salonen JT, Lakka TA, Lakka HM, Valkonen VP, Everson SA, Kaplan GA. Hyperinsulinemia is associated with the incidence of hypertension and dyslipidemia in middle-aged men. *Diabetes.* 1998;47:270-275.

8. Suzuki M, Kimura Y, Tsushima M, Harano Y. Association of insulin resistance with salt sensitivity and nocturnal fall of blood pressure. *Hypertension.* 2000;35:864-868.

9. Brett SE, Ritter JM, Chowienczyk PJ. Diastolic blood pressure changes during exercise positively correlate with serum cholesterol and insulin resistance. *Circulation.* 2000;101:611-615.

10. Phillips RA, Krakoff LR, Dunaif A, Finegood DT, Gorlin R, Shimabukuro S. Relation among left ventricular mass, insulin resistance, and blood pressure in nonobese subjects. *J Clin Endocrinol Metab.* 1998;83:4284-4288.

11. Thom T, Haase N, Rosamond W, et al. Heart disease and stroke statistics--2006 update: a report from the American Heart Association Statistics Committee and Stroke Statistics Subcommittee. *Circulation.* 2006; 113:e85-e151.

12. Kannel WB, Schwartz MJ, McNamara PM. Blood pressure and risk of coronary heart disease: the Framingham study. *Dis Chest.* 1969;56:43-52.

13. The Pooling Project Research Group. Relationship of blood pressure, serum cholesterol, smoking habit, relative weight and ECG abnormalities to incidence of major coronary events: final report of the pooling project. The pooling project research group. *J Chronic Dis.* 1978;31:201-306.

14. Kannel WB, Wolf P, Dawber TR. Hypertension and cardiac impairments increase stroke risk. *Geriatrics.* 1978;33:71-73.

15. Stamler J, Vaccaro O, Neaton JD, Wentworth D. Diabetes, other risk factors, and 12-yr cardiovascular mortality for men screened in the Multiple Risk Factor Intervention Trial. *Diabetes Care.* 1993;16:434-444.

16. MacMahon S, Peto R, Cutler J, et al. Blood pressure, stroke, and coronary heart disease. Part 1, Prolonged differences in blood pressure: prospective observational studies corrected for the regression dilution bias. *Lancet.* 1990;335:765-774.

17. Adler AI, Stratton IM, Neil HA, et al. Association of systolic blood pressure with macrovascular and microvascular complications of type 2 diabetes (UKPDS 36): prospective observational study. *BMJ*. 2000;321:412-419.

18. Chobanian AV, Bakris GL, Black HR, et al. The Seventh Report of the Joint National Committee on Prevention, Detection, Evaluation, and Treatment of High Blood Pressure: the JNC 7 report. *JAMA*. 2003;289:2560-2572.

19. Wolf PA, Kannel WB, Verter J. Current status of risk factors for stroke. *Neurol Clin*. 1983;1:317-343.

20. Wolf PA, D'Agostino RB, Belanger AJ, Kannel WB. Probability of stroke: a risk profile from the Framingham Study. *Stroke*. 1991;22:312-318.

21. Salonen JT, Puska P, Tuomilehto J, Homan K. Relation of blood pressure, serum lipids, and smoking to the risk of cerebral stroke. A longitudinal study in Eastern Finland. *Stroke*. 1982;13:327-333.

22. Abbott RD, Donahue RP, MacMahon SW, Reed DM, Yano K. Diabetes and the risk of stroke. The Honolulu Heart Program. *JAMA*. 1987;257:949-952.

23. Davis PH, Dambrosia JM, Schoenberg BS, et al. Risk factors for ischemic stroke: a prospective study in Rochester, Minnesota. *Ann Neurol*. 1987;22:319-327.

24. Hu G, Sarti C, Jousilahti P, et al. The impact of history of hypertension and type 2 diabetes at baseline on the incidence of stroke and stroke mortality. *Stroke*. 2005;36:2538-2543.

25. Bertoni AG, Hundley WG, Massing MW, Bonds DE, Burke GL, Goff DC Jr. Heart failure prevalence, incidence, and mortality in the elderly with diabetes. *Diabetes Care*. 2004;27:699-703.

26. Kannel WB. Epidemiology and prevention of cardiac failure: Framingham Study insights. *Eur Heart J*. 1987;8 (suppl F):23-26.

27. Haider AW, Larson MG, Franklin SS, Levy D. Systolic blood pressure, diastolic blood pressure, and pulse pressure as predictors of risk for congestive heart failure in the Framingham Heart Study. *Ann Intern Med*. 2003;138:10-16.

28. Iribarren C, Karter AJ, Go AS, et al. Glycemic control and heart failure among adult patients with diabetes. *Circulation*. 2001;103:2668-2673.

29. US Renal Data System. USRDS 2003 *Annual Data Report: Atlas of End-Stage Renal Disease in the United States*. Bethesda, MD: National Institutes of Health, National Institute of Diabetes and Digestive and Kidney Diseases; 2003

30. Humphrey LL, Ballard DJ, Frohnert PP, Chu CP, O'Fallon WM, Palumbo PJ. Chronic renal failure in non-insulin-dependent diabetes mellitus. A population-based study in Rochester, Minnesota. *Ann Intern Med*. 1989;111:788-796.

31. Brancati FL, Whelton PK, Randall BL, Neaton JD, Stamler J, Klag MJ. Risk of end-stage renal disease in diabetes mellitus: a prospective cohort study of men screened for MRFIT. Multiple Risk Factor Intervention Trial. *JAMA*. 1997;278:2069-2074.

32. Lee ET, Lee VS, Lu M, Lee JS, Russell D, Yeh J. Incidence of renal failure in NIDDM. The Oklahoma Indian Diabetes Study. *Diabetes*. 1994;43:572-579.

33. Klag MJ, Whelton PK, Randall BL, et al. Blood pressure and end-stage renal disease in men. *N Engl J Med*. 1996;334:13-18.

34. Fox CS, Larson MG, Leip EP, Culleton B, Wilson PW, Levy D. Predictors of new-onset kidney disease in a community-based population. *JAMA*. 2004;291:844-850.

35. Klein R, Klein BE. Diabetic eye disease. *Lancet*. 1997;350:197-204.

36. Leske MC, Wu SY, Hennis A, et al. Hyperglycemia, blood pressure, and the 9-year incidence of diabetic retinopathy: the Barbados Eye Studies. *Ophthalmology*. 2005;112:799-805.

37. Knowler WC, Bennett PH, Ballintine EJ. Increased incidence of retinopathy in diabetics with elevated blood pressure. A six-year follow-up study in Pima Indians. *New Engl J Med*. 1980;302:645-650.

38. Agardh E, Agardh CD, Koul S, Torffvit O. A four-year follow-up study on the incidence of diabetic retinopathy in older onset diabetes mellitus. *Diabetic Medicine*. 1994; 11:273-278.

39. Dowse GK, Humphrey AR, Collins VR, et al. Prevalence and risk factors for diabetic retinopathy in the multiethnic population of Mauritius. *Am J Epidemiol*. 1998; 147:448-457.

40. Teuscher A, Schnell H, Wilson PW. Incidence of diabetic retinopathy and relationship to baseline plasma glucose and blood pressure. *Diabetes Care*. 1988;11:246-251.

41. Janghorbani M, Jones RB, Murray KJ, Allison SP. Incidence of and risk factors for diabetic retinopathy in diabetic clinic attenders. *Ophthalmic Epidemiology*. 2001;8:309-325.

42. Tudor SM, Hamman RF, Baron A, Johnson DW, Shetterly SM. Incidence and progression of diabetic retinopathy in Hispanics and non-Hispanic whites with type 2 diabetes. San Luis Valley Diabetes Study, Colorado. *Diabetes Care*. 1998;21:53-61.

43. West KM, Ahuja MM, Bennett PH, et al. Interrelationships of microangiopathy, plasma glucose and other risk factors in 3583 diabetic patients: a multinational study. *Diabetologia* 1982;22:412-420.

44. Maser RE, Pfeifer MA, Dorman JS, Kuller LH, Becker DJ, Orchard TJ. Diabetic autonomic neuropathy and cardiovascular risk. Pittsburgh Epidemiology of Diabetes Complications Study III. *Arch Intern Med* 1990;150:1218-1222.

45. Forrest KY, Maser RE, Pambianco G, Becker DJ, Orchard TJ. Hypertension as a risk factor for diabetic neuropathy: a prospective study. *Diabetes*. 1997;46:665-670.

46. Tesfaye S, Chaturvedi N, Eaton SE, et al. Vascular risk factors and diabetic neuropathy. *N Engl J Med*. 2005;352:341-350.

47. Cohen JA, Jeffers BW, Faldut D, Marcoux M, Schrier RW. Risks for sensorimotor peripheral neuropathy and autonomic neuropathy in non-insulin-dependent diabetes mellitus (NIDDM). *Muscle Nerve*. 1998;21:72-80.

48. Sands ML, Shetterly SM, Franklin GM, Hamman RF. Incidence of distal symmetric (sensory) neuropathy in NIDDM. The San Luis Valley Diabetes Study. *Diabetes Care*. 1997;20:322-329.

49. Department of Veterans Affairs. Office of Quality and Performance. Diabetes mellitus: clinical practice guideline. 2003.

50. Borhani NO, Applegate WB, Cutler JA, et al. Systolic Hypertension in the Elderly Program (SHEP). Part 1: Rationale and design. *Hypertension*. 1991;17:II2-II15.

51. Prevention of stroke by antihypertensive drug treatment in older persons with isolated systolic hypertension. Final results of the Systolic Hypertension in the Elderly Program (SHEP). SHEP Cooperative Research Group. *JAMA*. 1991;265:3255-3264.

52. Curb JD, Pressel SL, Cutler JA, et al. Effect of diuretic-based antihypertensive treatment on cardiovascular disease risk in older diabetic patients with isolated systolic hypertension. Systolic Hypertension in the Elderly Program Cooperative Research Group. *JAMA*. 1996;276:1886-1892.

53. Amery A, Birkenhager W, Bulpitt CJ, et al for Syst-Eur. A multicentre trial on the treatment of isolated systolic hypertension in the elderly: objectives, protocol, and organization. *Aging (Milano.)* 1991;3:287-302.

54. Staessen JA, Fagard R, Thijs L, et al. Randomised double-blind comparison of placebo and active treatment for older patients with isolated systolic hypertension. The Systolic Hypertension in Europe (Syst-Eur) Trial Investigators. *Lancet*. 1997;350:757-764.

55. Tuomilehto J, Rastenyte D, Birkenhager WH, et al. Effects of calcium-channel blockade in older patients with diabetes and systolic hypertension. Systolic Hypertension in Europe Trial Investigators. *N Engl J Med*. 1999;340:677-684.

56. Hansson L. The Hypertension Optimal Treatment study (the HOT study). *Blood Pressure*. 1993;2:62-68.

57. Hansson L, Zanchetti A, Carruthers SG. Effects of intensive blood-pressure lowering and low-dose aspirin in patients with hypertension: principal results of the Hypertension Optimal Treatment (HOT) randomised trial. *Lancet*. 1998;351:1755-1762.

58. Zanchetti A, Hansson L, Clement D, et al. Benefits and risks of more intensive blood pressure lowering in hypertensive patients of the HOT study with different risk profiles: does a J-shaped curve exist in smokers? *J Hypertens*. 2003;21:797-804.

59. UKPDS Study Group. Tight blood pressure control and risk of macrovascular and microvascular complications in type 2 diabetes: UKPDS 38. UK Prospective Diabetes Study Group. *BMJ*. 1998;317:703-713.

60. Holman RR, Paul SK, Bethel MA, Neil HA, Matthews DR. Long-term follow-up after tight control of blood pressure in type 2 diabetes. *N Engl J Med*. 2008;359:1565-1576.

61. Schrier RW, Estacio RO, Jeffers B. Appropriate Blood Pressure Control in NIDDM (ABCD) Trial. *Diabetologia* 1996;39:1646-1654.

62. Estacio RO, Jeffers BW, Hiatt WR, Biggerstaff SL, Gifford N, Schrier RW. The effect of nisoldipine as compared with enalapril on cardiovascular outcomes in patients with non-insulin-dependent diabetes and hypertension. *N Engl J Med*. 1998;338:645-652.

63. Estacio RO, Jeffers BW, Gifford N, Schrier RW. Effect of blood pressure control on diabetic microvascular complications in patients with hypertension and type 2 diabetes. *Diabetes Care*. 2000;23 (suppl 2):B54-B64.

64. Patel A, MacMahon S, Chalmers J, et al. Effects of a fixed combination of perindopril and indapamide on macrovascular and microvascular outcomes in patients with type 2 diabetes mellitus (the ADVANCE trial): a randomised controlled trial. *Lancet*. 2007;370:829-840.

65. de Galan BE, Perkovic V, Ninomiya T, et al. Lowering blood pressure reduces renal events in type 2 diabetes. *J Am Soc Nephrol*. 2009;20:883-892.

66. Howard BV, Roman MJ, Devereux RB, et al. Effect of lower targets for blood pressure and LDL cholesterol on atherosclerosis in diabetes: the SANDS randomized trial. *JAMA*. 2008;299:1678-1689.

67. Goff DC Jr, Gerstein HC, Ginsberg HN, et al. Prevention of cardiovascular disease in persons with type 2 diabetes mellitus: current knowledge and rationale for the Action to Control Cardiovascular Risk in Diabetes (ACCORD) trial. *Am J Cardiol*. 2007;99:4i-20i.

68. Cushman WC, Grimm RH Jr, Cutler JA, et al. Rationale and design for the blood pressure intervention of the Action to Control Cardiovascular Risk in Diabetes (ACCORD) trial. *Am J Cardiol*. 2007;99:44i-55i.

69. Buse JB, Bigger JT, Byington RP, et al. Action to Control Cardiovascular Risk in Diabetes (ACCORD) trial: design and methods. *Am J Cardiol*. 2007;99:21i-33i.

70. Psaty BM, Lumley T, Furberg CD, et al. Health outcomes associated with various antihypertensive therapies used as first-line agents: a network meta-analysis. *JAMA*. 2003;289:2534-2544.

71. Blood Pressure Lowering Treatment Trialists' Collaboration. Effects of different blood-pressure-lowering regimens on major cardiovascular events: results of prospectively-designed overviews of randomised trials. *Lancet*. 2003;362:1527-1535.

72. Turnbull F, Neal B, Algert C, et al. Effects of different blood pressure-lowering regimens on major cardiovascular events in individuals with and without diabetes mellitus: results of prospectively designed overviews of randomized trials. *Arch Intern Med*. 2005;165:1410-1419.

73. ALLHAT Collaborative Research Group. Diuretic versus alpha-blocker as first-step antihypertensive therapy: final results from the Antihypertensive and Lipid-Lowering Treatment to Prevent Heart Attack Trial (ALLHAT). *Hypertension* 2003;42:239-246.

74. Barzilay JI, Davis BR, Bettencourt J, et al. Cardiovascular outcomes using doxazosin vs. chlorthalidone for the treatment of hypertension in older adults with and without glucose disorders: a report from the ALLHAT study. *J Clin Hypertens* (Greenwich). 2004;6:116-125.

75. ALLHAT Collaborative Research Group. Major outcomes in high-risk hypertensive patients randomized to angiotensin-converting enzyme inhibitor or calcium channel blocker vs diuretic: The Antihypertensive and Lipid-Lowering Treatment to Prevent Heart Attack Trial (ALLHAT). *JAMA*. 2002;288:2981-2997.

76. Whelton PK, Barzilay J, Cushman WC, et al. Clinical outcomes in antihypertensive treatment of type 2 diabetes, impaired fasting glucose concentration, and normoglycemia: Antihypertensive and Lipid-Lowering Treatment to Prevent Heart Attack Trial (ALLHAT). *Arch Intern Med*. 2005;165:1401-1409.

77. Rahman M, Pressel S, Davis BR, et al. Renal outcomes in high-risk hypertensive patients treated with an angiotensin-converting enzyme inhibitor or a calcium channel blocker vs a diuretic: a report from the Antihypertensive and Lipid-Lowering Treatment to Prevent Heart Attack Trial (ALLHAT). *Arch Intern Med*. 2005;165:936-946.

78. Wing LMH, Reid CM, Ryan P, et al and the Second Australian National Blood Pressure Study Group. A comparison of outcomes with angiotensin-converting-enzyme inhibitors and diuretics for hypertension in the elderly. *New Engl J Med*. 2003;348:583-592.

79. Dahlof B, Sever PS, Poulter NR, et al. Prevention of cardiovascular events with an antihypertensive regimen of amlodipine adding perindopril as required versus atenolol adding bendroflumethiazide as required, in the Anglo-Scandinavian Cardiac Outcomes Trial-Blood Pressure Lowering Arm (ASCOT-BPLA): a multicentre randomised controlled trial. *Lancet*. 2005;366:895-906.

80. Marre M, Chatellier G, Leblanc H, Guyene TT, Menard J, Passa P. Prevention of diabetic nephropathy with enalapril in normotensive diabetics with microalbuminuria. *BMJ*. 1988;297:1092-1095.

81. Flack JR, Molyneaux L, Willey K, Yue DK. Regression of microalbuminuria: results of a controlled study, indapamide versus captopril. *J Cardiovasc Pharmacol*. 1993;22 (suppl 6):S75-S77.

82. Hallab M, Gallois Y, Chatellier G, Rohmer V, Fressinaud P, Marre M. Comparison of reduction in microalbuminuria by enalapril and hydrochlorothiazide in normotensive patients with insulin dependent diabetes. *BMJ*. 1993;306:175-182.

83. Ravid M, Savin H, Jutrin I, Bental T, Lang R, Lishner M. Long-term effect of ACE inhibition on development of nephropathy in diabetes mellitus type II. *Kidney Int Suppl*. 1994;45:S161-S164.

84. Sano T, Kawamura T, Matsumae H, et al. Effects of long-term enalapril treatment on persistent micro-albuminuria in well-controlled hypertensive and normotensive NIDDM patients. *Diabetes Care*. 1994;17:420-424.

85. Trevisan R, Tiengo A. Effect of low-dose ramipril on microalbuminuria in normotensive or mild hypertensive non-insulin-dependent diabetic patients. North-East Italy Microalbuminuria Study Group. *Am J Hypertens*. 1995;8:876-883.

86. Crepaldi G, Carraro A, Brocco E, et al. Hypertension and non-insulin-dependent diabetes. A comparison between an angiotensin-converting enzyme inhibitor and a calcium antagonist. *Acta Diabetol*. 1995;32:203-208.

87. Velussi M, Brocco E, Frigato F, et al. Effects of cilazapril and amlodipine on kidney function in hypertensive NIDDM patients. *Diabetes* 1996;45:216-222.

88. Sano T, Hotta N, Kawamura T, et al. Effects of long-term enalapril treatment on persistent microalbuminuria in normotensive type 2 diabetic patients: results of a 4-year, prospective, randomized study. *Diabet Med*. 1996;13:120-124.

89. Ravid M, Lang R, Rachmani R, Lishner M. Long-term renoprotective effect of angiotensin-converting enzyme inhibition in non-insulin-dependent diabetes mellitus. A 7-year follow-up study. *Arch Intern Med*. 1996;156:286-289.

90. Donnelly R, Molyneaux LM, Willey KA, Yue DK. Comparative effects of indapamide and captopril on blood pressure and albumin excretion rate in diabetic microalbuminuria. *Am J Cardiol*. 1996;77:26B-30B.

91. Pinol C, Cobos A, Cases A, et al. Nitrendipine and enalapril in the treatment of diabetic hypertensive patients with microalbuminuria. *Kidney Int Suppl*. 1996;55:S85-S87.

92. Schnack C, Hoffmann W, Hopmeier P, Schernthaner G. Renal and metabolic effects of 1-year treatment with ramipril or atenolol in NIDDM patients with microalbuminuria. *Diabetologia* 1996;39:1611-1616.

93. Ahmad J, Siddiqui MA, Ahmad H. Effective postponement of diabetic nephropathy with enalapril in normotensive type 2 diabetic patients with microalbuminuria. *Diabetes Care* 1997;20:1576-1581.

94. Ravid M, Brosh D, Levi Z, Bar-Dayan Y, Ravid D, Rachmani R. Use of enalapril to attenuate decline in renal function in normotensive, normoalbuminuric patients with type 2 diabetes mellitus. A randomized, controlled trial. *Ann Intern Med* 1998;128:982-988.

95. Mogensen CE, Neldam S, Tikkanen I, et al. Randomised controlled trial of dual blockade of renin-angiotensin system in patients with hypertension, microalbuminuria, and non-insulin dependent diabetes: the candesartan and lisinopril microalbuminuria (CALM) study. *BMJ* 2000;321:1440-1444.

96. Deerochanawong C, Kornthong P, Phongwiratchai S, Serirat S. Effects on urinary albumin excretion and renal function changes by delapril and manidipine in normotensive type 2 diabetic patients with microalbuminuria. *J Med Assoc Thai*. 2001;84:234-241.

97. Parving HH, Lehnert H, Brochner-Mortensen J, Gomis R, Andersen S, Arner P. The effect of irbesartan on the development of diabetic nephropathy in patients with type 2 diabetes. *N Engl J Med*. 2001;345:870-878.

98. Tutuncu NB, Gurlek A, Gedik O. Efficacy of ACE inhibitors and ATII receptor blockers in patients with microalbuminuria: a prospective study. *Acta Diabetol*. 2001;38:157-161.

99. Bakris GL, Smith AC, Richardson DJ, et al. Impact of an ACE inhibitor and calcium antagonist on microalbuminuria and lipid subfractions in type 2 diabetes: a randomised, multi-centre pilot study. *J Hum Hypertens*. 2002;16:185-191.

100. Tan KC, Chow WS, Ai VH, Lam KS. Effects of angiotensin II receptor antagonist on endothelial vasomotor function and urinary albumin excretion in type 2 diabetic patients with microalbuminuria. *Diabetes Metab Res Rev*. 2002;18:71-76.

101. Viberti G, Wheeldon NM. Microalbuminuria reduction with valsartan in patients with type 2 diabetes mellitus: a blood pressure-independent effect. *Circulation*. 2002;106:672-678.

102. Sasso FC, Carbonara O, Persico M, et al. Irbesartan reduces the albumin excretion rate in microalbuminuric type 2 diabetic patients independently of hypertension: a randomized double-blind placebo-controlled crossover study. *Diabetes Care* 2002;25:1909-1913.

103. Fogari R, Preti P, Zoppi A, et al. Effects of amlodipine fosinopril combination on microalbuminuria in hypertensive type 2 diabetic patients. *Am J Hypertens*. 2002;15:1042-1049.

104. Zandbergen AA, Baggen MG, Lamberts SW, Bootsma AH, de Zeeuw D, Ouwendijk RJ. Effect of losartan on microalbuminuria in normotensive patients with type 2 diabetes mellitus. A randomized clinical trial. *Ann Intern Med* 2003;139:90-96.

105. Marre M, Puig JG, Kokot F, et al. Equivalence of indapamide SR and enalapril on microalbuminuria reduction in hypertensive patients with type 2 diabetes: the NESTOR Study. *J Hypertens*. 2004;22:1613-1622.

106. Jerums G, Allen TJ, Campbell DJ, et al. Long-term renoprotection by perindopril or nifedipine in non-hypertensive patients with Type 2 diabetes and microalbuminuria. *Diabet Med*. 2004;21:1192-1199.

107. Ruggenenti P, Fassi A, Ilieva AP, et al. Preventing microalbuminuria in type 2 diabetes. *N Engl J Med*. 2004;351:1941-1951.

108. Dalla VM, Pozza G, Mosca A, et al. Effect of lercanidipine compared with ramipril on albumin excretion rate in hypertensive Type 2 diabetic patients with microalbuminuria: DIAL study (diabete, ipertensione, albuminuria, lercanidipina). *Diabetes Nutr Metab*. 2004;17:259-266.

109. Rossing K, Christensen PK, Jensen BR, Parving HH. Dual blockade of the renin-angiotensin system in diabetic nephropathy: a randomized double-blind crossover study. *Diabetes Care*. 2002;25:95-100.

110. Lewis EJ, Hunsicker LG, Clarke WR, et al. Renoprotective effect of the angiotensin-receptor antagonist irbesartan in patients with nephropathy due to type 2 diabetes. *N Engl J Med*. 2001;345:851-860.

111. Matos JP, de Lourdes RM, Ismerim VL, Boasquevisque EM, Genelhu V, Francischetti EA. Effects of dual blockade of the renin angiotensin system in hypertensive type 2 diabetic patients with nephropathy. *Clin Nephrol*. 2005;64:180-189.

112. Hansson L, Lindholm LH, Niskanen L, et al. Effect of angiotensin-converting-enzyme inhibition compared with conventional therapy on cardiovascular morbidity and mortality in hypertension: the Captopril Prevention Project (CAPPP) randomised trial. *Lancet*. 1999;353:611-616.

113. Niklason A, Hedner T, Niskanen L, Lanke J. Development of diabetes is retarded by ACE inhibition in hypertensive patients--a sub-analysis of the Captopril Prevention Project (CAPPP). *J Hypertens*. 2004;22:645-652.

114. The Heart Outcomes Prevention Evaluation Study Investigators. Effects of an angiotensin-converting-enzyme inhibitor, ramipril, on cardiovascular events in high-risk patients. *New Engl J Med*. 2000;342:145-153.

115. Bosch J, Yusuf S, Gerstein HC, et al. Effect of ramipril on the incidence of diabetes. *N Engl J Med*. 2006;355:1551-1562.

116. Dahlof B, Devereux RB, Kjeldsen SE, et al. Cardiovascular morbidity and mortality in the Losartan Intervention For Endpoint reduction in hypertension study (LIFE): a randomised trial against atenolol. *Lancet*. 2002;359:995-1003.

117. Olsen MH, Fossum E, Hoieggen A, et al. Long-term treatment with losartan versus atenolol improves insulin sensitivity in hypertension: ICARUS, a LIFE substudy. *J Hypertens*. 2005;23:891-898.

118. Kostis JB, Wilson AC, Freudenberger RS, Cosgrove NM, Pressel SL, Davis BR. Long-term effect of diuretic-based therapy on fatal outcomes in subjects with isolated systolic hypertension with and without diabetes. *Am J Cardiol*. 2005;95:29-35.

119. Ernst ME, Carter BL, Goerdt CJ, et al. Comparative antihypertensive effects of hydrochlorothiazide and chlorthalidone on ambulatory and office blood pressure. *Hypertension*. 2006;47:352-358.

120. Tuomilehto J, Lindstrom J, Eriksson JG, et al. Prevention of type 2 diabetes mellitus by changes in lifestyle among subjects with impaired glucose tolerance. *N Engl J Med*. 2001;344:1343-1350.

121. Knowler WC, Barrett-Connor E, Fowler SE, et al. Reduction in the incidence of type 2 diabetes with lifestyle intervention or metformin. *N Engl J Med*. 2002;346:393-403.

122. Appel LJ, Moore TJ, Obarzanek E, et al. A clinical trial of the effects of dietary patterns on blood pressure. DASH Collaborative Research Group. *N Engl J Med*. 1997;336:1117-1124.

123. Centers for Disease Control and Prevention. National Center for Chronic Disease Prevention and Health Promotion. National Estimates on Diabetes. Available at http://www.cdc.gov/diabetes/pubs/estimates05.htm#prev. Accessed May 5, 2009.

Chapter 10: Diabetic Dyslipidemia

Gissette Soffer, MD
Henry N. Ginsberg, MD

Contents

1. Introduction

Diabetes mellitus is associated with a 3- to 4-fold increase in risk for coronary heart disease (CHD).[22] The increase in risk is particularly evident in younger age groups and in women: females with type 2 diabetes (T2DM) appear to lose a great deal of the protection that characterizes females without T2DM. Furthermore, patients with T2DM have 50% greater in-hospital mortality and a 2-fold increased rate of death within 2 years of surviving a myocardial infarction (MI). Older patients with diabetes, and those with T2DM for more than 10 years who have not had a CHD event, have the same risk for CHD as those without diabetes who have not had a CHD event. Overall, CHD is the leading cause of death in individuals with diabetes who are over the age of 35 years.

Although a significant portion of this increased risk is associated with the presence of well-characterized risk factors for CHD, including hypertension and hypercholesterolemia, a significant proportion of the increased risk remains unexplained. Patients with diabetes, particularly those with T2DM, have a characteristic dyslipidemia, with increased plasma triglyceride levels, decreased levels of high density lipoprotein (HDL) cholesterol and cholesteryl ester-depleted, small low-density lipoproteins (LDL). These abnormalities are 2-3 times more likely to be present in patients with T2DM than in those without diabetes. These same alterations in plasma lipids are commonly seen in patients with insulin resistance and/or the Metabolic Syndrome. Patients with poorly controlled type 1 diabetes can also have a dyslipidemic pattern, although this is much less common, and probably occurs on a background of insulin resistance or the Metabolic Syndrome. Several large clinical trials have shown that reductions in the levels of LDL cholesterol and plasma triglycerides, and/or increases in the levels of HDL cholesterol, are associated with reduced rates of CHD events. There is now strong evidence that health care professionals caring for patients with diabetes should treat lipid abnormalities aggressively.

This review will provide a brief pathophysiological basis for the dyslipidemia commonly present in patients with diabetes, and then review the clinical trial evidence available to direct various treatment approaches. Because of the greater prevalence of lipid abnormalities in T2DM, most of the emphasis in this review will focus on that group of patients.

2. Lipoprotein Structure

Lipoproteins are spherical, macromolecular complexes carrying various lipids and proteins in plasma.[13] The hydrophobic triglyceride and cholesteryl ester molecules comprise the core of the lipoproteins, and this core is covered by amphipathic (both hydrophobic and hydrophilic) phospholipids and proteins. Hundreds to thousands of triglyceride and cholesteryl ester molecules are carried in the core of different lipoproteins. Apolipoproteins are the proteins on the surface of the lipoproteins. They help to solubilize the core lipids and play critical roles in the regulation of plasma lipid and lipoprotein transport. Apolipoprotein (apo) B100 is required for the secretion of hepatic-derived, very low density lipoproteins (VLDL) and LDL. Apo B48 is a truncated form of apoB-100, that is produced by editing of the mRNA for apoB in the intestine. ApoB48 is required for secretion of chylomicrons from the small intestine. Apo A-I is the major structural protein in HDL and is required for the generation of mature HDL particles in the circulation. Other apolipoproteins will be discussed in the context of their roles in lipoprotein metabolism.

3. Metabolism in Diabetes

Abnormal Chylomicron Metabolism

Dietary fat (triglyceride) and cholesterol are absorbed into the cells of the small intestine and are incorporated into the core of nascent chylomicrons, which traverse the lymphatic system and enter the circulation via the thoracic duct at the superior vena cava. In the capillary beds of adipose tissue and muscle, chylomicrons interact with the enzyme lipoprotein lipase (LpL) and the chylomicron core triglyceride is hydrolyzed. ApoC-II is the necessary activator of LpL, while apoC-III inhibits this enzyme. ApoC-III, whose production is increased in individuals with insulin resistance, probably plays a very important role in the dyslipidemia of T2DM. A very recently discovered apolipoprotein, apoA-V, facilitates LpL activity and appears to be an important determinant of population triglyceride levels. The fatty acids that are liberated from chylomicron triglycerides are mostly taken up locally by fat cells, where they are made back into triglyceride, or by muscle cells, where they can be used for energy. Some of the liberated fatty acids can travel to the liver. Chylomicron remnants, products of this lipolytic process that have lost ~75%-85% of the triglyceride, interact with several receptor pathways on hepatocytes, and are removed from the circulation by the liver. Hepatic lipase (HL), which hydrolyzes chylomicron remnant triglycerides, also plays a role in remnant removal.

Several defects in chylomicron and chylomicron remnant metabolism have been observed in patients with T2DM. First, studies in diabetic hamsters suggest increased production of apoB48, leading to increased numbers of chylomicrons being secreted; this finding has recently been confirmed in humans with T2DM.[10] Importantly, LpL may be modestly reduced in patients with T2DM, even when glycemic control is adequate; thus there will be less than optimal LpL activity available to process increased numbers of chylomicrons. Furthermore, although chylomicron remnant clearance is impaired, defects in hepatic LDL or LDL-related protein receptors, which are both active in removing chylomicron remnants, do not seem to be common in T2DM. The role of HL in the defective chylomicron metabolism in T2DM is also unclear; HL is often increased in hypertriglyceridemic, insulin-resistant individuals. Recent studies indicate that heparin sulfate proteoglycans on the hepatocyte surface play a key role in remnant lipoprotein uptake by the liver, and their production may be reduced in T2DM. Patients with well-controlled type 1 diabetes usually have normal fasting and postprandial triglyceride levels. In uncontrolled type 1 diabetes, however, LpL can be significantly reduced and marked postprandial lipemia has been observed. In most of these cases, however, a partial genetic defect in LpL synthesis or function, or genetic alterations in other genes involved in LpL action (apoC-III or apoA-V) probably played key roles, together with insulin deficiency. It is important to realize that if fasting levels of VLDL triglycerides are elevated, postprandial triglycerides will also be elevated, as they compete for many of the same metabolic pathways (see below).[15]

Abnormal VLDL Metabolism

The liver is the site of VLDL assembly. The core of the VLDL is comprised of triglycerides and cholesteryl esters. ApoB-100 (1 per particle), free (unesterified) cholesterol and phospholipids form the surface of VLDL. The *purpose* for VLDL production may be to remove excess energy, in the form of triglycerides, from the liver. There are several abnormalities in lipid metabolism that are likely contributors to the increased production of hepatic triglyceride-rich VLDL in T2DM. Increased flow of fatty acids to the liver from insulin-resistant adipose tissue, particularly during the postprandial period when increased plasma insulin levels normally inhibit adipose tissue lipolysis, hepatic uptake of triglyceride-enriched chylomicron and VLDL remnants (see below), and increased fatty acid synthesis from glucose (*de novo* lipogenesis) in the liver, can all stimulate the assembly and secretion of triglyceride-rich VLDL (Figure 1). It is important to remember that the liver can secrete both increased numbers of VLDL particles and particles with more TG on them (larger particles). Abnormalities of cholesterol metabolism, with excess hepatic cholesterol synthesis, may also contribute to the overproduction of VLDL; in this instance, depending on the availability of hepatic triglyceride, increased cholesterol in the liver may cause secretion of triglyceride-depleted lipoproteins, such as intermediate density lipoproteins (IDL) or LDL.

Figure 1

Substrate driving forces

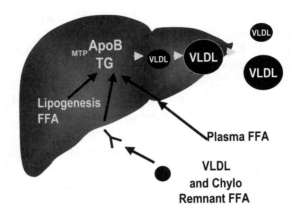

Substrate driving forces for the assembly and secretion of apoB-lipoproteins. Fatty acids released from the peripheral adipose tissue, VLDL and chylomicron remnants carrying triglyceride, and *de novo* synthesis in the liver of fatty acids all contribute to the formation of VLDL that are secreted by the liver. In insulin resistance and T2DM, more fatty acids are released from insulin-resistant fat cells, slightly lower LpL in the peripheral fat tissue leads to triglyceride-enriched remnant lipoproteins that are taken up by the liver, and more *de novo* synthesis of fatty acids in the liver all stimulate the assembly and secretion of VLDL.

Once in the plasma, VLDL triglyceride is hydrolyzed by LpL, generating smaller and denser VLDL, and then VLDL remnants, also called IDL. Small VLDL and IDL are similar to chylomicron remnants, except that VLDL remnants, in addition to removal by the liver, can undergo further plasma catabolism to become LDL. As in the case of chylomicron metabolism, LpL activity plays an important role for normal functioning of the metabolic cascade from VLDL to remnants to LDL; apoC-II, apoC-III and apoA-V are important for LpL interaction with VLDL. However, LpL activity is usually only mildly reduced (if at all) in patients with T2DM. Once the remnants have been formed, HL, apoE (another surface apolipoprotein that interacts with both the LDL receptor and the LDL receptor-related protein or LRP) and LDL receptors play important roles in remnant removal. As noted above for chylomicrons, heparin sulfate proteoglycans on the surface of hepatocytes probably also play a role in remnant removal.[4] Regulation of the process, whereby VLDL remnants and IDL are either taken up by the liver or converted to LDL, is poorly defined. In normal individuals, 50%-70% of VLDL are converted to LDL; in patients with hypertriglyceridemia, this conversion is less efficient. Once LDL is generated, apoB-100, the sole protein on its surface, is the ligand for the LDL receptor; apoB-100 does not interact with LRP. The concentration of LDL in plasma is determined by both the production of LDL and the availability of LDL receptors (Figure 2).

People with T2DM commonly have increased plasma levels of triglyceride, which equates to increased numbers of larger VLDL particles. In population studies, levels of triglyceride greater than the 90th percentile for individuals without T2DM are 2-3 times more common in individuals with T2DM. Overproduction of VLDL, with increased secretion of both triglyceride and apoB-100, seems to be the common etiology of the increased plasma VLDL levels. Individuals with type 1 diabetes, who are in good glycemic control, usually have average or better than average plasma triglyceride levels. This may be due in part to the ability of insulin to inhibit apoB-100 secretion from the liver, or to increase LpL. As noted above, decreased LpL-mediated hydrolysis of VLDL triglycerides may contribute significantly to elevated triglyceride levels, particularly in patients with either type 1 or 2 diabetes who have poor glycemic control. Obesity and insulin resistance are important contributors to the hypertriglyceridemia of T2DM.

Regulation of plasma levels of LDL cholesterol in T2DM is complex. In the presence of hypertriglyceridemia, small, dense, cholesterol-depleted, triglyceride-enriched LDL are present (Figure 3). This means that there will be more LDL particles for any LDL cholesterol level, compared with people who have LDLs of normal size and composition. Removal of LDL, mainly via LDL receptor

Figure 2

Normal metabolism of VLDL and LDL

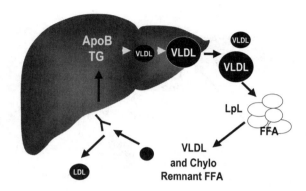

VLDL delivers much of its triglyceride as fatty acids to adipose (and muscle) after interacting with LpL in the capillaries beds of the tissue. The resulting IDL/VLDL remnant can be either taken up by the liver, delivering the rest of their triglycerides, or be further modified, mainly by HL, to become LDL. Chylomicron remnants, which are generated from the interaction of chylomicrons with LpL (thereby delivering dietary triglycerides to tissues) are all taken up by the liver. LDL can be taken up by the liver or by peripheral tissues, delivering cholesterol to those organs and tissues.

pathways, can be increased, normal or reduced in T2DM. Glycosylated and/or oxidatively modified lipoproteins, which can be present in increased amounts in the blood of patients with either type 1 or 2 diabetes, interact less efficiently with the LDL receptor, and have the potential to increase plasma LDL levels. On the other hand, modified LDLs can be removed from plasma by alternative metabolic pathways, including retention in the arterial wall or uptake by macrophages. Insulin also plays a role in stimulating the expression of the gene for LDL receptors; severe insulin deficiency in poorly controlled type 1 or T2DM may be associated with reduced LDL receptor function and increased LDL cholesterol levels.

Figure 3

VLDL and LDL metabolism in insulin resistance and T2DM

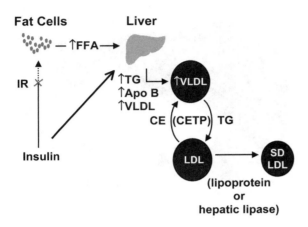

Increased VLDL in the circulation, in the presence of CETP, will stimulate increased exchange of LDL cholesteryl esters for VLDL triglycerides. This will deplete LDL of cholesterol. Additionally, hepatic lipase and/or lipoprotein lipase will hydrolyze the TG in LDL, producing small, dense LDL.

Abnormal HDL Metabolism

Of all of the lipoprotein classes, HDL may be the most complex. The majority of HDL are formed by the coalescence of individual apolipoproteins, including apo A-I, A-II and A-IV, with phospholipids. The resulting nascent, disc-like HDL, also called pre-beta HDL, function as acceptors of cellular-free cholesterol and are the initial HDL particles involved in reverse cholesterol transport (the movement of cholesterol from peripheral tissues to the liver for excretion from the body). The movement of cellular-free cholesterol to apo A-I is mediated via a protein, ABCA1. This is a transmembrane protein that appears to form a channel, through which apo A-I can interact with phospholipids and free cholesterol from the cell. Conversion of the free cholesterol to cholesteryl ester, by the addition of a fatty acid in a reaction catalyzed by lecithin cholesterol acyl transferase (LCAT), produces HDL_3. HDL_3 continues to accumulate cholesteryl ester and becomes HDL_2, which can deliver cholesteryl ester and free cholesterol (there is always some on the surface of

HDL) to the liver, via a process called selective uptake. A recently identified second membrane protein, ABCG1, also moves cell cholesterol to HDL; ABCG1, however, delivers free cholesterol to mature HDL_3 and HDL_2. The selective uptake of cholesteryl esters from HDL to several organs, including the liver (without catabolism of the entire HDL particle), was demonstrated to be the result of the HDL interaction with a receptor called scavenger receptor B-1 (SR-B1). Whole HDL particle uptake into cells can also occur, but those pathways are presently undefined. Finally, plasma HDL cholesteryl esters can move from the HDL particle into VLDL, and chylomicron particles in the presence of the cholesteryl ester transfer protein (CETP). The latter process is regulated by the level of triglycerides and the number of triglyceride-rich lipoproteins in the circulation. Thus, LpL activity can modulate HDL levels by influencing plasma levels of triglyceride in VLDL or chylomicrons. HL can affect HDL levels by breaking down phospholipids on the surface of the particles; this leads to dissolution of the HDL and loss of apo A-I from the circulation.

T2DM patients almost always have low levels of plasma HDL cholesterol. CETP-mediated transfer of cholesteryl ester from HDL into VLDL and chylomicrons, both of which are increased in most patients with T2DM, plays a key role in reducing HDL cholesterol concentrations (Figure 4). Low HDL levels in T2DM can also be present in the absence of fasting hypertriglyceridemia, and the mechanism for this is undefined, although it may reflect high postprandial triglyceride levels or some direct effect of insulin resistance on HDL metabolism. HDL levels are normal or even increased in patients with well-controlled type 1 diabetes, and this seems to be related to the effects of insulin treatment, possibly through suppression of HL or stimulation of LpL. High, ambient insulin levels might also reduce the livers secretion of VLDL, thereby lowering plasma triglyceride levels.

Figure 4

Clearance of free apo A-I

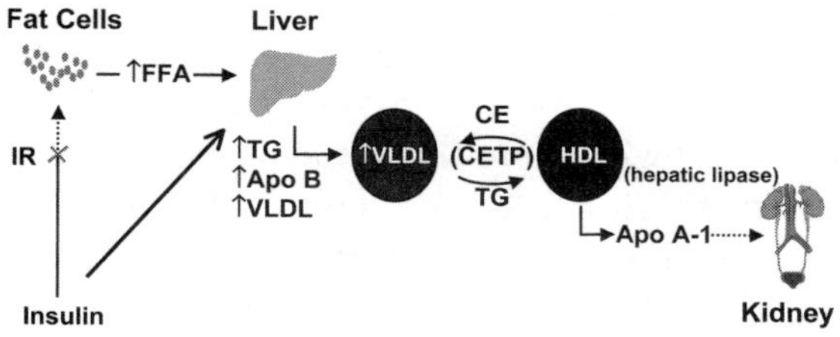

Increased VLDL in the circulation, in the presence of CETP, will stimulate increased exchange of HDL cholesteryl esters for VLDL triglycerides. This will deplete HDL of cholesterol. Additionally, hepatic lipase in the capillary bed of the liver will hydrolyze the TG and the phospholipid in HDL, the HDL will become smaller and apo A-I will dissociate. Free apo A-I will be cleared much faster than normal from the circulation, leading to fewer HDL in the blood.

4. Therapeutic Approaches to Diabetic Dyslipidemia

Dietary Therapy

Weight loss and diet modification are critical components to any plan for the treatment of diabetes, irrespective of the absence or presence of dyslipidemia. However, the presence of dyslipidemia increases the rationale for intensive diet intervention. It is important to remember that improvements in plasma triglyceride and total cholesterol levels during dietary intervention can be observed, even in the absence of weight loss. Thus, reductions in dietary saturated fat intake, along with reduced cholesterol consumption, can improve the lipid profile even if caloric intake is unchanged.

There is, however, a longstanding and continuing controversy concerning the composition of the *optimal diet* for patients with diabetes. When treating type 1 diabetes, there is no doubt that careful management of carbohydrate intake is very important for the development of a stable regimen of insulin administration. In the treatment of patients with T2DM, the issue of how much carbohydrate and fat to include in a diet plan is less certain, and open to debate. Specific recommendations for the approach to medical nutrition therapy for glycemic control in T2DM is outlined in Chapter 6 in this manual.

Certainly, reducing dietary saturated fat and cholesterol intake is central to lipid-lowering. Such changes will lower LDL ~10%; this may not seem like much, but this degree of reduction is equivalent to almost 2 doublings of an HMG-CoA reductase inhibitor (see below) once the starting dose has been initiated. The optimal replacement for saturated fat is the focus of the controversy. The issue of whether poly- or monounsaturated fats, rather than carbohydrates, should replace saturated fats has become much larger than it deserves based on the data. There is no doubt that high-fiber (not just *complex*) carbohydrates should be consumed, and even then, high-fiber carbohydrates are not a panacea. A diet that is varied in poultry and fish, with many vegetables and legumes, and with skim or 1% dairy products, should be recommended for patients with diabetes needing plasma lipid modification. Most importantly, because almost all individuals with T2DM usually need weight loss, removing saturated fat from the diet, without replacing it, is the optimal approach, at least initially. A simple approach is to focus on reducing calories, by whatever means is most efficacious for a particular patient, and when significant weight loss has occurred, turn attention to the types of calories consumed. Since most physicians are both ill-equipped and lacking in the time to do nutritional counseling, they should depend on registered dietitians.[2]

Weight Loss

Weight reduction is an essential part of dietary therapy in individuals with T2DM; it has not typically been a specific focus in patients with type 1 diabetes, although this is changing as many more patients with type 1 diabetes become overweight and develop obesity.[33] Weight loss has been shown not only to improve glycemic control and reduce insulin resistance (see Chapters 6 and 7), but to favorably affect lipoprotein patterns as well. Several groups of investigators have shown that when weight reduction is achieved and maintained in T2DM, there is a sustained decrease in triglyceride levels. Most, but not all, studies show an increase in HDL cholesterol as well with weight loss. It is important to remember that while weight loss is actively ongoing, HDL cholesterol can actually fall; however, it will rise to levels above baseline after weight stabilization (at a new lower weight) occurs. The optimal weight loss diet in individuals with diabetes is controversial. As stated above, determining the eating habits of individual patients and then removing calories in the most effective way is the goal; the kinds of calories removed, in the short-term, is less important. The only caveat here is that saturated fats should either be removed or exchanged for unsaturated fats.

Glycemic Control

Treatment of patients with T2DM with either insulin or oral insulin secretagogues usually has modest, if any, effect on their dyslipidemia. This is almost certainly because the lipid abnormalities are more closely related to insulin resistance than to insulin deficiency, and those agents have little or no effect on insulin sensitivity. Therapeutic approaches to type 2 diabetes that effect insulin sensitivity, such as metformin and thiazolidinediones (peroxisome proliferator-activated receptor-γ or PPARγ agonists), should theoretically lower

VLDL secretion from the liver by reducing plasma fatty acid concentrations and improving hepatic insulin sensitivity. In a recent study of pioglitazone therapy in patients with T2DM and hyperlipidemia, reductions in triglycerides of 25% were not associated with any reductions in VLDL secretion, but instead with improvements in the efficiency of triglyceride clearance from plasma.[28] The latter appeared to be due to a combination of increased LpL mass and decreased secretion of apoC-III from the liver. Rosiglitazone does not affect triglyceride concentrations in plasma, despite having equal potency, compared to pioglitazone, as an insulin sensitizer. The basis for the difference in the mechanism of action of these 2 PPARγ agonists remains to be determined. The effects of the 2 thiazolidinediones on plasma LDL cholesterol have been variable, although rosiglitazone seems to increase LDL cholesterol 5%-10%, whereas pioglitazone raises LDL 0%-5%. Both agents increase the average size of LDL particles; the ability of rosiglitazone to do this is interesting in light of its lack of effect on VLDL triglyceride levels. Metformin lowers plasma triglyceride concentrations ~5%, possibly because its insulin-sensitizing effects are limited to the liver, and do not occur in the peripheral tissues. Metformin also reduces LDL 5%-10%. Intensive insulin treatment (in patients with type 1 diabetes) lowers triglyceride and LDL cholesterol levels.

HDL cholesterol levels have only modest correlation with the level of control of hyperglycemia in patients with T2DM. Therapy with sulfonylureas does not increase HDL cholesterol concentrations. On the other hand, modest increases in HDL cholesterol levels, concomitant with modest decreases in triglyceride concentrations, have been observed with metformin therapy. Thiazolidinediones have been shown to raise HDL cholesterol levels in patients with T2DM. Of interest, although rosiglitazone and pioglitazone appear to differ in their effects on plasma triglyceride levels, they raise HDL cholesterol concentrations similarly, with pioglitazone being modestly better in a recent head-to-head trial. The mechanism for thiazolidinedione-mediated increases in HDL cholesterol and apo A-I levels is unclear.

While improved glycemic control, particularly if thiazolidinediones or other PPARγ agonists are used, can improve dyslipidemia in individuals with T2DM, direct lipid-altering therapy will almost always be necessary to achieve optimal control of dyslipidemia. Of particular interest are the many non-glycemic, non-lipid effects that have been observed with PPARγ agonists; they lower inflammatory markers like C-reactive protein, they improve the coagulation/fibrinolysis profile and they may have direct effects at the vessel wall. A recent study of more than 5000 patients with T2DM and known CVD, treated with either pioglitazone or placebo, demonstrated a favorable trend toward reductions in a wide-ranging primary endpoint of coronary, cerebrovascular and peripheral vascular events, and a modest but significant reduction in the cluster of total mortality, non-fatal MI and stroke (16%; P=0.027). Pioglitazone has also shown benefit in trials where carotid intimal medial thickening (IMT) or coronary atherosclerosis assessed by intravascular ultrasound (IVUS) were the endpoints. Several small studies indicate that rosiglitazone may reduce carotid IMT progression as well; results of larger outcome studies are awaited. There has been substantial controversy over the past 3 years regarding the cardiovascular safety of PPARγ agonists, particularly for rosiglitazone. Although it is not clear (and may never be) if rosiglitazone reduces cardiovascular events, the evidence that it increases CVD risk remains quite limited. On the other hand, the studies noted above support the conclusion that pioglitazone is beneficial with regard to cardiovascular outcomes,[27] particularly in patients with advanced CVD.[9] Providers should be aware that both of these drugs increase sodium retention by the kidneys, and congestive heart failure incidences rises with their use.

Lipid-lowering Drugs

If therapeutic goals for plasma lipids have not been achieved after an adequate trial of glycemic control, diet, weight loss and exercise, drug therapy should be considered. The length of time devoted to lifestyle changes should depend on the initial presentation of the patient, the severity of the dyslipidemia, and the presence of CHD or risk factors for CHD. Patients with modifiable lifestyle habits and/or poorly controlled glucose levels may

Table 1

American Diabetes Association Dyslipidemia Treatment Goals and Recommendations for Adults with Diabetes[34]

- Statin therapy should be added to lifestyle therapy, regardless of baseline lipid levels, for diabetic patients:

    * with overt CVD

    * without CVD who are over the age of 40 years and have 1 or more other CVD risk factors

- For patients at lower risk than those mentioned above (eg, without overt CVD and under the age of 40 years), statin therapy should be considered in addition to lifestyle therapy, if LDL cholesterol remains above 100 mg/dl or in those with multiple CVD risk factors

- In individuals without overt CVD, the primary goal is an LDL cholesterol <100 mg/dl (2.6 mmol/l)

- In individuals with overt CVD, a lower LDL cholesterol goal of <70 mg/dl (1.8 mmol/l), using a high dose of a statin, is an option

- If drug-treated patients do not reach the above targets on maximal-tolerated statin therapy, a reduction in LDL cholesterol of 30%-40% from baseline is an alternative therapeutic goal

- Triglyceride levels <150 mg/dl (1.7 mmol/l), and HDL cholesterol >40 mg/dl (1.0 mmol/l) in men and >50 mg/dl (1.3 mmol/l) in women, are desirable. However, LDL cholesterol-targeted statin therapy remains the preferred strategy

- If targets are not reached on maximally tolerated doses of statins, combination therapy using statins and other lipid-lowering agents may be considered to achieve lipid targets, but this has not been evaluated in outcome studies for either CVD outcomes or safety

require more time devoted to those problems before initiation of specific lipid-altering drug treatment. It is clear that lipid-lowering agents will be less efficacious, or actually ineffective, if these related factors are not addressed. In contrast, when patients are severely dyslipidemic, and/or have very high risk for CVD, earlier progression to pharmacotherapy is prudent. In patients with clinically significant CHD or other vascular disease, drug treatment to lower LDL cholesterol levels should nearly always be initiated along with lifestyle interventions. The severity of the dyslipidemia, independent of glycemic control, is an indicator of the presence of other genetic causes of lipid abnormalities, and this can also be taken into account when considering initiation of specific lipid-lowering therapy. Clearly, physicians cannot wait forever to control plasma glucose or achieve significant weight loss before moving on to specific lipid-altering treatment.[12,19]

The American Diabetes Association (ADA) recommendations for management of dyslipidemia vary based on age, duration of diabetes, risk for CVD or the presence of CVD (Table 1). In general, the ADA guidelines suggest initiation of therapy to lower LDL cholesterol for all patients who are older than 40 years of age, regardless of risk status, and initiation of therapy in patients at high risk or with CVD at any prevalent LDL cholesterol level. The goal in all patients, once lipid-altering drugs are initiated, is an LDL cholesterol <100 mg/dl. An optional goal of <70 mg/dl is offered for individuals with diabetes and overt CVD, or multiple risks for CVD. Goals for triglycerides and HDL cholesterol are less well-defined, but it is reasonable to try to reach a triglyceride level <150 mg/dl for all patients, and an HDL cholesterol concentration >40 mg/dl in men. Women should attempt to raise their HDL cholesterol level to >50 mg/dl. The National Cholesterol Education Program (NCEP) Adult Treatment Panel III guidelines equate the presence of diabetes with the presence of CHD. NCEP recommends that all patients with diabetes mellitus have drug therapy initiated when their LDL cholesterol level is >100 mg/dl, with a goal for LDL cholesterol that is <100 mg/dl. There are no specific guidelines for treatment of either triglycerides or HDL cholesterol levels in ATP III; a triglyceride level >200 mg/dl is considered high, while an HDL cholesterol level of <40 mg/dl is considered low (no gender differential). However, the definition of the Metabolic Syndrome in ATP III uses a triglyceride of 150 mg/dl, and HDL cholesterol levels of 40 mg/dl (men) and 50 mg/dl (women) as criteria for the diagnosis.

HMG-CoA Reductase Inhibitors (Statin Therapy)

During the past 2 decades, the treatment of hypercholesterolemia has undergone a revolution with the introduction of potent, safe HMG-CoA reductase inhibitors, known as statins. Lovastatin, pravastatin, fluvastatin, simvastatin, atorvastatin and rosuvastatin are available drugs in this category in the U.S. These agents work by competitively inhibiting HMG-CoA reductase, the rate-limiting enzyme in cholesterol synthesis, and this treatment results in both decreased hepatic production of apoB-100–containing lipoproteins and up-regulation of LDL receptors. The overall effect is a dramatic lowering of LDL cholesterol. VLDL triglyceride concentrations may also be reduced in subjects with moderate hypertriglyceridemia, including patients with T2DM. The reduction of triglycerides is directly related to the reduction of LDL cholesterol achieved. At their starting doses, which now range between 5 and 40 mg/day, statins lower LDL cholesterol by 25%-40%. The most potent statins (simvastatin, atorvastatin and rosuvastatin), at high doses, can lower LDL cholesterol by up to 45%-55% and lower triglycerides 20%-45%. The reduction in triglycerides achieved at these high levels of LDL cholesterol reduction will also depend on the starting triglyceride level; higher baseline triglycerides can be lowered more. Statins can raise HDL cholesterol by up to 5%-10%, but are not considered as first-line HDL-raising drugs.

The most important potential side effect associated with statin therapy is myositis, characterized by diffuse severe muscle tenderness and weakness, and elevated levels of CPK (usually >1000 IU/ml). In severe cases, rhabdomyolysis and concomitant myoglobinemia can place patients at risk for renal failure due to myoglobinuria. This is a risk, particularly in patients with diabetes who have preexisting nephropathy. However, the incidence of myositis when statins are used as monotherapy is

~1 in about 3000 patients, and careful patient instruction about the signs and symptoms, with advice to stop the medication and consume large volumes of liquids if symptoms occur, should obviate more serious outcomes. About 1%-3% of patients complain of myalgias with statin use, but have normal CPK levels; the basis for their symptoms is unclear. Unfortunately, many of these patients choose to discontinue therapy because of their symptoms. Statins can also cause non-clinically significant elevations in liver function tests in 1%-2% of patients, generally at higher doses. It is important for physicians and patients to realize that, despite labeled warnings and the requirement for liver function testing at initiation of treatment, statins are not generally hepatotoxic; clinically significant hepatotoxicity is, in fact, extremely rare.

Multiple clinical trials have demonstrated a reduction in CVD events and death in patients with T2DM treated with statins.[16, 29] In the Heart Protection Study, there was a significant reduction in CVD events in high risk/secondary prevention patients with diabetes on simvastatin 40 mg/day vs. placebo.[7] In that trial, there were enough patients with what was classified as type 1 diabetes to demonstrate a benefit in that group, similar to that seen in the overall study. The CARDS study,[6] which compared atorvastatin 10 mg/day with placebo, demonstrated significant reductions in CVD events in patients with diabetes without prior CVD. Furthermore, a subgroup analysis of patients with T2DM in the TNT showed significant reductions in events with atorvastatin 80 mg/day vs. 10 mg/day.[32] On the other hand, the ASPEN study,[25] with a similar design, did not show benefit of higher dose atorvastatin; the differences between ASPEN and TNT are not well-understood.

Overall, these studies provide strong support for statins as the first-line therapy for patients with diabetes with isolated elevation of LDL cholesterol, combined hyperlipidemia, or with moderate hypertriglyceridemia and an LDL cholesterol level above goal. Thus, despite the fact that the most common lipid abnormality in diabetes is a dyslipidemia characterized by high triglycerides and low HDL cholesterol levels, with average or slightly elevated LDL cholesterol concentrations,

statins are generally considered as the first agents to be used.

Although the use of statins is widespread, these very effective agents are still underused. More importantly, the proportion of patients reaching LDL goals is well below optimal, particularly when the goal is an LDL cholesterol <100 mg/dl, as it is for patients with diabetes. Titrating the statin is an important priority if trying to reach goal LDL levels, and physicians must realize that statins are extremely safe drugs with proven benefits.[26] In the Heart Protection Study, benefit was observed at all levels of baseline LDL, including initial LDL cholesterol levels <100 mg/dl.[20]

Bile Acid–binding Resins

Cholestyramine, colestipol and colesevelam are resins that bind bile acids in the intestine, interrupting the enterohepatic recirculation of those molecules. A reduction in the concentration of bile acids returning to the liver results in increased conversion of hepatic cholesterol to bile acids, which results in a diminution of a regulatory pool of hepatic cholesterol and up-regulation of the gene for hepatic LDL receptors. These changes lead to decreased plasma LDL concentrations. Usual doses of bile acid-binding resins are 8-24 g/day for cholestyramine, 10-30 g/day for colestipol (both as granular powders) and 3.75 g/day for colesevelam. Cholestyramine is mixed with sucrose, but there is a light form that is made with NutraSweet. Colestipol is also available in 1 g tablets. At full doses, cholestyramine and colestipol can reduce LDL levels ~25%; however, compliance is usually low and, in most patients, only mid-level doses are achieved. At 6 tablets per day, colesevelam lowers LDL cholesterol by 15%-20% and compliance is significantly better. Bile acid-binding resins are not absorbed, and therefore have no common systemic toxicity. The major drawback to the use of bile acid-binding resin in patients with diabetes is an increase in hepatic VLDL triglyceride production; as such elevations in plasma triglyceride levels may occur. An additional adverse effect of these agents is bloating and constipation, which may pose a significant problem in the patients with gastroparesis; this is much less common with colesevelam. Resins can also interfere with the absorption of other oral medications, although this problem has also been significantly reduced with colesevelam. With the availability of HMG-CoA reductase inhibitors, the need for resins has been markedly reduced. However, they can add greatly to LDL-lowering when added to statins, and are very useful in statin-intolerant patients. Recent studies demonstrated that colesevelam lowers HbA1C in the range of 0.5%, and the FDA approved an indication for colesevelam in diabetes.[3] The mechanism for this effect, which may or may not be common to all bile acid sequestrants, is unclear.

Ezetimibe

Ezetimibe is the first of a class of drugs that inhibit cholesterol absorption in the small intestine.[8] A receptor that is similar to a protein involved in intracellular transport of cholesterol has been identified as the target for ezetimibe. At the dose of 10 mg/day, ezetimibe reduces LDL cholesterol about 15%-20%, with little or no effects on HDL cholesterol or triglyceride concentrations. Ezetimibe is a useful addition to statin therapy when the LDL goal has not been reached, despite titration to maximal dose of any statin. It may also be useful in patients who are statin-intolerant. Ezetimibe is available in a combination with simvastatin, across the full dose range of the latter. Recent clinical trials have raised questions related to both efficacy and safety of ezetimibe, alone or in combination with statins. First, the ENHANCE trial failed to show benefit of ezetimibe plus simvastatin vs. simvastatin alone on carotid IMT in patients with familial hypercholesterolemia, despite the expected 16% greater reduction in the combination therapy group.[23] However, these patients had normal carotid IMT at baseline, and both groups had very low rates of progression during the study. In the SEAS trial, ezetimibe plus simvastatin was compared with double placebo. As to effects on progression of aortic stenosis; there was no benefit on the primary endpoint, but there was a significant increase in cancer incidence and mortality. Due to the relatively small sample of this trial (1800 participants), the significance of these cancer findings remains uncertain. However, because of concern, 2 very large trials reported interim safety data that suggested no increase in cancer incidence, but increased cancer mortality. Until these 2 trials (IMPROVE-IT and SHARP) are completed, with

over 20,000 people followed for several years, prudence should prevail, and ezetimibe use should be reserved for patients on maximally tolerated statins who are still above the goal LDL. Providers should also increase their consideration of bile acid sequestrants as an alternative therapy.

Fibric Acid Derivatives

Fibric acid derivatives are peroxisome proliferator-activated receptor-a (PPARa) agonists that have potent lipid-altering effects and are useful in patients with diabetes. In general, fibrate use in patients with T2DM results in lowering of triglycerides from 25%-40% and increases in HDL cholesterol from 10%-20%. These results have been observed in small trials; in large clinical trials, with observations over 3-5 years, the changes in triglycerides and HDL cholesterol are more modest; 20%-25% and 4%-8%, respectively. Fenofibrate and gemfibrozil are presently available in the U.S., with several other agents also available in Europe and Canada. Although their mechanism of action is unclear, these agents appear to work by both decreasing hepatic VLDL production and increasing the activity of LpL. The former effect probably results from fibrate-induced increases in genes for enzymes involved in fatty acid oxidation. These are PPARα-regulated genes, and their induction leads to diversion of fatty acids to oxidative pathways and away from TG synthesis. The effect on LpL is probably a direct action of a PPARα agonist on the LpL gene.

Fibrates effects on LDL cholesterol can vary: they can have LDL-lowering effect, no effect or even an LDL-raising effect in patients with more significant hypertriglyceridemia. The basis for these variable outcomes is complex and has to do with the efficiency with which VLDL is converted to LDL, how efficiently LDL is removed from plasma and the cholesteryl ester content of LDL. In the latter instance, fibrate treatment, with concomitant triglyceride lowering, usually converts small, dense, cholesteryl ester-depleted LDL into more normal cholesterol-enriched LDL. The usual dose is 600 mg of gemfibrozil BID and 145 mg QD for micronized fenofibrate. The FDA recently approved fenofibric acid, 130 mg/day; this is the active metabolite of fenofibrate. These agents are lithogenic and, therefore, contraindicated in patients with gallstones, and because they are tightly bound to plasma proteins, levels of other drugs (eg, warfarin) should be monitored carefully.

Fibrates do not significantly affect glycemic control and the side effect profile of fibrates is quite limited, making them well-tolerated therapy. As noted above, there is an increased risk of gallstone formation, but the overall incidence is very low. The fibrates have been reported to cause a myositis that clinically is similar to that associated with statin use; the incidence is between 1:1000 and 1:2000 patients.

The rise in LDL cholesterol concentration that can accompany triglyceride-lowering during fibrate therapy must be viewed in the context of clinical trials of fibrate therapy that included patients with diabetes. In the Helsinki Heart Study, the 2 groups with hypertriglyceridemia (with and without concomitant elevations in LDL cholesterol) had increases or no change in LDL cholesterol levels during gemfibrozil therapy, and yet achieved the same reduction in CHD events as the group with isolated LDL elevations, in which LDL cholesterol levels fell 10%-12% with treatment. The 2 groups in which LDL had little change or no change at all included the majority of participants with diabetes (a small number overall). A more recent study, the Veterans Administration HDL Intervention Trial,31 showed that gemfibrozil was efficacious in a group of men who had CHD and a mean baseline LDL cholesterol that was low (111 mg/dl) and did not change during the trial. The treated group did show a 7% increase in HDL cholesterol and a 25% reduction in triglycerides; these changes were associated with a 22% reduction in CHD events. In the 25% of the subjects in this trial who had diabetes (almost certainly T2DM), relative benefit was equal to that seen in the non-diabetic cohort. The subjects with diabetes had, as expected, higher absolute rates of events in both the placebo and the treatment group. In the DAIS trial, coronary angiograms were done at baseline and after 2 years of treatment with either fenofibrate or placebo. Fenofibrate therapy was associated with less progression of coronary disease.

When statins have been compared with fibrates in patients with T2DM, statins produced much greater LDL-lowering, while the fibrates lowered triglycerides and raised HDL cholesterol more than the statins. Importantly, several recent studies of combination treatment of patients with T2DM have shown the additive effects of combination treatment on the dyslipidemic pattern. It appears that combination therapy of statin and fibrate may have a major positive effect on CVD risk. The use of this combination has, however, been limited by evidence that the risk of myositis is significantly higher with combination therapy, possibly affecting up to 1:100 individuals. Recent evidence suggests, however, that fenofibrate is different from gemfibrozil in this regard. While gemfibrozil significantly increases blood concentrations of all of the statins except pravastatin, fenofibrate does not. As a result, the combination of statin and fenofibrate likely has the same low risk of myositis as either drug alone.[11]

The recent FIELD trial,[24] in which 9795 subjects with T2DM were randomized to fenofibrate or placebo, did not significantly lower rates of fatal CVD and non-fatal MI. A secondary endpoint that added stroke and revascularization procedures was of borderline significance. However, in both instances, the difference in events was only about 11%. The study's lack of significance may have resulted from the unbalanced introduction of statin therapy during the trial; non-study physicians placed their patients on statin in a 2:1 ratio of placebo: the fenofibrate treatment group. Additionally, the overall event rates in FIELD were much lower than expected (about 1.2% per year in the placebo group compared to a rate of almost 7% per year in diabetes patients treated with placebo in VA HIT), thus reducing the power of the study. The ACCORD trial lipid study, in which fenofibrate plus simvastatin is being compared to simvastatin alone, will be completed later in 2009 and should provide definitive data regarding the potential benefit of combination fenofibrate statin therapy in patients with T2DM.

Nicotinic Acid (Niacin)
As noted previously, the most common lipid abnormalities present in patients with diabetes are elevated triglycerides and low HDL cholesterol levels. Niacin, when used in pharmacological doses (1-3 g/day), has the ability to potently lower

triglycerides (25%-40%) and raise HDL cholesterol (10%-25%). Niacin also lowers LDL cholesterol (15%-20%), and this adds to its potential efficacy in a high-risk population. Niacin, as monotherapy, reduced non-fatal MI in the Coronary Drug Project, a secondary prevention trial. A long-term follow-up of that study showed reduced total mortality in the niacin-treated group. Niacin has been shown, in combination with bile acid resins or statins, to reduce angiographic evidence of coronary atherosclerosis. A recent study suggested similar beneficial effects of the combination for carotid intimal medial thickening.

The mechanism of action is generally thought to be through lowering hepatic VLDL apoB-100 production and increasing the synthesis of apo A-I. The molecular basis for these effects is unknown, although the recent discovery of a G-protein coupled receptor that binds niacin in adipose tissue should offer new avenues for research.[36] Niacin has several side effects that often limit its utility in non-diabetic individuals: niacin produces a prostaglandin-mediated flush that occurs ~30 min after ingestion and can last as long as 1 hour; patients turn red and feel hot. Niacin can cause gastric irritation and can exacerbate peptic ulcer disease, has been associated with dry skin, causes hyperuricemia, can precipitate gouty attacks and is associated with elevations of hepatic transaminases in ~3%-5% of patients. Rarely, regular short-acting niacin can also cause a clinically significant hepatitis.

All of these side effects can occur in anyone using niacin, but in patients with type 2 diabetes, hyperuricemia is more common given the higher baseline risk. Some studies have demonstrated that niacin therapy may worsen diabetes control, likely by inducing insulin resistance. This finding is interesting at a theoretical level, because niacin's ability to inhibit lipolysis and lower plasma-free fatty acid levels after a single dose might be expected to improve insulin sensitivity. 2 studies, 1 using regular short-acting niacin[5] and the other an intermediate-release formulation of niacin (Niaspan),[17] demonstrated that niacin was efficacious in T2DM, with modest but manageable effects on glycemic control in most cases. If a clinician is faced with persistently low HDL and/or

significant hypertriglyceridemia despite statin treatment, or with statin plus fibrate therapy, addition of niacin in either of the available forms should be considered. 2 major studies, Aim High and Heart Protection Study 2, should provide important new data regarding the efficacy of niacin in combination with statin vs. statin alone in patients with T2DM. Results are expected in 3-4 years.

Of note, "long-acting, no flush" niacin preparations can cause severe hepatotoxicity and should not be used. Gel matrix niacin (Niaspan) appears to have the same safety profile as short-acting niacin. There are some "no-flush", short-acting niacin preparations available (ie, niacin inositol), but their efficacy is not well-documented.

Omega-3 Fatty Acid Supplements

Fatty fish from the northern oceans are enriched in n-3 (omega-3) fatty acids, docosahexanoic acid and eicosapentanoic acid. Epidemiologic studies have suggested lower rates of cardiovascular disease in individuals who ingest higher doses of omega-3 fatty acids. Diets rich in plant sources of the n-3 fatty acid, α-linolenic acid, have also been associated with reduced cardiovascular events. n-3 fatty acids provided as supplements, in doses of 3-6 g/day, are potent triglyceride-lowering agents and can be useful in diabetes patients with triglyceride levels >500 mg/dl, especially those not responsive to other drug therapies.

The question of whether lower doses of n-3 fatty acids, as supplements, should be given to patients with type 2 diabetes remains incompletely answered. In the GISSI Prevention Trial,[18] 1 g of an n-3 fatty acid supplement significantly reduced a combined endpoint of death, fatal and nonfatal MI, and stroke in both nondiabetic individuals and subjects with diabetes. The major benefit within the combination of endpoints was on total mortality and cardiovascular mortality. A prevailing theory is that these fatty acids reduce arrhythmic sudden death, although this has not been proven definitively. The use of 1 g per day of n-3 fatty acids is not associated with alterations of glycemic control, but their use with aspirin therapy could increase the risk of bleeding. All patients with diabetes should be advised to eat fish several times each week. The American Heart Association (AHA) has recommended concentrated fish oil capsules as an alternative in people who cannot consume enough fish.

Hormone Replacement Therapy

The issue of whether postmenopausal women with diabetes should be on hormone replacement therapy (HRT) remains incompletely understood. Oral estrogen given alone raises HDL levels by 10%-20%, by increasing apo A-I synthesis and decreasing hepatic lipase activity. Estrogen alone also lowers LDL cholesterol ~20% by increasing LDL receptor number on cells, particularly in the liver. Another benefit relates to the ability of estrogen to lower lipoprotein (a) levels ~20%. A potentially negative effect of estrogen administration on diabetic dyslipidemia is the increase in plasma triglycerides that occurs via increased hepatic secretion of VLDL. Severe hyperlipidemia and pancreatitis have been observed in women with preexisting hypertriglyceridemia who were receiving oral estrogen treatment. The addition of a progestational agent has been associated with reduced HDL-raising effects, but also lesser triglyceride raising, compared with estrogen therapy alone; micronized progesterone appears to have less of these effects.

However, the results of major studies, such as HERS (Heart and Estrogen/Progestin Replacement Study),[21] WAVE (Women's Angiographic Vitamins and Estrogen) and WHI (Women's Health Initiative),[35] showed that there is no significant cardiovascular benefit in women with or without prior MI who receive combined therapy with equine conjugated estrogens (Premarin) plus low-dose medroxyprogesterone (Provera)[30] or with estrogen alone.[1] In fact, total cardiovascular events were increased with HRT therapy in active phase of WHI, as was the incidence of breast cancer. Additionally, stroke and total cardiovascular disease events were increased with estrogen therapy alone in WHI. Based on these results, HRT is generally not recommended to reduce cardiovascular risk in diabetes. Indeed, women with diabetes who require hormone replacement therapy for hot flashes or other non-treatable symptoms of sys-temic estrogen deficiency (osteoporosis should be treated with drugs specific for that problem) should understand that there may be an increased risk for cardiovascular events and breast cancer.

5. Conclusion

The patient with diabetes and hyperlipidemia can be effectively managed through a combination of lifestyle interventions and pharmacotherapy. Close guidance and monitoring is needed, however, in choosing the proper approach. A variety of options are available to improve plasma lipids and thus reduce risk of CHD. Fortunately, if lifestyle changes are not adequate, the physician has effective and safe agents from which to choose. Despite the fact that the characteristic diabetic dyslipidemia is one of higher triglycerides, lower HDL cholesterol and average or slightly higher than average LDL cholesterol levels, the evidence from clinical trials indicates clearly that lowering LDL cholesterol should be a central priority. Treatment with statins, regardless of initial LDL cholesterol levels will, based on numerous clinical trials, reduce event rates significantly. Whether statin therapy should always be first is a question that cannot be answered with full confidence, but it seems prudent to say that at least 90% of patients with diabetes (and essentially of patients with diabetes who have LDL cholesterol levels above 100 mg/dl) should get a statin as part of their overall cardioprotective therapy.

When isolated hypertriglyceridemia and low HDL cholesterol (with an LDL cholesterol <100 mg/dl) are the presenting abnormalities, fibric acid derivatives could be an alternative as the first choice for drug therapy. In some cases, fibric acid derivatives will be all that is necessary. If the LDL cholesterol increases during fibrate treatment and goes above 100 mg/dl, the physician has several choices. First, a bile acid-binding resin could be added to the fibrate: this would lower LDL cholesterol without significantly affecting triglyceride levels. The second alternative would be to either switch to an HMG-CoA reductase inhibitor; this would be the logical choice if the triglyceride elevation (before or during fibrate treatment) was only moderate (<200 mg/dl). Finally, the physician could add a statin to the fibrate. The latter combination is effective in correcting severe combined hyperlipidemia, but carries an increased risk of myositis. We believe that this combination can be used successfully, particularly if the patient knows clearly that he or she must stop the medications, drink large quantities of liquids and call a physician if diffuse, symmetric muscle pain occurs.

Based on recent studies, that fenofibrate will be much safer in combination with statins than was gemfibrozil. However, gemfibrozil monotherapy greatly reduced cardiovascular events in VA HIT, while fenofibrate did not show significant benefit in FIELD; these data have created a conundrum for health care workers. The patient should have liver function tests obtained regularly with the use of fibrates or reductase inhibitors, alone or in combination. A baseline CK level will be helpful if the patient later complains of muscle symptoms. The final choice, nicotinic acid, could be used in patients with severe, combined hyperlipidemia or extremely low levels of HDL cholesterol. Both short-acting and intermediate-release niacin preparations are efficacious when used with a statin, and the risk of myositis is extremely low with this combination. If the diabetes is well-controlled, addition of niacin may have only a minimal-to-modest effect on HbA1c levels in most patients; any such change could be managed with modifications in glycemic medications.

In those patients who present with combined elevations of both LDL cholesterol and plasma triglycerides, an HMG-CoA reductase inhibitor is probably the most effective single agent. Again, niacin could also be used as a sole drug, with caution taken as described above. A fibric acid derivative or n-3 fatty acid supplements could be added if triglycerides are not sufficiently reduced by either of those drugs alone.

Therapy for the diabetic patient with an isolated reduction in HDL cholesterol is not clearly defined. Fibrates have not been demonstrated to be very effective in raising HDL cholesterol levels in nondiabetic individuals with isolated reductions in HDL, although no similar studies have been carried out in patients with diabetes. Niacin may be more effective in elevating HDL cholesterol concentrations when they are low in the absence of hypertriglyceridemia, but all of the caveats of niacin use in diabetes would apply here as well. An alternative to raising HDL in these subjects would be to more aggressively treat LDL cholesterol levels, with the goal of reducing them to much less than 100 mg/dl. It must be clear, however, that there are no endpoint trials supporting any approach to isolated reductions in HDL cholesterol, either in non-diabetic individuals or patients with diabetes.

Finally, in those patients with diabetes who have isolated high levels of LDL cholesterol, either a bile acid resin or an HMG-CoA reductase inhibitor may be used primarily. The combination of these 2 agents has been shown to be effective in those individuals with extremely high levels of LDL cholesterol who are resistant to monotherapy. Triglyceride levels need to be observed closely in those patients placed on resins. The recent availability of ezetimibe, either alone or in combination with a statin, adds significantly to our ability to lower LDL cholesterol levels. However, as noted above, recent studies should be used as a guide to usage of ezetimibe.

6. References

1. Anderson GL. Effects of conjugated equine estrogen in postmenopausal women with hysterectomy: the Women's Health Initiative randomized controlled trial. *JAMA.* 2004;291:1701-1712.

2. ADA. Management of dyslipidemia in adults with diabetes (Position Statement). *Diabetes Care.* 1999;22 (suppl 1):S56-S59.

3. Bays HE, Goldberg RB, Truitt KE, Jones MR. Colesevelam hydrochloride therapy in patients with type 2 diabetes mellitus treated with metformin. *Arch Intern Med.* 2008;168:1975-1983.

4. Bishop JR, Stanford KI, Esko JD. Heparan sulfate proteoglycans and triglyceride-rich lipoprotein metabolism. *Curr Opin Lipidology.* 2008;19:307-313.

5. Chesney CM, Elam MB, Herd JA, et al. Effect of niacin, warfarin, and antioxidant therapy on coagulation parameters in patients with peripheral arterial disease in the Arterial Disease Multiple Intervention Trial (ADMIT). *Am Heart J.* 2000;140:631-636.

6. Colhoun HM, Betteridge DJ, Durrington PH, et al and the Cards Investigators. Primary prevention of cardiovascular disease with atorvastatin in type 2 diabetes in the Collaborative Atorvastatin Diabetes Study (CARDS): multicentre randomized placebo-controlled trial. *Lancet.* 2004;364:685-696.

7. Collins R, Armitage J, Parish S, Sleigh P, Peto R. MRC/BHF heart protection study of cholesterol-lowering with simvastatin in 5963 people with diabetes: a randomized placebo-controlled trial. *Lancet.* 2003;361:2005-2016.

8. Davidson MH. Ezetimibe: a novel option for lowering cholesterol. *Expert Rev Cardiovasc Ther.* 2003;1:11-21.

9. Dormandy JA, Charbonnel B, Eckland DJ, et al and the PROactive Investigators. Secondary prevention of macrovascular events in patients with type 2 diabetes in the PROactive Study (PROspective pioglitazone Clinical Trial In macrovascular Events): a randomized controlled trial. *Lancet*. 2005;366(9493):1279-1289.

10. Duez H, Pavlic M, Lewis GF. Mechanism of intestinal lipoprotein overproduction in insulin resistant humans. *Atheroscler Suppl*. 2008;9:33-38.

11. Ellen RLB, McPherson R. Long-term efficacy and safety of fenofibrate and a statin in the treatment of combined hyperlipidemia. *Am J Cardiol*. 1998;81:60B-65B.

12. Expert Panel on Detection, Evaluation, and Treatment of High Blood Cholesterol in Adults. Executive summary of the third report of the National Cholesterol Education Program (NCEP) Expert Panel on Detection, Evaluation, and Treatment of High Blood Cholesterol in Adults (Adult Treatment Panel III). *JAMA*. 2001;285:2486-2497.

13. Ginsberg HN. Lipoprotein physiology. In: Hoeg J, ed. *Endocrinology and Metabolism Clinics of North America*. Philadelphia, PA: WB Saunders; 1998.

14. Ginsberg HN, Illingworth DR. Postprandial dyslipidemia: an atherogenic disorder common in patients with diabetes mellitus. *Am J Cardiol*. 2001;88:9H-15H.

15. Goldberg RB, Kendall DM, Deeg MA, et al and the GLAI Study Investigators. A comparison of lipid and glycemic effects of pioglitazone and rosiglitazone in patients with type 2 diabetes and dyslipidemia. *Diabetes Care*. 2005;28:1547-1554.

16. Goldberg RB, Mellies MJ, Sacks FM, et al. Cardiovascular events and their reduction with pravastatin in diabetic and glucose-intolerant myocardial infarction survivors with average cholesterol levels: subgroup analysis in the Cholesterol and Recurrent Events (CARE) trial. *Circulation*. 1998;98:2513-2519.

17. Grundy SM, Vega GL, McGovern ME, et al. Diabetes Multicenter Research Group: efficacy, safety, and tolerability of once-daily niacin for the treatment of dyslipidemia associated with type 2 diabetes: results of the assessment of diabetes control and evaluation of the efficacy of niaspan trial. *Arch Intern Med*. 2002;22:1568-1576.

18. Gruppo Italiano per lo Studio della Sopravvivenza nell'Infarto miocardico (GISSI Investigators). Dietary supplementation with n-3 polyunsaturated fatty acids and vitamin E after myocardial infarction: results of the GISSI-Prevenzione trial. *Lancet*. 1999;354:447-455.

19. Haffner SM. Management of dyslipidemia in adults with diabetes (Technical Review). *Diabetes Care*. 1998;21:160-178.

20. Heart Protection Study Collaborative Group. MRC/BHF Heart Protection Study of cholesterol lowering with simvastatin in 20,536 high-risk individuals: a randomised placebo-controlled trial. *Lancet*. 2002;360:7-22.

21. Hulley S, Grady D, Bush T, et al. Randomized trial of estrogen plus progestin for secondary prevention of coronary heart disease in postmenopausal women: Heart and Estrogen/progestin Replacement Study Research Group. *JAMA*. 1998;280:605-613.

22. Kannel WB, D'Agostino RB, Wilson PWF, Bleanger AJ, Gagnon DR. Diabetes, fibrinogen, and risk of cardiovascular disease: the Framingham experience. *Am Heart J*. 1990;120:672-676.

23. Kastelein JJ, Akdim F, Stroes ES, et al. Simvastatin with or without ezetimibe in familial hypercholesterolemia. *N Engl J Med*. 2008;358:1431-1443.

24. Keech A, Simes RJ, Barter P, et al and the FIELD Study Investigators. Effects of long-term fenofibrate therapy on cardiovascular events in 9795 people with type 2 diabetes mellitus (the FIELD study): randomised controlled trial. *Lancet*. 2005;366:1849-1861.

25. Knopp RH, D'Emden M, Smilde JG, Pocock SJ. The atorvastatin study for prevention of coronary heart disease endpoints in non-insulin dependent diabetes mellitus (ASPEN). *Diabetes Care* 2006;20:1478-1485.

26. LaRosa JC, Grundy SM, Waters DD, et al and the Treating to New Targets (TNT) Investigators. Intensive lipid lowering with atorvastatin in patients with stable coronary disease. *N Engl J Med*. 2005;352:1425-1435.

27. Mazzone T, Meyer PM, Feinstein SB, et al. Effect of pioglitazone compared with glimepiride on carotid intima-media thickness in type 2 diabetes: a randomized trial. *JAMA*. 2006;296:2572-2581.

28. Nagashima K, Lopez C, Donovan D, et al. Effects of the peroxisome proliferator-activated receptor gamma agonist, pioglitazone, on lipoprotein metabolism in patients with type 2 diabetes mellitus. *J Clin Invest*. 2005;115:1323-1332.

29. Pyorala K, Pedersen TR, Kjekshus J, Faegerman O, Olsson AG, Thorgeirsson G. Cholesterol lowering with simvastatin improves prognosis of diabetic patients with coronary artery disease: a subgroup analysis of the Scandinavian Simvastatin Survival Study. *Diabetes Care*. 1997;20:614-620.

30. Rossouw JE, Anderson GL, Prentice RL, et al for the Writing Group for the Women's Health Initiative Investigators. Risks and benefits of estrogen plus progestin in healthy post-menopausal women: principal results From the Women's Health Initiative randomized controlled trial. *JAMA*. 2002;288:321-333.

31. Rubins HB, Robins SJ, Collins D, et al. Gemfibrozil for the secondary prevention of coronary heart disease in men with low levels of high-density lipoprotein cholesterol: Veterans Affairs High-Density Lipoprotein Cholesterol Intervention Trial Study Group. *N Engl J Med*. 1999;341:410-418.

32. Shepherd J, Barter P, Carmena R, et al. Effect of lowering LDL cholesterol substantially below currently recommended levels in patients with coronary heart disease and diabetes: the Treating to New Targets (TNT) study. *Diabetes Care*. 2006;29:1220-1226.

33. Sibley SD, Palmer JP, Hirsch IB, Brunzell JD. Visceral obesity, hepatic lipase activity, and dyslipidemia in type 1 diabetes. *J Clin Endocrinol Metab*. 2003;88:3379-3384.

34. ADA. Standards of Medical Care in Diabetes, 2009. *Diabetes Care*. 2009;32:S13-S61.

35. Writing Group for the Women's Health Initiative. Risks and benefits of estrogen plus progestin in healthy postmenopausal women: principal results from the Women's Health Initiative randomized controlled trial. *JAMA*. 2002;288:321-333.

36. Zhang Y, Schmidt RJ, Foxworthy P, et al. Niacin mediates lipolysis in adipose tissue through its G-protein coupled receptor HM74A. *Biochem Biophys Res Commun*. 2005;334:729-732.

Chapter 11: Pre-diabetes and the Prevention of Diabetes

A. Melissa Solum MD
John B Buse MD, PhD
Thomas O'Connell, MD

Contents

1. Introduction

For several decades, there has been an emerging epidemic of overweight and obesity. From 1960 to 2004, the prevalence of overweight increased from 44.8%-66% in US adults age 20-74; the prevalence of obesity doubled, from 13.3% to 32.1%, with most of the rise occurring since 1980.[1] A staggering 33% of Americans are now obese (body mass index or BMI ≥30 kg/m²) and 6.6% are morbidly obese (BMI ≥40 kg/m²).[2] Coexistent with the increase in obesity has been a dramatic rise in the incidence of diabetes and earlier disorders of glucose metabolism. There are approximately 150 million people worldwide with diabetes. In the United States, there are 24.1 million people with diabetes and an estimated 1/4 are undiagnosed.[3] There are another 57 million in the U.S. and 314 million worldwide with *pre-diabetes*, in whom the risk of progression to overt type 2 diabetes is high.[4]

Pre-diabetes represents a state of glucose dysregulation that falls between normal glucose metabolism and type 2 diabetes. Some have objected to the term *pre-diabetes*, as not all people with this condition go on to develop overt diabetes. From the perspective of health risk communication between the lay public and health care professionals however, pre-diabetes remains as a useful term. The more precise laboratory categories of glucose metabolism—impaired fasting glucose (IFG) and impaired glucose tolerance (IGT)—do not adequately convey the seriousness of the condition. IFG is defined by fasting plasma glucose (FPG) between 100-125 mg/dl after a fast of at least 8 hours. IGT is defined based on glucose levels achieved during the 75 gram oral glucose tolerance test (OGTT). To be performed correctly, an OGTT requires at least 3 days of an unrestricted carbohydrate diet (>250 g carbohydrate per day) for adequate preparation. Patients present for testing after at least an 8-hour fast and generally have a baseline and 2-hour plasma glucose drawn. The presence of a 2-hour post-challenge level between 140 and 199 mg/dl is termed IGT.[5] Studies suggest that between 25% and 40% of people with pre-diabetes will progress to overt type 2 diabetes over 3-5 years.[6,7] Given more time, however, up to 70% may eventually develop type 2 diabetes.[8] The intermediate term risk of progression to type 2 diabetes is greatest for those with both IFG and IGT (~15% per year), intermediate risk for those with isolated IGT without IFG (~10% per year) and least for those with isolated IFG without IGT (~5% per year). Obviously, those with glucose values closest to the cut point for diabetes, fasting glucose ≥126 mg/dl and 2-hour glucose ≥200 mg/dl are at highest risk of progression to diabetes.

Cardiovascular disease risk is also modestly increased in those with pre-diabetes, and is markedly increased in those with overt diabetes.[9-11] It has been argued that the excess cardiovascular risk among people with pre-diabetes is minimal if they never develop diabetes. Interestingly, microvascular disease (retinopathy, neuropathy and nephropathy) has been documented in people with pre-diabetes,[12] though the development of advanced microvascular complications in the absence of diabetes is exceptionally rare. There appears to be a fairly linear relationship between the level of glucose dysregulation and risk of complications from hyperglycemia.

The high prevalence of pre-diabetes along with the significant risk of progression to overt type 2 diabetes, and heightened risk of both micro- and macrovascular disease, has generated tremendous interest in diabetes prevention and the management of pre-diabetes. Multiple studies investigating both intensive lifestyle modification and pharmacologic therapy have been completed, and there are a number of additional studies ongoing at present.

2. Screening for Pre-diabetes: Current Recommendations

The first step in a program of diabetes prevention is to determine who to screen for diabetes. Many professional and advocacy groups (ADA, AACE, AHA, ACC) recommend routine screening for diabetes, starting at age 35-45 years, independent of risk factors and repeating screening at least every 3-5 years. Most groups recommend earlier and more frequent screening in patients who are overweight (BMI ≥25 kg/m²) and/or with other risk factors. Not all recommendations are identical, however, and there are no randomized trials of screening protocols to determine the relative costs and benefits of any particular strategy. The current screening recommendations of the ADA are presented in Table 1. In primary care practice, a large proportion of adult patients will meet screening criteria.

Type 2 diabetes in children is an emerging problem, with similar frequency to type 1 diabetes and associated with classical risk factors. A smaller number of children in primary care practice will meet currently recommended criteria for screening for type 2 diabetes and pre-diabetes presented in Table 2.

Table 1

Criteria for Testing for Pre-diabetes and Diabetes in Asymptomatic Adult Individuals

1. Testing should be considered in all adults who are overweight (BMI ≥25 kg/m²)[a] and have additional risk factors:

   - Physical inactivity
   - First-degree relative with diabetes
   - Members of a high-risk ethnic population (eg, African American, Latino, Native American, Asian American, Pacific Islander)
   - Women who delivered a baby weighing >9 pounds or were diagnosed with gestational diabetes
   - Hypertension (≥140/90 mm Hg or on therapy for hypertension)
   - HDL cholesterol level <35 mg/dl (0.90 mmol/l) and/or a triglyceride level >250 mg/dl (2.82 mmol/l)
   - Women with polycystic ovarian syndrome (PCOS)
   - IGT or IFG on previous testing
   - Other clinical conditions associated with insulin resistance (eg, severe obesity, acanthosis nigricans)
   - History of CVD

2. In the absence of the above criteria, testing for pre-diabetes and diabetes should begin at age 45 years

3. If results are normal, testing should be repeated at least at 3-year intervals, with consideration of more frequent testing depending on initial results and risk status

[a]At-risk BMI may be lower in some ethnic groups (eg, Asians)

Adapted from: ADA. Standards for medical care in diabetes – 2009. Diabetes Care. 2009;32(suppl 1): s13-s61.

Table 2

Testing for Type 2 Diabetes in Asymptomatic Children

Criteria: Overweight (BMI >85th percentile for age and sex, weight for height >85th percentile, or weight >120% of ideal for height) – Plus – any two of the following risk factors:

- Family history of type 2 diabetes in first- or second-degree relative

- Race/ethnicity (Native American, African American, Latino, Asian American, Pacific Islander)

- Signs of insulin resistance or conditions associated with insulin resistance (acanthosis nigricans, hypertension, dyslipidemia, PCOS or small-for-gestational-age birthweight)

- Maternal history of diabetes or gestational diabetes during the child's gestation

Age of initiation: age 10 years or at onset of puberty, if puberty occurs at a younger age

Frequency: every 3 years

Test: FPG preferred

Adapted from: ADA. Standards for medical care in diabetes – 2009. Diabetes Care. 2009;32 (suppl 1): s13-s61.

Lifestyle Intervention for Prevention of Diabetes

Several studies have examined the effect of lifestyle programs on the risk of development of type 2 diabetes in people with pre-diabetes (Table 3). One of the first was a study conducted in the industrial city of DaQing, China. Participants were screened for IGT at clinical centers and then cluster-randomized by clinic into 4 arms: diet, exercise, combined diet and exercise, and no intervention (control).[13] The interventions were practical, with modest individualization, and generally conducted in group visits. After 6 years, diet alone, exercise alone, and combined diet and exercise all substantially reduced the risk of developing diabetes, in both normal weight and overweight individuals, respectively 31%, 46%, and 42% reduction from control. Subsequent 20-year follow-up without intervening intervention demonstrated that the benefit with respect to diabetes prevention was largely maintained with trends towards benefits with respect to all-cause mortality and CVD.[14] The Finnish Diabetes Prevention Study (Finnish DPS) found similar results amongst a group of 522 overweight subjects who had 2 OGTTs with a mean 2-hour value in the IGT range.[15] With fairly intensive individualized counseling addressing both nutrition and physical activity, the intervention participants were able to achieve a 58% decrease in their risk of developing diabetes in just 3 years.

In the United States, the Diabetes Prevention Program (DPP) enrolled 3234 participants with impaired glucose tolerance and a fasting glucose between 95 and 125 mg/dl.[7] The lifestyle intervention group underwent an intensive individualized program of nutrition, physical activity, and behavioral counseling and support, aimed to achieve and maintain at least a 7% loss of body weight, with at least 150 minutes of moderately vigorous exercise weekly in addition to a healthy low-calorie, low-fat diet. The study participants randomized to this lifestyle modification arm had a 58% reduction in the risk of developing diabetes over an average of about 3 years, as compared to the placebo group who received a placebo tablet and routine lifestyle counseling.

These studies convincingly and consistently demonstrate that comprehensive lifestyle programs

Table 3

Diabetes Prevention Trials

Study	N	Inclusion criteria	Duration of Intervention (years)	Intervention	Relative Risk Reduction	Number Needed to Treat (NNT)
Da Qing[13]	577	IGT	6	Lifestyle	46%	4.3
Finnish DPS[15]	522	IGT, BMI >25 kg/m^2	3	Lifestyle	42%	9.5
DPP–lifestyle[7]	2161	IGT, FPG 95-125 mg/dl, BMI >24 kg/m^2	3	Lifestyle	58%	6.9
DPP-metformin[7]	2155	IGT, FPG 95-125 mg/dl, BMI >24 kg/m^2	3	Metformin	31%	13.9
EDIT[18]	631	IGT	6	Acarbose	34%	n/a[a]
STOP-NIDDM[19]	1368	IGT	3	Acarbose	25%	10
DREAM[6]	5269	IFG and/or IGT	3	Rosiglitazone	60%	6.9
ACT-NOW[23]	602	IFG	3	Pioglitazone	81%	n/a[a]
XENDOS[25]	3305	IGT and BMI >30 kg/m^2	4	Orlistat	45%	10

---

[a]*Incompletely reported at this time*

aimed at producing moderate weight loss (5%-10% body weight) administered by specially trained personnel with consistent follow-up over 3-6 years can either prevent of delay the development of diabetes. Such a comprehensive lifestyle program for patients with pre-diabetes is recommended by various professional and advocacy groups.

Pharmacologic Intervention

At present there are no medications approved by the FDA for the treatment of pre-diabetes or for diabetes prevention. The American College of Endocrinology recommends consideration of medications in certain individuals with pre-diabetes, particularly those with pre-existing or strong risk factors for cardiovascular disease.[16] The ADA recommends use of metformin, and reserves this recommendation for those who are at highest risk, based on having both IGT and IFG, and who are likely to respond well to metformin based on subgroup analyses of the DPP (under 60 years of age with a BMI of 30 kg/m^2 or higher and at least one other risk factor for diabetes: either family history of diabetes in a first degree relative, high triglycerides, low HDL, hypertension or an A1C over 6%).[8]

While there are no medications approved for the treatment of pre-diabetes, several clinical trials have demonstrated the potential benefit of medical therapies for diabetes prevention. In the DPP, a portion of the participants were randomized to receive standard lifestyle advice combined with metformin 850 mg twice daily or matching placebo. There was a 31% reduction in the risk of progressing to diabetes with metformin, with this benefit being greater in those with fasting plasma glucose >110 mg/dl, less than 60 years of age and with a BMI >30 kg/m^2.[7] A smaller study performed in overweight Asians from India confirmed that metformin can reduce the risk of diabetes.[17] However, the Early Diabetes Intervention Trial (EDIT) failed to demonstrate any benefit to metformin therapy in an older, less overweight, less hyperglycemic group.[18] These trials together provide the rationale for the details surrounding the ADA recommendations regarding the use of metformin to prevent/delay the onset of diabetes in high-risk individuals.

Acarbose has also been evaluated for diabetes prevention. The STOP-NIDDM trial (Screening TO Prevent NIDDM trial), randomized 1368 individuals with IGT and IFG to the α-glucosidase inhibitor, acarbose 100 mg TID vs. placebo.[19] Acarbose demonstrated a 25% relative risk reduction and a higher probability of reverting to normal glucose tolerance than placebo. Though the number of CVD events in the STOP-NIDDM study was small, there was a statistically significant reduction.[20] EDIT also had a study arm using acarbose 50 mg TID. Amongst the trial participants who had IGT, there was a risk reduction of 66% of developing diabetes compared to those given placebo.[18]

Thiazolidinediones have also been examined for their ability to prevent or delay diabetes. Troglitazone was removed from the global market due to concerns regarding liver toxicity but was the subject of 2 trials which demonstrated not only efficacy to prevent diabetes but durability of response after the drug was withdrawn.[21,22] The 2 remaining agents from this class have also been studied for their effect in preventing progression to type 2 diabetes in high-risk individuals. The Diabetes Reduction Assessment with Ramipril and Rosiglitazone Medication (DREAM) trial studied over 5000 individuals who had IFG and/or IGT[6] who were randomized to placebo or rosiglitazone 8 mg daily. After 3 years or average follow-up, the

rosiglitazone group had a 60% relative risk reduction on rates of developing diabetes, as defined by OGTT. However, in DREAM, there were numerically more major cardiovascular events in the participants randomized to rosiglitazone. This, along with other data raising concern over the safety of rosiglitazone, has slowed adoption of this treatment for prevention. The as-yet unpublished study, ACT NOW (ACTos NOW for the Prevention of Diabetes) randomized 602 obese individuals with IGT and IFG to pioglitazone 45 mg daily or placebo. After an average follow-up of almost 3 years, there was a substantial 81% reduction in the risk of conversion to diabetes despite mean weight gain of 3.9 kg with pioglitazone. Importantly, the investigators reported no increase in CVD events associated with pioglitazone use.[23]

Other diabetes prevention studies utilizing diabetes medications to be reported over the next few years include the ORIGIN (Outcome Reduction with Initial Glargine Intervention) trial examining the effect of basal insulin (vs. usual care) and the NAVIGATOR (Nateglinide And Valsartan in Impaired Glucose Tolerance Outcomes Research) trial examining the short-acting, sulfonylurea-receptor agonist nateglinide. These studies also contain secondary randomizations that explore the effects of fish oil (omega-3 supplementation) and the angiotensin receptor blocker valsartan on diabetes risk.

Other medications without primary indications for hyperglycemia have been examined for effects to prevent/delay diabetes. In the DREAM trial, the angiotensin converting enzyme inhibitor ramipril at a dose of 10 mg QD was studied in a second randomization and not found to have an effect on the risk of progression to diabetes.[24] The XENDOS (XENical in the prevention of Diabetes in Obese Subjects) trail examined the effects of orlistat, an intestinal lipase inhibitor indicated for the treatment of overweight and obesity,[25] in preventing diabetes. It randomized 3305 obese volunteers who did not have diabetes by OGTT to orlistat 120 mg or placebo TID in addition to a lifestyle program. Over the course of the 4-year study, 48% in the orlistat group and 66% in the placebo group were lost to follow-up. Mean weight loss of all participants was 5.8 kg in the orlistat group and

3.0 kg in the placebo group. Subgroup analyses revealed that in the patients with impaired glucose tolerance at baseline, there was a 45% risk reduction for the development of diabetes. The importance of the observation has been criticized due to the large proportion of people lost to follow-up. Importantly, it was also demonstrated that in those participants who did not have IGT at baseline, there was essentially no effect of the intervention in reducing the risk, largely because the risk of developing diabetes was so low.

The incidence and prevalence of diabetes is dramatically on the rise. This trend and the high cost and health care utilization of people with diabetes threatens the viability of health care systems worldwide. People at high risk for the development of diabetes are logical targets for intervention to reduce the burden of diabetes. The enormous number of people with abnormal levels of fasting glucose and oral glucose tolerance tests (over 3 times the population of people with diagnosed diabetes) is daunting, raising the issue of how best to screen for people at high risk for diabetes and in whom to intervene.

Current recommendations suggest that all individuals over the age of 45, and those younger who are overweight with other risk factors for diabetes, should be screened at least every 3 years, as long as risk factors remain.

Recently, numerous groups have suggested screening and diagnosing diabetes based on the glycated hemoglobin A1C assay, as the test does not have to be performed in the fasting state and as its accuracy and precision at least matches, and usually exceeds, those of glucose assays. People with hemoglobinopathies and abnormal red cell turnover can have spurious results and should not have A1C measured. Nevertheless, an A1C of 6.5% or higher is being examined as a diagnostic cut point for diabetes.[26] As risk for the development of diabetes is a continuous function of fasting plasma glucose, 2-hour glucose or A1C, people have called for abolishing the term pre-diabetes and describing those with non-diabetic measures of glycemia which are higher than average, particularly in combination with other risk markers, as being at "high risk for diabetes". Those with an A1C above the upper limits of the normal range (6%) would certainly be at high risk for developing diabetes over an intermediate time scale (less than 5 years), and excepting those with limited life expectancy, comprehensive lifestyle intervention, combining physical activity, medical nutrition therapy and behavioral approaches should be initiated; this would be a subgroup in whom medication therapy should also be considered. People with risk factors and A1C over 5% are also at lower but nevertheless increased risk to develop diabetes on a somewhat longer time scale

(3-10 years). Arguably lifestyle intervention should be initiated according to clinical judgment based on risk factors, such as overweight, dyslipidemia, hypertension, non-alcoholic hepatic steatosis or other problems, amenable to weight loss.

Among pharmacologic therapies which have been tested for their effect to reduce the risk of developing diabetes, metformin 850 mg BID has, by consensus, emerged as having optimal safety and proven efficacy, particularly for patients with fasting glucose ≥110 mg/dl under the age of 60 with a BMI ≥30 kg/m^2. Other agents have demonstrated efficacy, but problems with tolerability, adverse clinical effects or incomplete reporting of results have limited consensus regarding their appropriateness for diabetes prevention. Patients at high risk for diabetes under treatment should be assessed for progression every 6-12 months and treatment intensified if A1C rises, particularly to 6.5%-7% or higher.

With comprehensive lifestyle modifications, the incidence of diabetes can be reduced by 40%-60%. Similarly, various medications have demonstrated 25%-81% reduction in diabetes. There are, however, no medications currently FDA-approved for the prevention of diabetes. Long-term follow-up of the largest studies of diabetes prevention should accumulate enough clinically relevant endpoints over the next few years to address the issue of whether these approaches provide for benefits with respect to diabetes complications and mortality. Much greater research is needed to fully appreciate the cost-effectiveness and clinical efficacy of prevention approaches for type 2 diabetes.

5. References

1. National Center for Health Statistics. Chartbook on Trends in the Health of Americans. Health, United States, 2006. Hyattsville, MD: Public Health Service; 2006.

2. Ogden CL, Carroll MD, McDowell MA, Flegal KM. Obesity among adults in the United States – no change since 2003—2004. NCHS data brief no 1. Hyattsville, MD: National Center for Health Statistics; 2007.

3. Centers for Disease Control. Number of people with diabetes increases to 24 million. http://www.cdc.gov/media/pressrel/2008. Posted June 24, 2008.

4. International Diabetes Federation. Diabetes Atlas: Prevalence. http://www.eatlas.idf.org/Prevalence.

5. Genuth S, Alberti KH, Bennett p, Buse j, et al. Expert Committee on the Diagnosis and Classification of Diabetes Mellitus: follow-up report on the Diagnosis of diabetes mellitus. *Diabetes Care*. 2003;26:3160-3167.

6. The Dream Trial Investigators. Effect of Rosiglitazone on the Frequency of Diabetes in Patients with Impaired Glucose Tolerance or Impaired Fasting Glucose: a Randomised Controlled Trial. *Lancet*. 2006;368(9541):1096-1105.

7. Diabetes Prevention Program Research Group. Reduction in the Incidence of Type 2 Diabetes with Lifestyle Intervention or Metformin. *N Engl J Med*. 2002;346(6):393-403.

8. Nathan DM, Davidson MB, DeFronzo RA, et al. Impaired Fasting Glucose and Impaired Glucose Tolerance: Implications for care. *Diabetes Care*. 2007;30(3):753-759.

9. Coutinho M, Gerstein HC, Wang Y, Yusuf S. The relationship between glucose and incident cardiovascular events: a metaregression analysis of published data from 20 studies of 95,783 individuals followed for 12.4 years. *Diabetes Care*. 1999;22:233-240.

10. Barzilay JI, Spiekerman CF, Wahl PW, et al. Cardiovascular disease in older adults with glucose disorders: comparison of American Diabetes Association criteria for diabetes mellitus with WHO criteria. *Lancet*. 1999;354:622-625.

11. Meigs JB, Nathan DM, D'Agostino RB Sr, William PW. Fasting and post-challenge glycemia and cardiovascular disease risk: the Framingham Offspring Study. *Diabetes Care*. 2002;25:1845-1850.

12. Wong TY, Liew G, Tapp RJ, et al. Relation between fasting glucose and retinopathy for diagnosis of diabetes: three population-based cross-sectional studies. *Lancet*. 2008:371:736-743.

13. Pan XR, Li GW, Hu YH, et al. Effects of Diet and Exercise in Preventing NIDDM in People with Impaired Glucose Tolerance. The Da Qing IGT and Diabetes Study. *Diabetes Care*. 1997:20(4):537-544.

14. Li G, Zhang P, Wang J, et al. The long-term effect of lifestyle interventions to prevent diabetes in the China Da Qing Diabetes Prevention Study: a 20-year follow-up study. *Lancet*. 2008;371:1783-1789.

15. Tuomilehto J, Lindstrom J, Eriksson JG, et al. Prevention of Type 2 Diabetes by Changes in Lifestyle among Subjects with Impaired Glucose Tolerance. *N Engl J Med*. 2001;344(18):1343-1350.

16. Diagnosis and Management of Prediabetes in the Continuum of Hyperglycemia-When do the risks of Diabetes Begin? A Consensus Statement from the American College of Endocrinology and the American Association of Clinical Endocrinologists. *Endocrine Practice*. 2008;14 (No. 7):1-14.

17. Ramachandran A, Snehalatha C, Mary S, Mukesh B, Bhaskar AD, VijayV. The Indian Diabetes Prevention Programme shows that lifestyle modification and metformin prevent type 2 diabetes in Asian Indian subjects with impaired glucose tolerance (IDPP-1). *Diabetologia*. 2006; 49:289-297.

18. Holman R, Blackwell L, Stratton IM, Manley SE, Tucker L, Frighi V. Six-year Results from the Early Diabetes Intervention Trial (EDIT). *Diabetic Med*. 2003;S2:15.

19. Chiasson JL, Josse RG, Gomis R, Hanefeld M, Karasik A, Laakso M; STOP-NIDDM Trail Research Group. Acarbose for prevention of type 2 diabetes mellitus: the STOP-NIDDM randomised trial. *Lancet*. 2002;359:2072-2077.

20. Chiasson JL, Josse RG, Gomis R, Hanefeld M, Karasik A, Laakso M; STOP-NIDDM Trial Research Group. Acarbose treatment and the risk of cardiovascular disease and hypertension in patients with impaired glucose tolerance: the STOP-NIDDM trial. *JAMA*. 2003;290(4):486-494.

21. Buchanan TA, Xiang AH, Peters RK, et al. Preservation of Pancreatic β-Cell Function and Prevention of Type 2 Diabetes by Pharmacologic Treatment of Insulin Resistance in High-Risk Hispanic Women. *Diabetes*. 2002;51:2796-2803.

22. Knowler WC, Hamman RF, Edelstein SL, et al; Diabetes Prevention Program Research Group. Prevention of type 2 diabetes with troglitazone in the Diabetes Prevention Program. *Diabetes*. 2005;54:1150-1156.

23. ACT NOW presentation. 68th Scientific Sessions of the American Diabetes Association. San Francisco, California. June 2008.

24. DREAM Trial Investigators, Bosch J, Yusuf S, et al. Effect of ramipril on the incidence of diabetes. *N Engl J Med*. 2006;355:1551-1562.

25. Togerson JS, Blodrin MN, Hauptman J, Sjostrom L. XENical in the Prevention of Diabetes in Obese Subjects (XENDOS) Study. *Diabetes Care*. 2004;27(1):155-161.

26. Saudek CD, Herman WH, Sacks DB, Bergenstal RM, Edelman D, Davidson MB. A new look at screening and diagnosing diabetes mellitus. *J Clin Endocrinol Metab*. 2008;93(7):2447-2453.

Chapter 12: Hospital Management of Diabetes

Robert Cuddihy, MD

Contents

1. Introduction

The importance of good glycemic control in the inpatient hospital setting has been documented in multiple venues.

van den Berghe's initial landmark study demonstrated that tight glycemic control reduced morbidity and mortality in the surgical ICU. Improved glycemic control also resulted in reduced rates of infections, renal failure, critical illness polyneuropathy and decreased the need for blood transfusions. Improved glycemic control has resulted in an ~50% reduction in the mortality, and reduced the rate of infections by two-thirds following coronary artery bypass grafting. Intensified efforts to control hyperglycemia resulted in 30% reduction at 1 year following an acute myocardial infarction (MI).

However, the link between tight glycemic control and these beneficial outcomes has not been without controversy.

There have been less dramatic results in some recent studies and concerns that the risk-benefit ratio of tight glycemic control in some settings (eg, sepsis in the ICU) is outweighed by hypoglycemia. However, some of these studies had significant methodological flaws that raise questions as to the validity of their results.

In addition, the recently published NICE-SUGAR study demonstrated no added benefit and slightly increased mortality (odds ratio =1.14 compared to standard group) in individuals within the ICU with extremely tight glycemic control (glucoses 81-108 mg/dL, mean 115 mg/dL) vs. modestly tight glycemic control (glucose <180 mg/dl, mean 144 mg/dL). The group with intensive glycemic control had a rate of severe hypoglycemia (defined as glucose <40 mg/dL) that was almost 14-fold elevated over the control group. Even the control group in this study had far better glycemic control than has typically been seen in many hospitalized patients whose blood sugars continue to run well in the 200's mg/dL and above.

In general, the need for improvement of glycemic control has been widely accepted by diabetes and hospitalists' specialty organizations, including the American Association of Clinical Endocrinologists (AACE), American Diabetes Association (ADA) and Society of Hospital Medicine (SHM). Each of these organizations have their own guidelines seeking to drive improvements in glycemic control.

Despite these efforts, control of hyperglycemia in many hospital settings remains suboptimal. Widespread use of oral diabetic agents or PRN sliding scale insulin remains common; leading to continued poor glycemic control and raising patient safety issues. Some oral agents for diabetes raise the concern for hypoglycemia in the face of erratic meal timing and content and unpredictable activity patterns. Hypoglycemic risks can also increase with sliding scale insulin, due to stacking of repeated doses.

It is generally agreed that most patients with diabetes, or previously undiagnosed, marked hyperglycemia, should be treated with a 3-component insulin program, utilizing a long- or intermediate-acting basal (or background) insulin, short- or rapid-acting bolus (mealtime), and corrective dose (supplemental) insulin.

2. Improved Glycemic Control Improves Outcomes in the Hospital Setting

The importance of improved blood glucose control first gained widespread attention in the setting of acute MI and in patients undergoing coronary artery bypass grafting.

In the original DIGAMI trial by Malmberg et al, an intravenous infusion of a glucose and insulin with maintenance of tighter glycemic control, followed by daily multiple subcutaneous insulin injections for 3 months led to a 30% reduction in mortality at 1 year, in individuals presenting with acute MI. In fact, mortality was reduced in the treated group by 11% at an average 3.4 years of follow-up (Figure 1).

Furnary et al demonstrated a greater than 50% reduction in mortality (from 5.3% to 2.5%) following coronary artery bypass grafting in individuals who received Glucose Insulin Potassium (GIK). These individuals also benefited from a 66% reduction in deep, sternal wound infections.

Other studies have since demonstrated increased risks of infection following coronary artery bypass grafting, while tight glycemic control reduces the risk of infections.

In a landmark study, van den Berghe demonstrated a 47% reduction in mortality in the surgical ICU (Figure 2) in individuals randomized to achieve tighter glycemic control, aiming for blood glucose ranging between 80-110 mg /dL compared to a control group with goal ranging around the more typical 180-200 mg/dL range. Individuals achieving tighter glycemic control also had lower rates of bacteremia, acute kidney failure, blood transfusions and critical illness polyneuropathy by 46%, 41%, 50% and 44%, respectively.

Figure 1

DIGAMI study

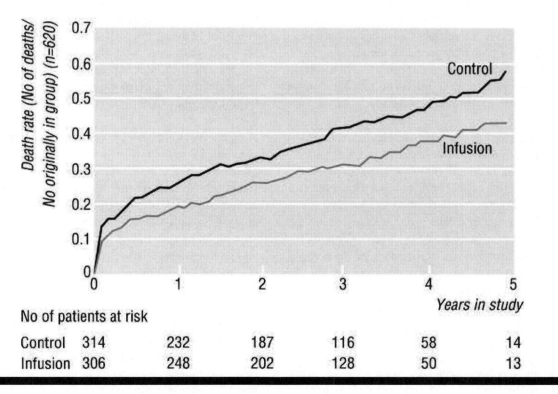

Figure 2

Intensive treatment vs. conventional treatment

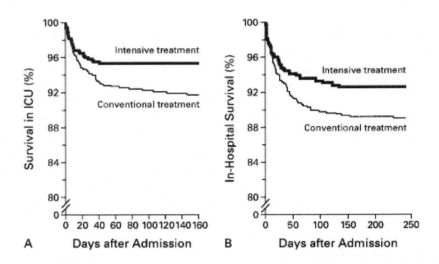

van den Berghe G, Wouters P, Weekers F, et al. Intensive insulin therapy in the critically ill patients. N Engl J Med. 2001;345:1359-1367.

However, not all studies have reached the same conclusions. DIGAMI-2 did not show benefits to intensifying glycemic control in acute MI, but suffered from several methodological flaws. The study was terminated by its steering committee because of slow recruitment after enrolling less than half the patients needed to adequately power the study. The study also did not achieve a significant difference between interventional and control groups in terms of glycemic control.

A second study by van den Berghe in a medical ICU did not demonstrate significantly decreased mortality in those individuals treated more intensively in terms of glycemic control. However, in this study, the decrease of glycemic levels achieved in the intensive group was less than that achieved in the prior study (111 vs. 103 mg/dL) and, thus, the glycemic differences between control and intensive groups was less. In addition, the patient population in this later study had a significantly higher baseline morbidity and acuity level than did the first.

The use of IV insulin protocols does come at a cost, and has been associated with increased risks of hypoglycemia. Brunkhorst et al demonstrated

that the use of IV insulin in critically ill patients with sepsis increased the risks of adverse events related to hypoglycemia. The Glucontrol trial in Europe was also stopped prematurely, due to unacceptable risks of hypoglycemia in this critically ill cohort of patients, many of whom (~50%) received steroids. A meta-analysis by Gandhi et al suggests that while perioperative insulin infusion protocols may reduce mortality, they increase hypoglycemia.

A recent meta-analysis by Wiener et al recently concluded that "in critically ill adult patients, tight glucose control is not associated with significantly reduced hospital mortality but is associated with an increased risk of hypoglycemia." However, this analysis included several "unpublished studies," making an assessment of its validity nearly impossible. Other meta-analyses have found benefit with the use of IV insulin protocols in critically ill patients.

The Normoglycemia Intensive Care Evaluation-Survival Using Glucose Algorithm Regulation (NICE-SUGAR) trial has shed light on risk vs. benefit of intensive glucose control in critical care units. This large multicenter, multinational study with over 6100 critically ill participants with anticipated admission to the ICU to extend beyond 3 days were randomized to either intensive glycemic control targeting 81-108 mg/dL or conventional glycemic control targeting BG <180 mg/dL (and discontinuation of insulin infusion if BG <144 mg/dL). The results demonstrate that patients treated in the intensive group had a 14% relative greater risk of dying compared to patients in the conventional glucose group. The mean BG achieved was 115 mg/dL and 144 mg/dL in the intensive and conventional glycemic control groups, respectively. Moreover, the risk of severe hyperglycemia defined as <40 mg/dL was nearly 14 times greater in the intensive group compared to the conventional group.

Some have argued that the benefit derived from IV insulin seen in the surgical ICU in van den Berghe's studies is a result of the effect of insulin on free fatty acids and lipids seen in patients who receive early total parenteral nutrition (TPN). Very early use of TPN is common in some areas of Europe, but not common in the U.S. If this is correct, one might expect differential effects from IV insulin use in these different locales.

What about the general medical surgical wards? There is much less known about the effects of tightening of glycemic control and outcomes on the general medical and surgical wards, as most of the studies to date have focused on the medical and surgical ICU or cardiac surgery patients. There is evidence that higher glucose values are associated with increased morbidity and mortality in the general hospital population. Recommendations based on "best available evidence" for target ranges of glucose control in non-ICU hospital patients have been outlined by the ADA, AACE and other organizations (see Table 1).

In both the ICU and non-ICU patient populations, those individuals with newly discovered marked hyperglycemia who were not previously known to have diabetes suffer from higher rates of morbidity and mortality than their diabetic counterparts. Thus, the issue of screening for occult hyperglycemia is gaining more interest. A study by Wexler et al at the Massachussetts General Hospital (MGH) in Boston documented that 18% of all admissions (excluding those with known diabetes) to MGH over the study period had elevated A1Cs, suggesting either occult diabetes of impaired glucose tolerance. Fish et al documented elevated blood sugars in 41% of patients admitted to the ICU without a history of known diabetes over a 10-month period, and more recently, a review at our hospital of patients with marked hyperglycemia with an index blood sugar >300 mg/dL documented 13.5% had no antecedent history of known diabetes.

Table 1

Target Ranges for Hospital Glucose Control

Population	ADA	AACE	IDC
ICU	Critically ill surgical patients close to 110 mg/dL and generally <140 mg/dL; critically ill non-surgical <140 mg/dL	Upper Limit 110 mg/dL	70-140 mg/dL
Non-ICU	fasting <126 and random <180-200	Preprandial 100 mg/dL Maximal 180 mg/dL	Fasting or Preprandial 70-140 mg/dL
			Post-meal 70-180 mg/dL

ADA - American Diabetes Association
AACE - American Association of Clinical Endocrinologists
IDC - International Diabetes Center Minneapolis, MN

3. Treatment Strategies for Tight Glycemic Control in the ICU Setting

The use of IV insulin infusions is quickly becoming the standard of care for most critically ill patients with significant hyperglycemia.

These protocols all share a common thread of utilizing regular human insulin (usually 100 units in 100 mL of 0.9% normal saline) delivered by an IV infusion pump allowing flow rates to be adjusted to deliver IV insulin in incremental rate changes of 0.5 units/hour.

It is important to remember to prime the IV bag and tubing prior to initiating insulin delivery to ensure accurate dosing rates once non-specific binding sites of insulin in the bag and tubing are saturated (by priming).

Most IV insulin protocols start with 2.0-5.0 units/hour and then adjust rates of insulin delivery based on the current levels of blood glucose, overall current insulin infusion rate, as well as the rate of change, in the recent blood glucose levels (Appendix I). The added burden on nursing staff in checking hourly finger-stick blood glucose levels and then inputting and using this data into an algorithm can be significant,, thus the ability to automate data input and therapeutic dosage calculations and alterations will likely result in greater acceptance among hospital support staff, improved efficiency and reduced possible dosing errors, which will cumulatively improve patient safety.

Many of these protocols are based on personal experience and best educated estimates of insulin requirements that can be generalized to a broad-based hospital ICU population. Interestingly, comparing different insulin dosing protocols can lead to potential clinically significant differences in insulin doses in the same patient. For example, a patient who has been started on an insulin drip which is currently running at 4 units/hour has his glucose drop from 350 mg/dL to 248 mg/dl over the next hour. By the Yale protocol (see Appendix I), the rate of infusion would be changed to 2 units/hour, while via the Portland protocol one would continue at 4 units/hr (a 100% increased insulin dosing rate).

It is unlikely there will be a clinical trial comparing the various protocols head to head in a similar patient population.

A typical pattern of blood glucose levels following initiation and titration of insulin infusion rates over 3-10 hours (assuming relative clinical stability) is one of decreasing glycemic variability with progressively smaller glucose excursions over time (Figure 3). Glycemic levels most commonly remain relatively stable over time, or can be quickly adjusted for changes in clinical condition or therapeutic alterations, such as initiation or discontinuation of steroids and change in nutrition. Once glycemic levels remain stable over repeated

Figure 3

Glucose levels correcting on IV insulin drip

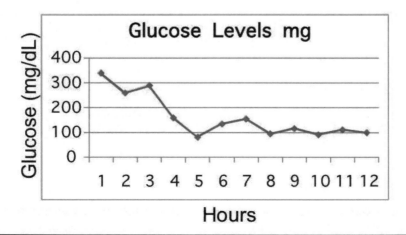

measures, over 2-3 hours time with no change in insulin infusion rate, the frequency of glucose monitoring can often safely be reduced to every 2 hours.

The next clinical challenge, in terms of ongoing glucose control, often occurs upon transferring the patient from an IV insulin protocol over to a subcutaneous (SC) insulin regimen with improvement in their condition or transfer out of the ICU to the general medical/surgical ward.

It is important to remember that the plasma half-life of regular human insulin delivered by IV is only 20 minutes. Therefore, insulin levels and therapeutic effect quickly dissipate following cessation of the IV insulin drip, and individuals can commonly develop rebounding hyperglycemic levels in short order. This is especially important in individuals with type 1 diabetes without any endogenous insulin production, who can quickly begin developing diabetic ketoacidosis (DKA) within an hour or so following discontinuation of the IV insulin drip. It may not be uncommon for patients to be without insulin coverage upon transferring out of an ICU to the general floor for a few hours if the IV is stopped in the ICU and it is assumed that the new SC insulin orders will be written by the accepting medical team once the patient arrives to the floor (general ward).

Staff should be clearly educated on the importance of overlapping SC insulin with the IV drip to ensure adequate insulin coverage. In general, it may take 4 hours for intermediate (NPH) or long-acting (LA) insulins (ie, detemir, glargine) to achieve adequate levels following their administration. Thus, an overlap of NPH or LA insulin given SC with the IV drip by approximately 4 hours, necessitating hourly glucose assessments and adjustment in the IV insulin infusion rate, should be standard practice. If short- (regular human) or rapid-acting (Lispro, Aspart, Glulisine) insulins are required (ie, for coverage meal or nutritional carbohydrate intake [enteral tube feed bolus]), the regular or SA insulin should be overlapped with the IV insulin drip by up to 30-60 minutes, with similar close monitoring.

4. Treatment Strategies for Tight Glycemic Control in the non-ICU Setting

While less than a third of the outpatient population with type 2 diabetes is treated with insulin, the vast majority of patients with type 2 diabetes and all patients with type 1 diabetes should be on insulin in the hospital.

The acuity levels of today's patients admitted to the hospital are higher than ever before, and the added physiologic stress of acute illness places excessive demands on the pancreas to overcome the counterregulatory hormone "stress" hormonal surge seen with serious illness.

Thus, most patients on oral agents for glucose control, and even many individuals that are strictly "diet controlled" in terms of their diabetes, will manifest stress-induced hyperglycemia in the hospital setting, necessitating insulin supplementation to achieve adequate glucose control and lower their risks.

Even in those few individuals where oral agents might suffice to adequately control glucose levels, there are major patient safety issues that arise with the use of oral agents in the hospital setting.

One of the most common oral agents is metformin, which entails a small risk of lactic acidosis, a potentially fatal adverse event. This risk is significantly increased in individuals with significantly diminished renal function, severe volume depletion or other "low flow" states (ie, decompensated cirrhosis or CHF, etc.), ischemia, hypoxemia or exposure to radiologic contrast dye loads. All these events are much more likely to occur in the hospital setting.

Thiazolidinediones (TZDs), such as pioglitazone or rosiglitazone, carry risks of volume retention/overload that can worsen CHF, edematous states and potential renal status in the hospital setting. The issue of cardiac risk with the use of rosiglitazone has also been raised and could raise a concern in the many patients with unstable cardiac conditions seen in today's hospitals.

The sulfonylurea agents (and meglitinides) meant to function a secretagogues-stimulating increased endogenous insulin, particularly in response to postprandial glucose excursions, raise the risks of

Figure 4

Normal insulin secretion with basal production and meal-related rises

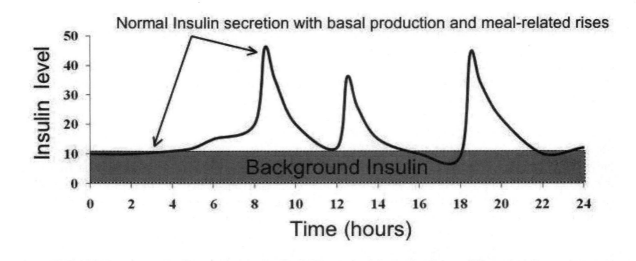

Normal Insulin secretion with basal production and meal-related rises

Figure 5

Bolus or mealtime insulin

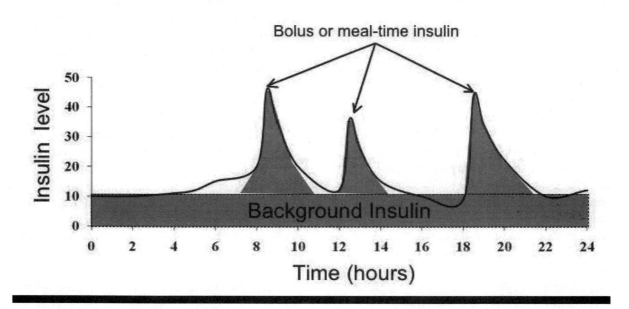

Bolus or meal-time insulin

severe hypoglycemia (particularly glyburide use in the elderly). Many of these agents are also dependent on properly functioning hepatic and renal clearance mechanisms that are often adversely affected by illness. With a high prevalence of GI disorders (both resulting in original need the for admission or nosocomially acquired), the use of agents with potential GI side effects, such as acarbose, metformin or incretins may be unwise.

In addition, to date we have little to no safety data on the use of the newest class of diabetes therapeutics, the incretins, within the hospital setting. Even a patient who is tolerating incretin therapy well as an outpatient may have increased risk with their use in the hospital setting, due to declining hepatic or renal function. The dipeptidyl peptidase-IV inhibitors (DDP-4) have been shown to increase stromal-derived factor-1 (sdf-1), an inflammatory chemokine in rodent models of rheumatoid arthritis (RA) and physiologically measurable increases in sdf-1 and substance P (a substance which mediates pain sensation) have been shown in humans. While these do not appear to be of much clinical relevance in the typical outpatient settings, such potential may raise concern in otherwise ill, compromised hospital patients.

It would appear that a strong argument can be made that all oral agents for glycemic control should be discontinued upon admission to the hospital. Insulin has a long track record with demonstrated safety and efficacy.

In using insulin in the hospital setting, one should try to replicate the situation seen under normal physiologic conditions, modified of course for the changes in meal and activity pattern, changes in underlying physiologic function and the added physiologic stress of illness.

As a starting point, insulin therapy should supply the background or basal insulin needs, duplicating the normal, continuous low level 24-hour insulin secretion that helps control hepatic glucose output in the fasting state (Figure 4). With the increase in insulin resistance seen with stress-induced changes in counterregulatory hormones, the requirements for background or basal insulin increase with illness.

If the patient is well enough to consume meals, or if nutritional support in the form of TPN or enteral tube feedings are to be given, then added insulin will be required to cover the expected rise in post-

Figure 6

Meal and corrective insulin

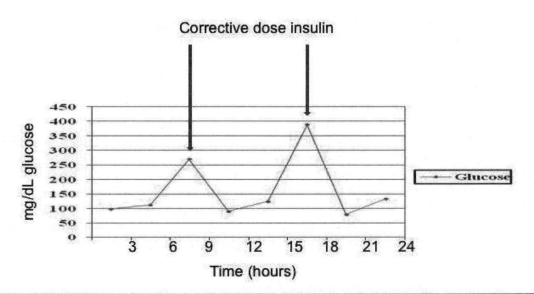

Figure 7

Stacking of second dose of RA insulin onto the first

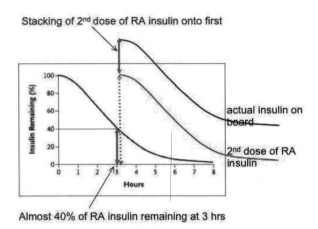

Stacking of 2nd dose of RA insulin onto first

actual insulin on board

2nd dose of RA insulin

Almost 40% of RA insulin remaining at 3 hrs

Modified from Hirsch IB. Insulin Analogues. N Engl J Med. 2005;352:174-183

prandial or meal-related glucose (Figure 4). By ordering this insulin based on the number of carbohydrate choices (15 gram) to be consumed, the order will be delivered when meals are eaten, but automatically held if the patient is NPO (nothing per oral/by mouth) (Figure 5).

Finally, the third component of a proper insulin regimen would be that of corrective dose or supplemental insulin, usually delivered before meals combined with the meal-related insulin if the patient is eating. The function of this component of the insulin regimen is intended to allow for transient treatment of persisting hyperglycemia, despite proper use of background (basal) and mealtime (bolus or prandial) insulin (Figure 6). The added dose of regular or rapid-acting insulin is meant to help bring down the elevated glucose levels back into the target range. Thus, it serves as a "correction dose" and is usually dosed as a specific number of units for each defined increment the blood glucose is over target (ie, 1 unit for every 50 mg/dL the blood glucose is over 150 mg/dL).

As a general rule of thumb, the corrective dose can initially be calculated by using the "rule of 1800." The rule utilizes the patient's total daily insulin dose (if known) or their insulin requirement over 24 hours, and divides 1800 by this number. For example, for a patient on a total of 60 units of insulin daily, this correction factor would be 1800/60 or 30 mg/dL, representing the expected drop in blood glucose an additional 1 unit of insulin would be anticipated to effect. Conversely, in a patient of twice as much total daily insulin of 120 units, the correction factor would be 1800/120 or 15 mg/dL. Not surprisingly, for individuals on this much insulin, the same additional 1 unit of insulin would be expected to drop the ambient blood glucose by only half as much, or 15 mg/dL.

Example:

- An individual in the hospital always has the same number of carbohydrates with each meal and is on 60 units total daily insulin (10 units before each meal and 30 units basal)

- Correction dose would be: 1800/60 = 30 or 1 unit for every 30 mg/dL over goal glucose levels

- If this person's premeal goals were glucose values between 80 and 120 mg/dL, but the premeal glucose was 240 mg/dL, this individual would need an additional corrective dose of 6 additional units of rapid- or short-acting insulin added to their usual 10 units of premeal insulin

- Excess glucose = 240 mg/dL – 120 mg/dL= 120mg/dL

- Corrective insulin = 120 mg/dL ÷ 30mg/dL = 4 extra units of insulin

- Total premeal dose = 14 units (10 units regularly scheduled, plus 4 extra units of correction)

If the patient is NPO, this corrective dose insulin can be delivered every 6 hours, but should typically not be given more frequently than this, to avoid insulin stacking and the risk of precipitating hypoglycemia (Figure 7).

At the International Diabetes Center at Park Nicollet and Methodist Hospital, we have settled upon a starting dose of insulin that balances the risk of hypoglycemia and willingness for nonspecialist generalists to accept and prescribe a complete (3-part) inpatient insulin regimen with the desire for tighter glycemic control. As such, in insulin-naïve patients, we begin with a total daily insulin dose at 0.4 units/Kg split evenly between background- (basal) and meal-related (bolus), or nutritional (enteral tube feed) insulins.

In patients receiving oral or intravenous steroids (>20 mg of prednisone or its equivalent), we begin at 0.6 units/Kg.

In patients previously on insulin, we use their outpatient total daily insulin requirement as a starting point and may modify this based on their current level of outpatient glycemic control (A1C). Because of irregular meal and activity patterns, we typically recommend converting patients on pre-mixed insulin regimens over to background/mealtime (basal/bolus) insulin regimens.

If patients then appear to be require significant doses of correction factor insulin (>20% of schedule total daily insulin dose), over the first 24 hours much of this added insulin can be incorporated into their scheduled insulin dosing by distributing it among the background/mealtime insulin doses, based on their glycemic patterns.

Transitions within the hospital, from ICU to general medical/surgical ward, or from hospital back to outpatient are fraught with potential for decompensation in levels of glycemic control. In patients receiving IV insulin drips in the ICU, cessation of the insulin drip prior to allowing adequate time for SC insulin to reach effective doses, glucose levels are likely to rise. In general, one should overlap SC regular or SA insulin by 30-60 minutes and intermediate LA insulins by 2-4 hours. More frequent blood glucose monitoring during periods of conversion may also be necessary to ensure a smooth transition.

Once a patient's condition has stabilized and they are ready for discharge from the hospital, several factors may impact their diabetes glucose treatment regimen upon returning to the outpatient setting. In general, if the patient was admitted to the hospital with evidence of long-standing poor glycemic control, such as an A1C >8% on 2 or more oral agents for glycemic control, the hospitalization should be taken as an opportunity to transition the patient to insulin therapy to achieve improved glycemic control and lower their long-term risks. This means that proper education and training should be provided to ensure the patient is capable and adherent with the regimen upon dismissal. It is of vital importance in these situations that good communication exist between the hospital diabetes team and the patient's primary care physician, explaining the reasoning behind the intensification of therapy, the specifics of the new insulin regimen should be communicated to the primary physician and the team should ensure appropriate follow-up is in place, including potential referral for further diabetes-related education and training.

In patients treated with medical nutritional therapy (MNT), or oral agents in whom the A1C is within reasonably good control (<8%) in the pre-hospital setting and upon admission, there is a good likelihood that they can be transitioned back to their outpatient regimen upon resolution of the physiologic stress from acute illness. However, in individuals with longer-term changes in their medical condition or therapy (ie, longer-term steroid therapy), insulin may continue to be required.

There are some special circumstances within the hospital setting that require unique insulin regimens.

In individuals receiving oral high-dose steroids with marked hyperglycemia, IV insulin protocol can be used, particularly within the first 24 hours, to help in gauging insulin requirements. However, many times these patients are on the general medical-surgical wards, where the increased nursing demands and decreased nurse-to-patient ratios make use of IV insulin protocols more difficult. In some circumstances, local hospital policy may in fact prohibit IV insulin use on the general wards. In such circumstances, SC insulin regimens will likely be required.

One of the more common steroid regimens is the use of a single AM dose of prednisone. Given that the half-life of oral prednisone is approximately 12 hours, this regimen leads to marked mid-day hyperglycemia, often with a slow return towards baseline glucose levels over the evening and nighttime hours. An AM dose of NPH insulin is frequently useful in these circumstances, as the time course of hyperglycemia and the time-action curve for NPH insulin are nicely matched. Thus, the effect of NPH insulin dissipates as the steroidal effect on glucose wanes. This same sequence can be repeated the following morning. Such a regimen may also work well for the occasional alternate day dosing of prednisone or other oral steroid that is occasionally used to attempt diminished adrenal suppression.

It is very important to closely link the insulin and steroid dosing, such that if the steroid dose is held or discontinued the insulin administration is held as well. Just as important would be a decreasing of the insulin dosing as the steroid dose is tapered.

In patients receiving TPN, it is often convenient to add the insulin to the bag which automatically links the insulin to the nutritional support it is meant to cover. Often, the daily requirement of insulin is first determined by an IV insulin infusion during the first 24 hours of continuous TPN. Then, if the patient's clinical condition and insulin requirements appear to remain stable, approximately 60% of the total daily insulin requirement can be add to the patient's TPN bag on the following day.

Finally, the use of enteral tube feedings can remain a challenge, as the typical regimen of SC regular or SA insulin to provide meal-related prandial or bolus coverage are not suited for this atypical presentation of oral carbohydrates and calories. One should try matching the expected time-course of the tube feeding with the appropriate insulin action time course (ie, NPH insulin for overnight tube feeds or twice daily NPH or LA insulin for continuous tube feeds). With such a program, it often remains difficult to maintain tight glycemic control without increased risk of hypoglycemia, unless one continues to utilize corrective dose SA insulin on a 4-6 hour PRN basis.

As noted above, if using corrective doses more frequently than every 6 hours, one must be especially vigilant in monitoring for stacking of the insulin doses with risk of hypoglycemia. The other major risk of hypoglycemia occurs when the enteral tube is accidentally dislodged or the tube feeds are stopped for any reason, as the nutritional insulin supplementation will also need to be curtailed.

If one is utilizing NPH or LA insulin and the enteral feeds are not quickly restarted, then more frequent glucose monitoring with added IV glucose supplementation may be required to avoid hypoglycemia.

6. New Hyperglycemia in Patients Without a Known Diagnosis of Diabetes in the Hospital Setting

Roughly one-third of all patients with diabetes remain undiagnosed . 57 million Americans have pre-diabetes and may become overtly hyperglycemic with the overt physiologic stress of acute illness or therapies (ie, steroids) in the hospital. The work of Umpierrez and others have clearly documented that this group with previously undiagnosed hyperglycemia in the hospital setting suffers from the greatest added morbidity and mortality of any group. This is true, even compared to the group with known diabetes with well-documented increased risk compared to non-diabetic individuals.

It is important to screen for occult hyperglycemia in the hospital setting, to identify these individuals and initiate appropriate insulin therapies to reduce their risks. Wexler and colleagues recently assessed A1C on the number of consecutive patients admitted to MGH and found elevated values (>6%) in 18%

Fortunately, many patients have glucose levels checked as part of routine laboratory assessments in the hospital, often a part of chemistry or metabolic panels, but action to track or treat such elevated glucoses is often missing. It is often useful to assess glucose upon admission to the ICU, as these patients are under the highest levels of physiologic stress. Patients receiving IV or oral steroids should be monitored after initiating steroids or increasing the dose. Monitoring anyone started on tube feeds or TPN is prudent.

It is likely that maintaining a high level of suspicion to find such individuals with occult hyperglycemia, and appropriately treating them with insulin to maintain tighter glycemic control, will help reduce their high levels of morbidity and mortality.

7. Conclusion

While the benefits of tight glycemic control in the hospital setting is still being debated in some circles, the evidence to date points to improved patient outcomes.

It should be remembered that while fear of hypoglycemia remains common, rates of marked hyperglycemia still far outweigh the low rates of clinically significant hypoglycemia, often by a factor of 10-fold or greater.

Major diabetes organizations, such as the ADA and AACE, have weighed the evidence and have outlined their glycemic targets for individuals with diabetes or hyperglycemia within the hospital setting (Table 1). The major hospital-accrediting organization, the Joint Commission on Accreditation of Healthcare Organizations (JCAHO), which accredits hospitals within the United States and has made improvements in diabetes care within the nation's hospitals a priority, now offers a hospital program for diabetes accreditation at http://www.jointcommission.org/CertificationPrograms/Inpatient+Diabetes.

While some debate as to the advantages of tight glycemic control in our hospitals is likely to continue, few would advocate a return to the days of "sliding scale" insulin, with its wide fluctuations in glycemic levels and increased patient safety concerns.

In the meantime, striving to control blood glucose in the hospital to as near normal as can reasonably be accomplished without exposing patients to excessive risk for severe hypoglycemia seems the prudent choice.

8. Appendix I

IV Example of Insulin Protocol
(Yale and Portland Protocols)

The following insulin infusion protocol is intended for use in hyperglycemic adult patients in an ICU setting, but is not specifically tailored for those individuals with diabetic emergencies, such as diabetic ketoacidosis (DKA) or hyperglycemic hyperosmolar states (HHS). When these diagnoses are being considered, or if BG≥ 500 mg/dL, an MD should be consulted for specific orders. Also, please notify an MD if the response to the insulin infusion is unusual or unexpected, or if any situation arises that is not adequately addressed by these guidelines.

Initiating an Insulin Infusion

1.) INSULIN INFUSION: Mix 1 U Regular Human Insulin per 1 cc 0.9 % NaCl. Administer via infusion pump (in increments of 0.5 U/hr).
2.) PRIMING: Flush 50 cc of infusion through all IV tubing before infusion begins (to saturate the insulin binding sites in the tubing).
3.) TARGET BLOOD GLUCOSE (BG) LEVELS: **100-139 mg/dL**
4.) BOLUS & INITIAL INSULIN INFUSION RATE: Divide initial BG level by 100, then round to nearest 0.5 U for bolus AND initial infusion rate.
  Examples: 1.) Initial BG = 325 mg/dL: 325 ÷ 100 = 3.25, round ↑ to 3.5: IV bolus 3.5 U + start infusion @ 3.5 U/hr.
  2.) Initial BG = 174 mg/dL: 174 ÷ 100 = 1.74, round ↓ to 1.5: IV bolus 1.5 U + start infusion @ 1.5 U/hr.

Blood Glucose (BG) Monitoring

1.) Check BG hourly until stable (3 consecutive values within target range). In hypotensive patients, capillary blood glucose (i.e., fingersticks) may be inaccurate and obtaining the blood sample from an indwelling vascular catheter is acceptable.
2.) Then check BG q 2 hours; once stable x 12-24 hours. BG checks can then be spaced to q 4 hours IF:
  a.) no significant change in clinical condition AND b.) no significant change in nutritional intake.
3.) If any of the following occur, consider the temporary resumption of hourly BG monitoring, until BG is again stable (2-3 consecutive BG values within target range):
  a.) any change in insulin infusion rate (i.e., BG out of target range)
  b.) significant changes in clinical condition
  c.) initiation or cessation of pressor or steroid therapy
  d.) initiation or cessation of renal replacement therapy (hemodialysis, CVVH, etc.)
  e.) initiation, cessation, or rate change of nutritional support (TPN, PPN, tube feedings, etc.)

Changing the Insulin Infusion Rate

If BG < 50 mg/dL:
D/C INSULIN INFUSION   Give 1 amp (25 g) D50 IV; recheck BG q 15 minutes.
⇒ When BG ≥ 100 mg/dL, wait 1 hour, then restart insulin infusion at 50% of original rate.

If BG 50-74 mg/dL:
D/C INSULIN INFUSION   If symptomatic (or unable to assess), give 1 amp (25 g) D50 IV; recheck BG q 15 minutes.
If asymptomatic, give 1/2 Amp (12.5 g) D50 IV or 8 ounces juice; recheck BG q 15-30 minutes.
⇒ When BG ≥ 100 mg/dL, wait 1 hour, then restart infusion at 75% of original rate.

If BG ≥ 75 mg/dL:
STEP 1: Determine the CURRENT BG LEVEL - identifies a COLUMN in the table:

BG 75-99 mg/dL	BG 100-139 mg/dL	BG 140-199 mg/dL	BG ≥ 200 mg/dL

STEP 2: Determine the RATE OF CHANGE from the prior BG level - identifies a CELL in the table - Then move right for INSTRUCTIONS:
[Note: If the last BG was measured 2-4 hrs before the current BG, calculate the hourly rate of change. Example: If the BG at 2PM was 150 mg/dL and the BG at 4PM is now 120 mg/dL, the total change over 2 hours is -30 mg/dL; however, the hourly change is -30 mg/dL ÷ 2 hours = -15 mg/dL/hr.]

BG 75-99 mg/dL	BG 100-139 mg/dL	BG 140-199 mg/dL	BG ≥ 200 mg/dL	INSTRUCTIONS*
		BG ↑ by > 50 mg/dL/hr	BG ↑	↑ INFUSION by "2Δ"
	BG ↑ by > 25 mg/dL/hr	BG ↑ by 1-50 mg/dL/hr OR BG UNCHANGED	BG UNCHANGED OR BG ↓ by 1-25 mg/dL/hr	↑ INFUSION by "Δ"
BG ↑	BG ↑ by 1-25 mg/dL/hr, BG UNCHANGED, OR BG ↓ by 1-25 mg/dL/hr	BG ↓ by 1-50 mg/dL/hr	BG ↓ by 26-75 mg/dL/hr	NO INFUSION CHANGE
BG UNCHANGED OR BG ↓ by 1-25 mg/dL/hr	BG ↓ by 26-50 mg/dL/hr	BG ↓ by 51-75 mg/dL/hr	BG ↓ by 76-100 mg/dL/hr	↓ INFUSION by "Δ"
BG ↓ by > 25 mg/dL/hr see below[†]	BG ↓ by > 50 mg/dL/hr	BG ↓ by > 75 mg/dL/hr	BG ↓ by > 100 mg/dL/hr	HOLD x 30 min, then ↓ INFUSION by "2Δ"

[†]D/C INSULIN INFUSION; √BG q 30 min; when BG ≥ 100 mg/dL, restart infusion @75% of most recent rate.

*CHANGES IN INFUSION RATE ("Δ") are determined by the current rate:

Current Rate (U/hr)	Δ = Rate Change (U/hr)	2Δ = 2X Rate Change (U/hr)
< 3.0	0.5	1
3.0 - 6.0	1	2
6.5 - 9.5	1.5	3
10 - 14.5	2	4
15 - 19.5	3	6
20 - 24.5	4	8
≥ 25	≥ 5	10 (consult MD)

Original Portland Protocol

Blood Glucose	Action
<75 mg/dL	Stop insulin. Give 25 cc dextrose 50% water (D50w) and recheck BG every 30 minutes. When BG reaches >150 mg/dL, restart at 50% of previous rate.
75 mg/dL to 100 mg/dL	Stop insulin. Recheck BG every 30 minutes. When levels reach >150 mg/dL, restart at 50% of previous rate unless the dose is less than 0.25 U/hr.
101 mg/dL to 125 mg/dL	If <10% lower than last BG, decrease rate by 0.5 U/hr. If >10% lower than last BG, decrease rate by 50%. If neither occurs, continue current rate.
126 mg/dL to 175 mg/dL	Same rate
176 mg/dL to 225 mg/dL	If lower than last BG, continue the same rate. If higher than last BG, increase rate by 0.5 U/hr.
>225 mg/dL	If >10% lower than last BG, continue same rate. If <10% lower than last BG or if higher than last BG, increase rate by 1 U/hr.

Source: The Portland Protocol for Continuous Intravenous Insulin Infusion in Post Operative Cardiac Surgery Patients.

Albert Starr Academic Center for Cardiac Surgery. The Portland Protocol for Continuous Intravenous Insulin Infusion in Post Operative Diabetic Cardiac Surgery Patients. March 2001. www.starrwood.com/research/insulin.html. Accessed March 17, 2004.

9. References

van den Berghe G, Wouters P, Weekers F, et al. Intensive insulin therapy in the critically ill patients. *N Engl J Med*. 2001;345:1359-1367.

Furnary AP, Zerr KJ, Grunkemeier GL, Starr A. Continuous intravenous insulin infusion reduces the incidence of deep sternal wound infection in diabetic patients after cardiac surgical procedures. *Ann Thorac Surg*. 1999;67:352-362.

Furnary AP, Gao G, Grunkemeier GL, et al. Continuous insulin infusion reduces mortality in patients with diabetes undergoing coronary artery bypass grafting. *J Thorac Cardiovascular Surg*. 2003;125:1007

Furnary AP, Wu Y, Bookin SO. Effect of hyperglycemia and continuous intravenous insulin infusions on outcomes of cardiac surgical procedures: the Portland Diabetic Project. *Endocr Pract*. 2004;10 (suppl 2):21-33.

Malmberg K, Norhammar A, Wedel H, Rydén L. Glycometabolic state at admission: important risk marker of mortality in conventionally treated patients with diabetes mellitus and acute myocardial infarction: long-term results from the Diabetes and Insulin-Glucose Infusion in Acute Myocardial Infarction (DIGAMI) study. *Circulation*. 1999;99:2626-2632.

Van den Berghe G, Wilmer A, Hermans G, et al. Intensive insulin therapy in the medical ICU. *N Engl J Med*. 2006;354:449-461.

Malmberg K. Prospective randomised study of intensive insulin treatment on long term survival after acute myocardial infarction in patients with diabetes mellitus. DIGAMI (Diabetes Mellitus, Insulin Glucose Infusion in Acute Myocardial Infarction) Study Group. *BMJ*. 1997;314:1512-1515.

Brunkhorst FM, Engel C, Bloos F, et al. Intensive insulin therapy and pentastarch resuscitation in severe sepsis. *N Engl J Med*. 2008;358:125-139.

Jaimes F, De La Rosa G, Morales C, et al. Unfractioned heparin for treatment of sepsis: A randomized clinical trial (The HETRASE Study). *Crit Care Med*. 2009;37(4):1185-1196.

Boord JB, Greevy RA, Braithwaite SS, et al. Evaluation of hospital glycemic control at US Academic Medical Centers. *J Hosp Med*. 2009;4:35-44.

Hirsch IB. Insulin Analogues. *N Engl J Med*. 2005;352:174-183.

Golden SH, Peart-Vigilance C, Kao WH, Brancati FL. Perioperative glycemic control and the risk of infectious complications in a cohort of adults with diabetes. *Diabetes Care*. 1999;22:1408-1414.

Kramer R, Groom R, Weldner D, et al. Glycemic control and reduction of deep sternal wound infection rates: a multidisciplinary approach. *Arch Surg*. 2008;143(5):451-456.

Gandhi GY, Murad MH, Flynn DN, et al. Effect of perioperative insulin infusion on surgical morbidity and mortality: systematic review and meta-analysis of randomized trials. *Mayo Clin Proc*. 83(4):418-430.

Wiener RS, Wiener DC, Larson RJ. Benefits and risks of tight glucose control in critically ill adults: a meta-analysis. *JAMA*. 2008;300(8):933-944.

Pittas AG, Siegel RD, Lau J. Insulin therapy for critically ill hospitalized patients: a meta-analysis of randomized controlled trials. *Arch Intern Med*. 2004;164:2005-2011.

NICE-SUGAR Study Investigators, Finfer S, Chittock DR, et al. Intensive versus conventional glucose control in critically ill patients. *N Engl J Med*. 2009;360:1283-1297.

Mesotten D, Swinnen JV, Vanderhoydonc F, Wouters PJ, Van den Berghe G. Contribution of circulating lipids to the improved outcome of critical illness by glycemic control with intensive insulin therapy. *J Clin Endocrinol Metab*. 2004;89:219-226.

Miles JM, McMahon MM, Isley WL. No, the glycaemic target in the critically ill should not be < or = 6.1 mmol/l. Diabetologia. 2008;51:916-920.

Umpierrez GE, Isaacs SD, Bazargan N, You X, Thaler LM, Kitabchi AE. Hyperglycemia: an independent marker of in-hospital mortality in patients with undiagnosed diabetes. J Clin Endocrinol Metab. 2002;87:978-982.

Cakir M, Altunbas H, Karayalcin U. Hyperglycemia: an independent marker of in-hospital mortality in patients with undiagnosed diabetes. J Clin Endocrinol Metab. 2003;88:1402.

Wexler T, Gunnell L, Omer Z, et al. Growth Hormone Deficiency is Associated with Decreased Quality of Life in Patients with Prior Acromegaly. J Clin Endocrinol Metab. 2009;93:4238-4244.

Fish LH, Moore AL, Morgan B, Anderson RL. Evaluation of admission blood glucose levels in the intensive care unit. Endocr Pract. 2007;13:705-710.

Davis ED, Harwood K, Midgett L, Mabrey M, Lien LF. Implementation of a new intravenous insulin method on intermediate-care units in hospitalized patients. Diabetes Educ. 2005;31:818-821.

Koro CE, Bowlin SJ, Bourgeois N, Fedder DO.. Glycemic control from 1988 to 2000 among U.S. adults diagnosed with type 2 diabetes: a preliminary report. Diabetes Care. 2004;27:17-20.

CDC National Diabetes Fact Sheet 2007. http://www.cdc.gov/diabetes/pubs/pdf/ndfs_2007.pdf. Accessed June 27, 2009.

Chapter 13: Diabetes in Children and Adolescents

Amy Criego, MD, MS
Betsy Schwartz, MD, MS

Contents

1. Type 1 Diabetes in Children and Adolescents

Historically, all childhood onset diabetes was considered to be the consequence of autoimmune destruction of beta cell mass. As such, type 1 diabetes was classically defined as onset in youth, while all diabetes with onset in adulthood was considered to be type 2 diabetes arising from the dual pathophysiology defects of insulin resistance and progressive beta-cell secretory dysfunction. However, it is now well-established that people of any age can develop either type 1 or type 2 diabetes. The increasing incidence of obesity and type 2 diabetes in the pediatric population will also be addressed, following the section on type 1 diabetes.

The American Diabetes Association (ADA) classifies type 1 diabetes into type 1A, indicating autoimmune beta cell failure, and type 1B, indicating non-immune medicated severe deficiency.[1] For the purposes of this review, type 1 diabetes will refer to autoimmune mediated type 1A insulin deficiency. Specifics regarding the pathogenesis and epidemiology of type 1 diabetes are detailed in the review by Gilliam and Hirsch and will be referenced where appropriate, while this chapter will focus on detailing the unique qualities of diabetes in the pediatric population.

2. Type 1 Epidemiology

Type 1 diabetes remains the most common form of diabetes diagnosed in the pediatric population, with variable reports regarding the current prevalence of type 2 diabetes. As noted earlier in the review by Gilliam and Hirsch, type 1 diabetes is most predominant in European and Middle Eastern populations, with the highest prevalence in northern Europe. Type 1 diabetes is less common in Africans, Asians and Native Americans, where the risk of type 2 diabetes is increased. The incidence of type 1 diabetes has been increasing for reasons that are not well understood or clearly defined. The incidence of type 1 diabetes mellitus has been increasing in the pediatric population, with the most vigorous increase noted in those under the age of 5 years.[2] With some countries reporting a doubling in the space of 2 generations, it has been estimated that the worldwide incidence of type 1 diabetes may be 40% higher in 2010 than in 1998.[3] Over the last 3 decades, the diagnosis of diabetes in children has become more complex as rates of obesity have continued to increase. While an increasing number of youth, especially in high-risk ethnic groups, are being diagnosed with type 2 diabetes, the presence of obesity and insulin resistance can also be seen in children with type 1 diabetes. This is identified by some as "double diabetes." Advancements in genetic testing have also increased the identification of monogenic forms of diabetes.[16]

3. Type 1 Diagnosis

The diagnosis of type 1 diabetes in children is typically made after symptoms of polyuria, polydypsia, polyphagia and weight loss occur. At this time, approximately 10%-20% of beta cells still remain, but these will also be destroyed over time. The diagnostic criterion for diabetes in children does not differ from adults, and includes a fasting plasma glucose ≥126 mg/dl or a random glucose ≥200 mg/dl. Diabetic ketoacidosis (DKA) is present in approximately 25% of patients at diagnosis, with younger children being at a higher risk for the development of DKA. Those with acidosis, dehydration and vomiting require hospitalization for medical stabilization and initiation of insulin, but the majority of patients can now be initially treated in the outpatient setting. Ambulatory insulin initiation programs have been well-established since the late 1980s and although not universally accepted, due in part to health care reimbursement issues, they have been shown to be both safe and effective, with a low risk of hospitalization. Initiation of insulin outside of the hospital setting requires close follow-up with experienced health care providers, but allows parents and children to immediately take ownership of this chronic disease and establish routines for successful self-management.

Following insulin initiation, residual beta cell mass rendered less functional by hyperglycemia may recover, and insulin doses often need to be decreased and, rarely, children will not require any exogenous insulin. This "honeymoon" period may last for a variable period of time, and may extend up to 6-12 months before complete destruction of beta cells and loss of insulin secretion occurs. During this time, it may be difficult for some children and adolescents to continue with their daily regimen. and it is important for health care teams to ensure that patients and families have realistic expectations regarding the eventual complete dissolution of endogenous insulin secretion. Daily blood glucose monitoring, insulin administration and clinic follow-up remain important, so that dose adjustments can be made in a timely manner to avoid worsening control over extended periods of time.

4. Type 1 Treatment Strategies

Uncontrolled type 1 diabetes in children can be associated with significant morbidity and mortality, including both acute metabolic complications (such as DKA) and a higher risk of chronic vascular complications. As described in the chapter of Wysham, the Diabetes Control and Complications Trial (DCCT) demonstrated a significant decrease in the risk of secondary microvascular complications with early intensive glycemic control, even in children.[9] The risk reductions for specific complications are again shown here:

- Primary retinopathy: 76% reduction

- Progression of retinopathy: 54% reduction

- Development of proliferative or severe retinopathy: 47% reduction

- Microalbuminuria: 39% reduction

- Frank albuminuria: 54% reduction

- Clinical neuropathy: 60% reduction

Complications of type 1 diabetes can occur early in the disease process and, therefore, prevention of long-term micro- and macrovascular complications must begin in the pediatric age group. Good glycemic control must be the goal from diagnosis, as there does not seem to be any "grace period," with early stages of complications seen 2-5 years after diagnosis. While the most common cause of death in youth with type 1 diabetes globally is lack of access to insulin, an analysis by the CDC suggested that a 10-year-old child developing diabetes in the year 2000 would live approximately 50-55 more years, losing about 18-20 years of life. This is indicative of the lack of metabolic control and complications that occur, even when access to treatment is available.[17]

Goals for diabetes control vary by age, due to a higher risk for severe hypoglycemia in younger children and the decreased likelihood of developing complications prior to puberty. Current treatment goals developed by the ADA based on age are listed in Table 1.

Table 1

American Diabetes Association Treatment Goals Based on Age

	Ages (years)			
	<6	**6–12**	**13–18**	**>18**
Hemoglobin A1c	7.5–8.5	<8.0	<7.5	<7.5
Preprandial glucose (mg/dl)	100–180	90–180	90–130	70–130
Bedtime/overnight glucose	110–200	100–180	90–150	

Appropriate diabetes care for children and adolescents also involves the entire family. Type 1 diabetes is self managed, and in younger children this often requires the training and assistance of parents and other family members, as well as school personnel and day care providers. In addition, multi-dose insulin regimens, improvements in blood glucose monitoring technology, the use of insulin analogs and advances in insulin delivery devices have increased the need for training on daily diabetes management. The benefit of these same advances includes greater flexibility and the promise of long-term health improvement. The patient's and family's knowledge, adherence and ongoing diabetes education are essential for these positive outcomes.

A diabetes team with physicians, diabetes nurse educators, nutritionists and mental health professionals is essential, with the patient and family being at the center of the team. Open lines of communication between all members, including school personnel, are necessary to optimize control. Additional caregivers will likely need diabetes education as well, and diabetes education for all involved must be updated periodically to keep up with the child's changing developmental needs

and ability to take on more responsibility. As children get older and take on the responsibility for blood glucose monitoring and insulin administration, feedback and motivation need to be provided by all team members, including physicians, nurse educators, dieticians and mental health providers. Adherence to the daily regimen is difficult, but essential to achieve good glycemic control. The frequency of self-monitoring of blood glucose has been shown to be associated with metabolic control.[18] Missed insulin doses, even occasionally, are frequent in adolescents and can significantly impact glycemic control.[19] Missed doses with insulin pump therapy are more easily identified with current technology.

Routine lab monitoring is also essential for the management of type 1 diabetes in children. Hemoglobin A1c values are recommended 4 times yearly. Additional studies, typically done annually, include: thyroid function studies, celiac antibody testing, lipids, urine microalbumin screening and dilated eye exams. Recommendations for screening and treatment of these complications in children/adolescents with type 1 diabetes are established by the ADA and are included in Table 2.[20]

Table 2

American Diabetes Assocation Recommendations for Screening and Treatment of Type 1 Diabetes in Children and Adolescents

	Timing for Initiation of Screening	Treatment Recommendations
Microalbuminuria	Annual screening for microalbuminuria, with a random spot urine sample for microalbumin-to-creatinine ratio, should be initiated once the child is 10 years of age and has had diabetes for 5 years	Confirmed, persistently elevated microalbumin levels on 2 additional urine specimens should be treated with an ACE inhibitor, titrated to normalization of microalbumin excretion if possible
Hypertension	Blood pressure assessed at quarterly clinic visits	• Treatment of high-normal blood pressure (systolic or diastolic blood pressure consistently between the 90th–95th percentile for age, sex and height) should include dietary intervention and exercise aimed at weight control and increased physical activity, if appropriate. If target blood pressure is not reached with 6-12 months of lifestyle intervention, pharmacologic treatment should be initiated • Pharmacologic treatment of high blood pressure (systolic or diastolic blood pressure consistently above the 95th percentile for age, sex and height, or consistently >130/80 mmHg for adolescents) should be initiated along with lifestyle intervention, as soon as the diagnosis is confirmed • ACE inhibitors should be considered for the initial treatment of hypertension • The goal of treatment is a blood pressure consistently <130/80 or below the 90th percentile for age, sex and height, whichever is lower

(continued)

Table 2

American Diabetes Assocation Recommendations for Screening and Treatment of Type 1 Diabetes in Children and Adolescents

	Timing for Initiation of Screening	**Treatment Recommendations**
Dyslipidemia	• If there is a family history of hypercholesterolemia (total cholesterol >240 mg/dl) or a cardiovascular event before age 55 years, or if family history is unknown, then a fasting lipid profile should be performed on children >2 years of age soon after diagnosis (after glucose control has been established). If family history is not of concern, then the first lipid screening should be performed at puberty (≥10 years). All children diagnosed with diabetes at or after puberty should have a fasting lipid profile performed soon after diagnosis (after glucose control has been established) • For both age-groups, if lipids are abnormal, annual monitoring is recommended. If LDL cholesterol values are within the accepted risk levels (<100 mg/dl [2.6 mmol/l]), a lipid profile should be repeated every 5 years	• Initial therapy should consist of optimization of glucose control and MNT, using a Step 2 AHA diet aimed at a decrease in the amount of saturated fat in the diet • After the age of 10, the addition of a statin is recommended in patients who, after MNT and lifestyle changes, have LDL >160 mg/dl (4.1 mmol/l) or LDL cholesterol >130 mg/dl (3.4 mmol/l) and 1 or more CVD risk factors. • The goal of therapy is an LDL cholesterol value <100 mg/dl (2.6 mmol/l)
Retinopathy	• The first ophthalmologic examination should be obtained once the child is ≥10 years of age and has had diabetes for 3-5 years • After the initial examination, annual routine follow-up is generally recommended. Less frequent examinations may be acceptable on the advice of an eye care professional	• Evaluation and treatment by retinal specialist

Table 2

American Diabetes Assocation Recommendations for Screening and Treatment of Type 1 Diabetes in Children and Adolescents

	Timing for Initiation of Screening	Treatment Recommendations
Thyroid Disease	• Patients with type 1 diabetes should be screened for thyroid peroxidase and thyroglobulin antibodies at diagnosis • TSH concentrations should be measured after metabolic control has been established. If normal, they should be rechecked every 1-2 years, or if the patient develops symptoms of thyroid dysfunction, thyromegaly or an abnormal growth rate. Free T4 should be measured if TSH is abnormal.	• Medication management for hypothyroidism • Medication or ablation for hyperthyroidism
Celiac Disease	• Patients with type 1 diabetes should be screened for celiac disease, by measuring tissue transglutaminase or anti-endomysial antibodies, with documentation of normal serum IgA levels, soon after the diagnosis of diabetes • Testing should be repeated if growth failure, failure to gain weight, weight loss or gastroenterologic symptoms occur • Consideration should be given to periodic rescreening of asymptomatic individuals	• Children with positive antibodies should be referred to a gastroenterologist for evaluation • Children with confirmed celiac disease should have consultation with a dietitian and be placed on a gluten-free diet

continued

Historically, insulin was administered in fixed doses and at specific times, significantly limiting the flexibility in children with type 1 diabetes. Although "sliding scale" doses were often given to account for elevated glucose values, this approach was reactive and non-physiologic. With the availability of analog insulin, insulin delivery has improved substantially, lending to more dietary and scheduling flexibility. This "basal-bolus" insulin regimen is now the standard of care for both children and adults with type 1 diabetes, and consists of 3 critical components:

- Background (basal) coverage: typically half of the insulin produced over a 24-hour period by a normal pancreas is background insulin. In people relying on exogenous insulin delivery, this can be done with insulin pump therapy, administering continuous doses of rapid-acting insulin (aspart, glulisine, lispro) or via injection once or twice daily with a long-acting insulin analog (glargine, detemir)

- Carbohydrate coverage: rapid-acting insulin can be administered based on estimated carbohydrates consumed. Based on age, body weight and individual insulin sensitivity, this dose is typically about 1 unit per 5-15 grams, although in younger children, insulin requirements may be much less, with some only needing 1 unit per 30-60 grams. As smaller doses are required, the needed for diluted insulin may become necessary. Fixed doses of insulin with set meal plans may be used, if carbohydrate intake is consistent or the concept of counting carbohydrates is too difficult. Ideally, this insulin is always administered prior to eating

- Correction doses: elevated blood glucose values require additional rapid-acting insulin, and this is typically administered prior to meals and at bedtime, but can be given every 2-3 hours, especially during illness. The correction dose is based on how much 1 unit will lower the blood glucose, and this scale is again affected by age, body weight and overall insulin sensitivity. For young children, 1 unit of insulin may lower the blood glucose 100-200 mg/dl, school-aged children typically require 1 unit to lower the blood glucose 50-100 mg/dl, and older children and

adolescents typically require 1 unit to lower their blood glucose only 25-50 mg/dl.

Whether insulin is administered via injection or insulin pump, blood glucose control benefits from consistent scheduling, frequent blood glucose monitoring and appropriate insulin administration prior to eating. Pediatric equipment such as short needles and 1/2 unit delivery devices are also necessary to achieve good diabetes control. As mentioned above, diluted insulin may be needed for very young children with minimal, but necessary, insulin requirements. Insulin pump therapy can offer additional flexibility and precise dose delivery.

Continuous glucose monitoring (CGM) sensors are a new and exciting technology introduced in the past few years, and these devices offer people with type 1 diabetes a unique approach to improving glucose control. Detail on the use of CGM is provided in Chapter 15.

CGM use in pediatrics offers unique advantages. The technique for use is similar in adults and children. The devices consist of a sensor inserted under the skin, which transmits interstitial fluid glucose levels to a receiver that allows users to follow trends in real time. Sensors do not replace finger-stick blood glucose monitoring, and these are an essential part of ensuring the sensor is giving accurate information. This technology allows patients and families to evaluate trends over time, in order to optimize insulin dose adjustments. While continuous sensor technology has not been shown to significantly improve hemoglobin A1c values in the pediatric population, this has mainly been attributed to the widely varied use of the CGM devices by age.[10] In children between the ages of 8-14, the average decrease in HbA1c was not significantly different in those using CGM vs. control groups; however, those in the CGM group were more likely to lower their HbA1c by at least 10% and achieve HbA1c levels below 7%.

15-24-year-old patients using CGM, as a group, also did not experience significant improvements in glucose control compared with the control group. Part of this observation may be that CGM use varied with age, averaging at least 6 days a week over the course of the trial in 83% of the patients 25 years and older, but dropping off to 30% of the 15-24-year-olds and 50% of the 8-14-year-olds (for whom CGM use typically involved their parents' assistance). Although glycemic control did not improve dramatically, additional advantages to using CGM included less frequent hypoglycemia and the use of trend information for dose adjustments.

5. Type 1 Factors Unique to the Pediatric Population

Newborns and Toddler

Children diagnosed with type 1 diabetes under the age of 5 years offer unique challenges for families and caregivers. Insulin doses may be minimal and require diluted insulin (U-10 or U-50) which is less stable and available far less commonly than U-100 insulin. Background analog insulins cannot be diluted, and diluents for rapid-acting insulin are not always available. Background insulin administered once daily in the morning may be a beneficial alternative in this age group, in order to provide adequate coverage during the daytime with doses wearing off overnight to avoid nocturnal hypoglycemia.

Irregular eating patterns in newborns and toddlers make it difficult to administer rapid-acting insulin prior to eating, although this type of administration is both more effective and more appropriate physiologically. Reactive insulin administration may lead to more blood glucose variability, and also increases the risk for hypoglycemia.

In addition to challenges of insulin administration, younger children may not be able to articulate symptoms of hypoglycemia, which in turn may increase the risk for severe hypoglycemia in this age group. Although glycemic goals are generally higher in this age group, it can still be a significant challenge and difficult balance for families, as a result of the erratic eating and activity patterns in these children. Of note, severe hypoglycemia in those under the age of 5 years has been shown to be associated with long-term cognitive effects, so efforts to reduce this risk are critical.

School Age

The majority of diabetes care in this age group will be managed or closely supervised by parents. School personnel are also closely involved, and need to be part of the diabetes care team and active in communication. As children get older, the transition to independence with daily diabetes cares needs to be achieved gradually with continued parental involvement. With extracurricular activities and increased time with peers, continued diabetes education focusing on the children's understanding is essential.

Adolescents

Adolescents with type 1 diabetes present numerous management challenges. As adolescents spend more time with peers and are exposed to social situations involving drugs and alcohol, they must be educated regarding the impact of these behaviors on diabetes control, some of which can be significantly detrimental or even life-threatening. Driving safely with type 1 diabetes must also be discussed, with emphasis on the importance of hypoglycemia avoidance and treatment, as well as monitoring of blood glucose prior to driving.

Disturbed eating behaviors have been shown to be very common in females with type 1 diabetes. A case-control prevalence study showed that eating disorders were twice as common in teenage girls with type 1 diabetes as in the general population (10% vs. 4.5%, respectively) with sub-threshold eating disorders being even more common, diagnosed in 14% of girls with type 1 diabetes and only 8% of the non-diabetic comparison group.[11] Although unintentional, diabetes management may be an iatrogenic factor that encourages dietary restraint and attention to food intake, that could trigger dietary dysregulation. This could lead to disturbed eating in vulnerable individuals. Disturbed eating in individuals with type 1 diabetes is associated with increases in the risk of DKA, and hospitalizations and complications, particularly retinopathy and neuropathy.[12-15] Attention to eating behaviors is essential to identify abnormalities early, so that appropriate evaluation and treatment can occur.

Although the daily management of type 1 diabetes can be onerous, contact with the diabetes team providing self-management tools can help children and adolescents, and the wide availability of insulin analogs, novel delivery devices and a broad array of monitoring tools can permit children with type 1 diabetes to live safe, normal, healthy lives. Regular follow-up with the health care team to monitor growth, development, educational needs and treatment adjustments significantly reduces the burden of care by providing support, and improving and updating diabetes care approaches over time. While the pathophysiology differs, children and adolescents with type 2 diabetes require essentially the same level of care. Details regarding type 2 diabetes in pediatrics will be addressed in the remainder of this chapter.

7. Type 2 Diabetes in Children and Adolescents

Prior to the 1990s, type 2 diabetes was rarely reported among children, and immune-mediated type 1 diabetes accounted for nearly all cases of diabetes in the pediatric population.[21] Corresponding with the rise in childhood obesity over the past 2 decades, the prevalence of type 2 diabetes in youth has increased dramatically, with type 2 diabetes representing 8%-45% of newly diagnosed diabetes in various North American pediatric centers.[22] Not unique to the United States, the increasing occurrence of type 2 diabetes in children has been reported in countries across the world, including Japan, Australia and the United Kingdom.[23-25]

8. Type 2 Epidemiology

The SEARCH for Diabetes in Youth Study is the largest effort to determine the prevalence of diabetes in youth in the United States to date.[26] In the year 2001, 6379 children and adolescents were diagnosed with diabetes among 6 participating centers. The overall prevalence of diabetes was estimated to be 1.82 per 1000 youth. Among children <10 years of age with diabetes, <1% were diagnosed with type 2 diabetes. In contrast, type 2 diabetes accounted for 15% of diabetes cases in adolescents aged 10-19-years-old. The proportion of type 2 diabetes varied greatly among race/ethnic groups, accounting for 6% of diabetes in Caucasians, 33% in African Americans, 22% in Hispanics and 76% in Native Americans in the adolescent age group (Table 3).

Table 3

Proportion of Type 2 Diabetes Among Prevalent Cases of Diabetes (type 1, type 2 and Other) According to Age Group and Race/Ethnicity

Race/Ethnicity	Ages 0-9 years	Ages 10-19 years
Non-Hispanic Caucasian	0.4	5.8
African American	0.1	32.7
Hispanic	1.3	21.9
Asian/Pacific Islanders	6.7	40.1
Native American	13.3	76.4

Adapted from SEARCH for Diabetes in Youth Study Group. The burden of diabetes mellitus among US youth: prevalence estimates from the SEARCH for Diabetes in Youth Study. Pediatrics. 2006;118:1510-1518.

9. Type 2 Pathophysiology

Similar to adults, the etiology of type 2 diabetes in youth results from the combination of 2 core physiologic defects: insulin resistance and impaired β-cell secretory function.[27, 28] In children, obesity is 1 of the most important contributors to insulin resistance.[29] Resistance of insulin-sensitive tissues, such as the liver and muscle, to the effects of insulin is an early abnormality in the development of type 2 diabetes. Peripheral insulin resistance leads to a compensatory increase in β-cell insulin secretory function, and this hyperinsulinemic response initially maintains normal glucose homeostasis.[30] Decreased insulin sensitivity and hyperinsulinemia coexist in obese children.[31, 32] The evolution from normal glucose tolerance to type 2 diabetes in youth occurs after a further decline in insulin sensitivity and impaired β-cell insulin secretion, in agreement with what is described in the adult literature.[28, 33, 34]

Metabolic studies investigating the specific underlying mechanisms in the development type 2 diabetes in youth are scarce. As with adults, the transition from normal to impaired glucose tolerance in obese youth is marked by a decline in first-phase insulin secretion, an early indicator of β-cell failure which occurs most commonly in the setting of impaired insulin sensitivity.[33] Adolescents with type 2 diabetes show a further decline in first-phase insulin secretion, as well as a defect in second-phase insulin secretion.[28, 32, 33] Of great concern is the rapid rate of deterioration to type 2 diabetes, found in 1 longitudinal study of 117 obese youth.[35] In only 2 years, 24% of subjects with impaired glucose tolerance developed diabetes. Compared to the progression described in adult studies, this suggests that β-cell failure may occur more rapidly in young individuals.[30, 36] Additional studies are necessary to establish that an accelerated progression to type 2 diabetes is common for youth with this disease.

10. Type 2 Established Risk Factors

Obesity

The prevalence of childhood obesity has tripled over the past 3 decades (Figure 1) and recent estimates show that 17% of children and adolescents in the United States are obese (defined as a BMI >95th percentile for age and gender).[37] Obesity is considered the most important risk factor for insulin resistance and type 2 diabetes in children. Impaired glucose tolerance has been found among 25% of obese children and 21% of obese adolescents.[32] Up to 85% of youth with type 2 diabetes are overweight or obese at the time of diagnosis.[38] Excessive weight gain has been shown to accelerate the progression to type 2 diabetes. In obese youth with impaired glucose tolerance, those who develop type 2 diabetes have a significantly higher BMI at baseline and gain more weight over time, when compared to those who do not develop type 2 diabetes.[35]

Figure 1

NHANES data on prevalence of obesity (BMI ≥95th percentile for age and gender) among children and adolescents from selected years 1971-1974 through 2003-2004

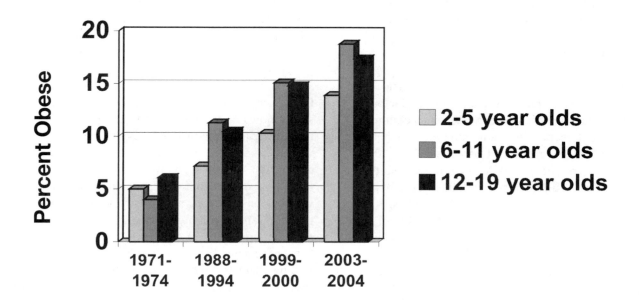

Adapted from NHANES data given on www.cdc.gov.

As with adults, it appears that central obesity and visceral fat, independent of BMI, correlate with insulin resistance in obese youth.[39, 40] There are a number of proposed mechanisms by which obesity causes insulin resistance. Elevated levels of free fatty acids can decrease insulin-stimulated peripheral glucose uptake and impaired insulin secretion, and can increase hepatic glucose production.[34] Adipose tissue also releases hormones and cytokines (such as leptin, c-reactive protein, tumor necrosis factor-α, visfatin and IL-6) which are associated with insulin resistance[21] and occur in higher levels in obese children and adolescents.[42-44] Other protective factors, such as adiponectin, are inversely correlated with insulin resistance in obese youth.[45]

Puberty

A transient insulin-resistant state occurs during puberty, and is a normal part of pubertal development. Insulin resistance, as measured by the euglycemic insulin clamp in a large cohort of children, increases at the beginning of puberty, peaks at mid-puberty and returns to prepubertal levels at the end of puberty.[46] Normal glucose homeostasis is generally maintained during puberty through compensatory hyperinsulinemia.[47] It is thought that growth hormone and IGF-1 contribute to this phenomena, and that the physiologic purpose for pubertal insulin resistance and hyperinsulinemia is to promote rapid growth, through the augmentation of protein anabolism.[48, 49]

While compensatory hyperinsulinemia during puberty allows most children to maintain normal glucose tolerance, this balance may decompensate when pubertal insulin resistance poses an additional burden to the glucose homeostasis of obese children with risk factors for type 2 diabetes. This may explain why type 2 diabetes is rarely seen in prepubertal children and the peak age at presentation corresponds with that of mid-puberty.[38]

Family History

A family history of type 2 diabetes in first- or second-degree relatives is a major risk factor for the development of type 2 diabetes in children and adolescents. Of youth with type 2 diabetes, 45%-80% have at least 1 parent and 74%-100% have a first- or second-degree relative with type 2 diabetes.[38] High-risk susceptibility genes have been identified, primarily in adult studies, and likely contribute to the strong heritability of type 2 diabetes.[50] In children, gene variants associated with impaired glucose metabolism have been found in genes coding for transcription factor 7-like 2 (TCF7L2), peroxisome proliferators-activated receptor (PPAR), insulin and ENPP1, a glycoprotein that interacts with the insulin receptor.[50, 51]

Race/Ethnicity — Higher Risk Population Groups

The prevalence of type 2 diabetes in the United States is highest among Native American youth, followed by Asian/Pacific Islanders, African American, Hispanic and then Caucasian youth (Table 3).[26] Over the past 3 decades, rates of obesity have increased to a greater degree among African American and Hispanic youth, when compared to Caucasian youth.[32] Despite this, studies have shown that African American and Hispanic children are more resistant to insulin than their Caucasian peers, even when adjusting for differences in body fat.[53] African American obese youth also appear to be at a greater risk for developing type 2 diabetes, when compared to Caucasian obese youth.[35] It is likely that the influence of race/ethnicity on developing type 2 diabetes is mediated by both genetic and environmental factors.[38]

Conditions Associated with Insulin Resistance (Metabolic Syndrome)

The metabolic syndrome refers to a common clustering of cardiovascular risk factors, including increased waist circumference, impaired glucose metabolism, hypertension and dyslipidemia. This syndrome is common in those with type 2 diabetes, prediabetes, and while the cluster occurs with increasingly higher frequencies, it does not represent a single disease or an established unifying pathogenesis.

Data from the SEARCH for Diabetes in Youth study show that 92% of youth with type 2 diabetes meet criteria for the metabolic syndrome, when defined as having 2 or more cardiovascular disease risk factors in addition to diabetes.[54] Polycystic ovary syndrome, a condition associated with insulin resistance and obesity, is commonly found in female youth with type 2 diabetes.[21] In addition, up to 90% of children with type 2 diabetes have acanthosis nigricans, a cutaneous finding characteristic of hyperinsulinemia and insulin resistance.[38]

Intrauterine and Early Life Factors Influencing Glucose Metabolism

Intrauterine and early life environments may influence risk for the later development of type 2 diabetes. Both low and high birth weight are associated with an increased risk of developing type 2 diabetes in child- and adulthood.[55, 56] Offspring of mothers with diabetes are also at a higher risk for later developing type 2 diabetes.[57] In fact, for Pima Indian youth, in utero exposure to diabetes has been found to be the strongest single risk factor for type 2 diabetes.[58] Breastfeeding in infancy appears to be protective and is associated with a reduced risk of type 2 diabetes later in life.[59] It is not known how such factors during fetal and early post-natal life impact later glucose metabolism, but it is possible that imprinting genes involved in adipocyte and pancreatic development may play a role.[50]

11. Screening for Type 2 Diabetes

In 2000, the ADA established guidelines for screening at-risk children for type 2 diabetes. Children who are overweight and have 2 additional risk factors (as detailed in Table 4) are advised to be screened for glucose intolerance, using a fasting blood glucose level. Screening should be considered at 10 years of age onward or earlier, to coincide with the onset of puberty. Testing should be performed every 2 years thereafter.[38] In 2007, the Expert Committee, a group of experts in childhood obesity formed by 15 national health care organizations, published their recommendations for the prevention, assessment and treatment of overweight and obese children and adolescents. Their screening recommendations for type 2 diabetes are similar to those of the ADA, however, the Expert Committee suggests screening obese children (BMI >95th percentile for age and gender), regardless of the presence of additional risk factors.[60]

Table 4

Screening Recommendations for Type 2 Diabetes in Children and Adolescents

Criteria: **Overweight** is defined by:

> BMI >85th percentile for age and gender

> Weight for height >85th percentile

> Weight >120th percentile of ideal (50th percentile) for height

Plus any 2 of the following risk factors:

> Family history of type 2 diabetes in first- or second-degree relatives

> Belong to high-risk race/ethnic group (Native American, African American, Hispanic, Asian/Pacific Islander)

> Signs/symptoms of insulin resistance (acanthosis nigricans, hypertension, PCOS, dyslipidemia)

Adapted from ADA. Type 2 diabetes in children and adolescents. Diabetes Care. *2000;23:381-389.*

12. Type 2 Diagnosis

The criteria for the diagnosis of diabetes in children are the same as in adults. A child with the classic symptoms of diabetes (polyuria, polydipsia and unexplained weight loss) and a random blood glucose level ≥200 mg/dl is defined as having diabetes. In addition, a child with a fasting blood glucose level ≥126 mg/dl or a blood glucose level ≥200 mg/dl 2 hours after ingestion of glucose during an oral glucose tolerance test is also defined as having diabetes.[38]

Children and adolescents presenting with type 2 diabetes should be distinguished from those with type 1 diabetes. In most patients, this classification can be made on the basis of typical clinical features. The majority of children presenting with type 2 diabetes are overweight or obese, whereas children with type 1 diabetes are usually thin or of normal weight.[21] Signs and conditions associated with insulin resistance are common in youth with type 2 diabetes. In fact, up to 90% of children presenting with type 2 diabetes have acanthosis nigricans.[38] Children with type 1 diabetes have a more acute presentation; ketonuria is usually present and up to 40% present with DKA. Type 2 diabetes has a more indolent course; 33% of youth with type 2 diabetes present with ketonuria and 5%-10% present with mild DKA. As discussed previously, youth with type 2 diabetes nearly always have a family history of type 2 diabetes. In contrast, only 5% of children with type 1 diabetes have a first- or second-degree relative with type 1 diabetes. Type 2 diabetes more commonly occurs in children with African American, Native American, Asian or Hispanic ancestry, whereas children with type 1 diabetes are usually Caucasian and of Northern European ancestry.[21,61]

However, distinguishing between type 1 and type 2 diabetes in youth is not always straightforward. With an increased prevalence of obesity among the general population, up to 25% of children diagnosed with type 1 diabetes may be overweight.[21] In addition, there is no definitive laboratory study that distinguishes type 1 and type 2 diabetes. β-cell autoantibodies are found in >90% of individuals with type 1 diabetes, and the absence of these antibodies was once considered a prerequisite for the diagnosis of type 2 diabetes.[38] Yet, at least 1 diabetes autoantibody is detected in up to 35% of children and adolescents diagnosed with type 2 diabetes.[62] An overlap, therefore, may exist between the clinical and laboratory findings of type 1 and type 2 diabetes. Children with a clinical phenotype of type 2 diabetes and evidence of autoimmunity have been described as having "type 1.5" or "double diabetes," a phenomena which appears to occur more commonly among minority youth.[63]

The goal of management of type 2 diabetes in children is not only to achieve glycemic control, but also to improve body weight through lifestyle modification and treating comorbid conditions, such as hypertension and hyperlipidemia. Ideally, a multidisciplinary team including a pediatric endocrinologist, diabetes nurse educator, dietician and behavioral specialist work together with the patient and his/her family to achieve these goals.

Initial treatment will depend on the clinical presentation and this can range from asymptomatic hyperglycemia to DKA and hyperosmolar nonketotic coma. For type 2 diabetes, DKA and hyperosmolar nonketotic coma occur infrequently at the time of diagnosis, but are associated with a high risk of morbidity and mortality in children.[38] Therefore, children in such crises require tertiary care under specialists experienced in the management of these disorders.

More commonly, children with type 2 diabetes are not acutely ill at diagnosis. Patients with mild hypoglycemia (blood glucose ≤200 mg/dl, HbA1C <8.5%) may be treated with metformin, the only oral agent which is FDA-approved for the treatment of type 2 diabetes in children and adolescents.[64] Metformin gained approval after a randomized, controlled study demonstrated safety and efficacy for the treatment of type 2 diabetes in children aged 10-16 years, at doses up to 1000 mg twice daily.[65] Children with more significant hyperglycemia (blood glucose >200 mg/dl, HbA1C >8.5%) and/or ketosis should be initially treated with insulin. Metformin may be considered once ketosis has resolved and insulin weaned, if normoglycemia is maintained (fasting blood glucose <126 mg/dl).[44] Glycosylated hemoglobin (HbA1C) should be measured every 3 months, with a goal of ≤7%.[38]

Lifestyle interventions should focus on changing dietary habits to reduce caloric intake, increasing physical activity and limiting sedentary behaviors. Ideally, the diabetes care team includes a nutritionist, mental health care provider and, if possible, an exercise physiologist to provide family-focused support for making lifestyle changes. An individualized approach where behaviors are changed gradually by making small, measurable and attainable goals at each visit, with input of the child and family, is recommended. For example, such goals may include discontinuing sweetened beverages, adding a fruit or vegetable to each meal or reducing fast food intake to once a month. Long-term goals are to improve body weight, instill life-long healthy habits and achieve glycemic control.[66]

Type 2 diabetes in children and adolescents is becoming a critical public health concern, particularly among minority youth. Like adults, youth with type 2 diabetes are at risk for serious complications, such as cardiovascular disease, retinopathy and nephropathy. Because of the longer duration of diabetes, young patients are at an even higher risk of developing such complications than adults with the disease.[67, 68] With the enormous impact of type 2 diabetes on the health and well-being of a growing population of children, it is imperative that prevention efforts targeting at-risk obese children become a shared priority for parents, health care providers, schools, food industries and governmental agencies.[64]

15. References

1. ADA. Report of the expert committee on the diagnosis and classification of diabetes mellitus. *Diabetes Care*. 1997;20:1183-1197.

2. Gale EA. The rise of childhood type 1 diabetes in the 20th century. *Diabetes*. 2002;51:3353-3361.

3. Onkamo P, Väänänen S, Karvonen M, Tuomilehto J. Worldwide increase in incidence of Type I diabetes—the analysis of the data on published incidence trends. *Diabetologia*. 1999;42:1395-1403.

4. Robles DT, Eisenbarth GS. Type 1A diabetes induced by infection and immunization. *J Autoimmun*. 2001;16:355-362.

5. Classen DC, Classen JB. The timing of pediatric immunization and the risk of insulin-dependent diabetes mellitus. *Infect Dis Clin Pract*. 1997;6: 449-454.

6. Scott FW. Cow milk and insulin-dependent diabetes mellitus: is there a relationship? *Am J Clin Nutr*. 1990;51:589-591.

7. Atkinson MA, Eisenbarth GS. Type 1 Diabetes: new perspectives on disease pathogenesis and treatment. *Lancet*. 2001;53:384-392.

8. Achenbach P, Warncke K, Reiter J, et al. Stratification of diabetes risk on the basis of islet autoantibody characteristics. *Diabetes*. 2004;53:384-392.

9. The DCCT Research Group. The effect of intensive treatment of diabetes on the development and progression of long-term complications in insulin-dependent diabetes mellitus. *N Engl J Med*. 1993;329:977-986.

10. The Juvenile Diabetes Research Foundation Continuous Glucose Monitoring Study Group. Continuous Glucose Monitoring and Intensive Treatment of Type 1 Diabetes. *N Engl J Med*. 2008;359:1464-1476.

11. Jones JM, Lawson ML, Daneman D, Olmsted MP, Rodin G.. Eating disorders in adolescent females with and without type 1 diabetes: cross sectional study. *BMJ*. 2000;320:1563-1566.

12. Biggs MM, Basco MR, Patterson G, Raskin P. Insulin withholding for weight control in women with diabetes. *Diabetes Care*. 1994;17:1186-1189.

13. Polonsky WH, Anderson BJ, Lohrer PA, Aponte JE, Jacobson AM, Cole CF. Insulin omission in women with IDDM. *Diabetes Care*. 1994;17:1178-1185.

14. Colas C. Eating disorders and retinal lesions in type 1 (insulin-dependent) diabetes women. *Diabetologia*. 1991;34:288.

15. Steel JM, Young RJ, Lloyd GG, Clarke BF. Clinically apparent eating disorders in young diabetic women: associations with painful neuropathy and other complications. *Br Med J (Clin Res Ed)*. 1987;294: 859-862.

16. Aanstoot HJ, Anderson BJ, Daneman D, et al. The global burden of youth diabetes: perspectives and potential: a charter paper. *Pediatr Diabetes*. 2007;8(suppl 8):1-42.

17. Narayan KM, Boyle JP, Thompson TJ, Sorensen SW, Williamson DF. Lifetime risk for diabetes mellitus in the United States. *JAMA*. 2003;290:1884-1890.

18. Haller M, Stalvey MS, Silverstein JH. Predictors of control of diabetes: monitoring may be the key. *J Pediatr*. 2004;139:197-203.

19. Olinder AL, Kernell A, Smide B. Missed olus doses: devastating for metabolic control in CSII-treated adolescents with type 1 diabetes. *Pediatr Diabetes*. 2009;10:142-148.

20. ADA. Standard of Medical Care In Diabetes – 2009. *Diabetes Care*. 2009;32:S13-S61.

21. Kaufman F. Type 2 diabetes in children and youth. *Endocrinol Metab Clin N Am*. 2005;34:659-676.

22. Fagot-Campagna A, Pettitt D, Engelgau M, et al. Type 2 diabetes among North American children and adolescents: An epidemiologic review and a public health perspective. *J Pediatr*. 2000;136(5):664-672.

23. Kitagawa T, Owada M, Urakami T, Yamauchi K. Increased incidence of non-insulin dependent diabetes mellitus among Japanese schoolchildren correlates with an increased intake of animal protein and fat. *Clin Pediatr*. 1998;37(2):111-115.

24. Braun B, Zimmermann M, Kretchmer N, Spargo R, Smith R, Gracey M. Risk factors for diabetes and cardiovascular disease in young Australian aborigines: a 5-year follow-up study. *Diabetes Care*. 1996;19:472-479.

25. Ehtisham S, Hattersley A, Dunger D, Barett T. First UK survey of paediatric type 2 diabetes and MODY. *Arch Dis Child*. 2004;89:526-529.

26. Liese A, D'Agostino R Jr, Hamman R, et al. The burden of diabetes mellitus among US youth: prevalence estimates from the SEARCH for Diabetes in Youth Study. *Pediatrics*. 2006;118(4):1510-1518.

27. Abdul-Ghani M, Tripathy D, DeFronzo RA. Contributions of beta-cell dysfunction and insulin resistance to the pathogenesis of impaired glucose tolerance and impaired fasting glucose. *Diabetes Care*. 2006;29:1130-1139.

28. Gungor N, Bacha F, Saad R, Janosky JE, Arslanian S. Youth type 2 diabetes: Insulin resistance, beta-cell function, or both? *Diabetes Care*. 2005;28:638-644.

29. Cali A, Caprio S. Prediabetes and type 2 diabetes in youth: an emerging epidemic disease? *Curr Opin Endocrinol Diabetes Obes*. 2008;15:123-127.

30. Weiss R, Gillis D. Patho-physiology and dynamics of altered glucose metabolism in obese children and adolescents. *Int J Pediatr Obesity*. 2008;3:15-20.

31. Caprio S, Bronson M, Sherwin RS, Rife F, Tamborlane WV. Co-existence of severe insulin resistance and hyperinsulinaemia in pre-adolescent obese children. *Diabetologia*. 1996;39:1489-1497.

32. Sinha R, Fisch G, Teague B, et al. Prevalence of Impaired Glucose Tolerance Among Children and Adolescents with Marked Obesity. *N Engl J Med*. 2002;346(11):802-810.

33. Weiss R, Caprio S, Trombetta M, Taksali SE, Tamborlane WV, Bonadonna RC. β-cell function across the spectrum of glucose tolerance in obese youth. *Diabetes*. 2005;54:1735-1743.

34. DeFronzo RA. Pathogenesis of type 2 diabetes mellitus. *Med Clin N Am*. 2004;88:787-835.

35. Weiss R, Taksali SE, Tamborlane WV, Burgert TS, Savoye M, Caprio S. Predictors of changes in glucose tolerance status in obese youth. *Diabetes Care*. 2005;28:902-909.

36. Edelstein S, Knowler W, Bain R, et al. Predictors of progression from impaired glucose tolerance to NIDDM: an analysis of six prospective studies. *Diabetes*. 1997;46:701-710.

37. Ogden C, Carroll M, Curtin L, McDowell M, Tabak C, Flegal K. Prevalence of Overweight and Obesity in the United States, 1999-2004. *JAMA*. 2006;295:1549-1555.

38. ADA. Type 2 diabetes in children and adolescents. *Diabetes Care*. 2000;23:381-389.

39. Bacha F, Saad R, Gungor N, Arslanian S. Are obesity-related metabolic risk factors modulated by the degree of insulin resistance in adolescents? *Diabetes Care*. 2006;29:1599-1604.

40. Lebovitz H, Banjerji M. Point: visceral adiposity is causally related to insulin resistance. *Diabetes Care*. 2005;28:2322-2325.

41. Nathan B, Moran A. Metabolic complications of obesity in childhood and adolescence: more than just diabetes. *Curr Opin Endocrinol Diabetes Obes*. 2008;15:21-29.

42. Aygun A, Gungor S, Ustundag B, Gurgoze M, Sen Y. Proinflammatory cytokines and leptin are increased in serum of prepubertal obese children. *Mediators Inflamm.* 2005;3:180-183.

43. Moran A, Steffen L, Jacobs DR, et al. Relation of C-reactiv protein to insulin resistance and cardiovascular risk factors in youth. *Diabetes Care.* 2005;28:1763-1768.

44. Haider D, Holzer G, Schaller G, et al. The adipokine visfatin is markedly elevated in obese children. *J Pediatr Gastroenterol Nutr.* 2006;43:548-549.

45. Shaibi G, Cruz ML, Weigensberg M, et al. Adiponectin independently predicts metabolic syndrome in overweight latino youth. *J Clin Endocrinol Metab.* 2007;92(5):1809-1813.

46. Moran A, Jacobs DR, Steinberger J, et al. Insulin resistance during puberty: results from clamp studies in 357 children. *Diabetes.* 1999;48:2039-2044.

47. Caprio S, Plewe G, Diamond M, et al. Increased insulin secretion in puberty: a compensatory response to reductions in insulin sensitivity. *J Pediatr.* 1989;114:963-967.

48. Caprio S, Cline G, Boulware S, et al. Effects of puberty and diabetes on metabolism of insulin-sensitive fuels. *Endocrinol Metab.* 1994;29:E885-E891.

49. Moran A, Rosenberg B. Puberty and insulin resistance. In: Daneman D, Hamilton J, eds. *Insulin Resistance in Children and Adolescents.* New York, NY: Nova Science Publishers, Inc.; 2005:87-101.

50. Kempf K, Rathmann W, Herder C. Impaired glucose regulation and type 2 diabetes in children and adolescents. *Diabetes Metab Res Rev.* 2008;24:427-437.

51. Korner A, Berndt J, Stumvoll M, Kiess W, Kovacs P. TCF7L2 gene polymorphisms confer an increased risk for early impairment of glucose metabolism and increased height in obese children. *J Clin Endocrinol Metab.* 2007;92:1956-1960.

52. Freedman DS, Khan L, Serdula M, Ogden C, Dietz WH. Racial and ethnic differences in secular trends for childhood BMI, weight, and height. *Obesity.* 2006;14(2):301-308.

53. Goran MI, Bergman RN, Cruz ML, Watanabe R. Insulin resistance and associated compensatory responses in African-American and Hispanic children. *Diabetes Care.* 2002;25:2184-2190.

54. Rodriguez B, Fujimoto W, Imperatore G, et al. Prevalence of cardiovascular disease risk factors in U.S. children and adolescents with diabetes: The SEARCH for Diabetes in Youth Study. *Diabetes Care.* 2006;29:1891-1896.

55. Wei J, Li H, Sung F, et al. Birth weight correlates differently with cardiovascular risk factors in youth. *Obesity.* 2007;15:1609-1616.

56. Harder T, Rodekamp E, Schellong K, Dudenhausen J, Plagemann A. Birth weight and subsequent risk of type 2 diabetes: a meta-analysis. *Am J Epidemiol.* 2007;165:849-857.

57. Dabelea D, Hanson R, Lindsay R, et al. Intrauterine exposure to diabetes conveys risks for type 2 diabetes and obesity: a study of discordant sibships. *Diabetes.* 2000;49:2208-2211.

58. Dabelea D, Hanson R, Bennett P, Roumain J, Knowler W, Pettitt D. Increasing prevalence of Type II diabetes in American Indian children. *Diabetologia.* 1998;41:904-910.

59. Owen C, Martin R, Whincup P, Smith G, Cook D. Does breastfeeding influence risk of tye 2 diabetes in later life? A quantitative analysis of published evidence. *Am J Clin Nutr.* 2006;84:1043-1054.

60. Barlow S. Expert committee recommendations regarding the prevention, assessment, and treatment of child and adolescent overweight and obesity: summary report. *Pediatrics*. 2007;120:S164-S192.

61. Jones KL. Role of obesity in complicating and confusing the diagnosis and treatment of diabetes in children. *Pediatrics*. 2008;121:361-368.

62. Hathout E, Thomas W, El-Shahawy M, Nahab F, Mace J. Diabetic autoimmune markers in children and adolescents with type 2 diabetes. *Pediatrics*. 2001;107:e102.

63. Libman IM, Pietropaolo M, Arslanian SA, LaPorte RE, Becker DJ. Evidence for heterogeneous pathogenesis of insulin-treated diabetes in black and white youth. *Diabetes Care*. 2003;26:2876-2882.

64. Libman IM, Arslanian SA. Prevention and treatment of type 2 diabetes in youth. *Horm Res*. 2007;67:22-34.

65. Jones KL, Arslanian S, Peterokova VA, Park J-S, Tomlinson MJ. Effect of metformin in pediatric patients with type 2 diabetes: a randomized controlled trial. *Diabetes Care*. 2002;25:89-94.

66. Corrales-Yauckoes K, Higgins L. Nutritional management of the overweight child with type 2 diabetes. *Pediatr Ann*. 2005;34:701-709.

67. Pavkov M, Bennett P, Knowler W, Krakoff J, Sievers M, Nelson R. Effect of youth-onset type 2 diabetes mellitus on incidence of end-stage renal disease and mortality in young and middle-aged Pima Indians. *JAMA*. 2006;296:421-426.

68. Hillier T, Pedula K. Complications in young adults with early-onset type 2 diabetes. *Diabetes Care*. 2003;26:2999-3005.

Chapter 14: Improving the Quality of Health Care: Focus on Diabetes

Gregg Simonson, PhD
Pam Tompos, MS, RD, LD
Jan Pearson, BAN, RN, CDE

Contents

Overview Health care in the United States is underperforming in many areas related to health outcomes, adherence to healthy behaviors and systems of care delivery. The cost of health care is high and increasing at alarming rates. The combination of underperformance and high cost is especially apparent for people with a chronic disease, such as diabetes. This information presented in this chapter is both timely and critical. The current U.S. administration placed health care reform at the top of the list as critical issues to address in the first year of the Obama presidency. President Obama addressed Congress, saying: "So let there be no doubt health care reform cannot wait, it must not wait, and it will not wait another year."

This chapter was written to highlight several models for improving health care and to describe what professional and national quality improvement organizations are doing to meet the challenge of our underperforming health care system. The chapter also explores potential drivers of performance improvement, including accountability through increased transparency of data and financial incentives through pay-for-performance (P4P). Group medical visits, a creative model for delivering health care at the patient level, are examined. Finally, consumer and employer trends are highlighted that describe major shifts in who pays for health care and how patients will access the health care system.

Diabetes is moving like a tidal wave, impacting people across the United States. 2007 statistics revealed there are 23.6 million people with diabetes and at least 57 million American adults with pre-diabetes. The number of cases of type 2 in young people, under 20 years of age, (previously rare) is increasing. Associated with diabetes and its comorbidities, comes a price tag of $174 billion direct and indirect costs.

How has the health care system organized to address this pandemic? An early model to provide a framework for management of diabetes was introduced by Dr. Donnell Etzwiler in 1994. In his *Blueprint for the Future,* he introduced a Chronic Disease Model recognizing the patient as the primary provider of the treatment team. With that acknowledgement, the model consisted of team/community care with the following components: education/training, available supplies and services, individualized care plans, standardized guidelines for care, ongoing monitoring and support, assessment and feedback with reward and recognition for both the patient and provider. Etzwiler's systems approach to diabetes management served as a historical precursor to the widely recognized chronic care model developed by Wagner.

Wagner recognized the need to further the work on a model for chronic care. After review of the literature, and with input from an advisory panel to the Group Health's MacColl Institute for Healthcare Innovation, the Chronic Care Model (CCM) was developed. A multi-dimensional approach to improving chronic care management, the CCM provides a framework to guide chronic care management in diverse health care settings. It is comprised of 6 key components that are interrelated:

1. Community and its resources and polices

2. Health systems to include payment systems, as well as provider organizations, large or small

3. Self-management support – so critical to the primary member of the care team – the patient

4. Delivery system design which promotes a team approach with a clear role definition for the practice team, physician and non-physician members

5. Decision support that includes evidence-based guidelines, as well as readily available specialist expertise

6. Clinical information systems that include reminders to ensure standards of care are being met, feedback to physicians on performance measures and diabetes registries for pre-/post-visit planning, as well as population-based care

Key in this model is the productive interactions that exist within the patient/practice team relationship (see Figure 1).

The Institute of Medicine (IOM) report, *Crossing the Quality Chasm,* released at approximately the same time as the CCM, reinforced the need for change in health care. It clearly noted that "the health care that we now have and the health care that we could have, lies not just in a gap, but a chasm." Critical to the report was the fact that current care systems cannot do the job; trying harder will not work, but changing the care system will. The report called for creative thinking and innovative designs, and set out 10 simple rules to guide development: 1.) Care is based on continuous healing relationships; 2.) Care is customized according to patient needs and values; 3.) The patient is the source of control; 4.) Knowledge is shared and information flows freely; 5.) Decision-making is evidence-based; 6.) Safety is a system property; 7.) Transparency is necessary; 8.) Needs are anticipated; 9.) Waste is continuously decreased, and; 10.) Cooperation among clinicians is a priority. Most of these very principles are at the core of Donnell Etzwiler's pioneering Chronic Disease Model.

Figure 1

The Chronic Care Model

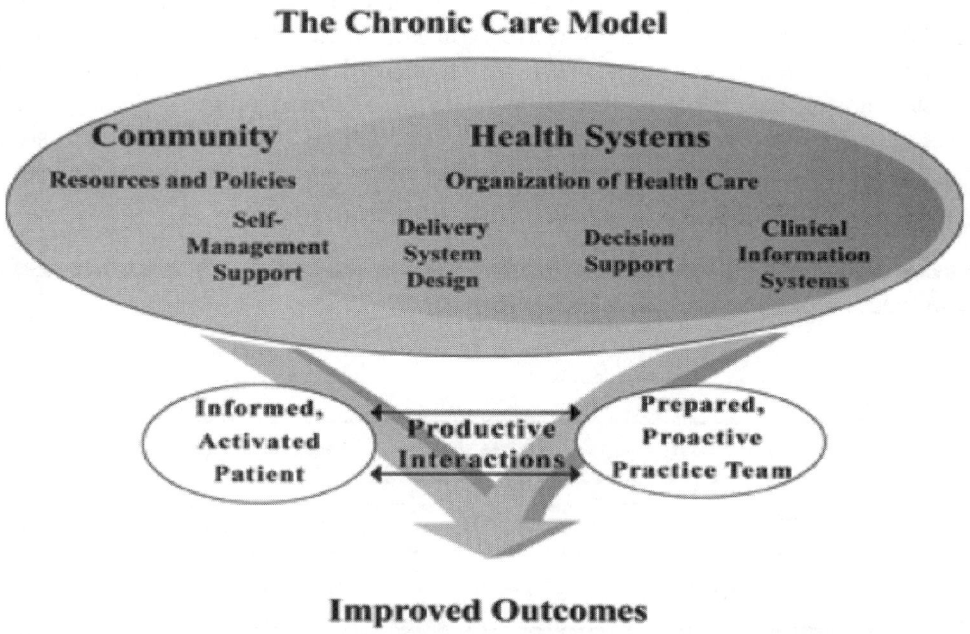

The Chronic Care Model

Community
Resources and Policies

Health Systems
Organization of Health Care

Self-Management Support

Delivery System Design

Decision Support

Clinical Information Systems

Informed, Activated Patient

Productive Interactions

Prepared, Proactive Practice Team

Improved Outcomes

Reprinted from Wagner EH. Chronic disease management: What will it take to improve care for chronic illness? Effective Clinical Practice. 1998;1:2-4., with permission.

Nearly a decade has passed since the release of the IOM report. How have we done in bridging the chasm? To answer this question, a systematic literature review was conducted, revealing 2 quality improvement models that appear to bridge the chasm: the Excellence Award Model (a blending of the Malcolm Baldridge Quality Award criteria and the European Foundation Quality Management [EFQM] Excellence Model) and the Chronic Care Model described above. The Excellence Award Model consists of these key components: *leadership, policy and strategy, management of people, partnership, resources and processes, key performance results and people, customer and society results.* 37 case studies were reviewed (16 in the Excellence Award Model and 21 in the Chronic Control Model). It was concluded that there is some evidence to support that implementing the Chronic Care Model may improve some processes or outcome performances. There was less evidence to demonstrate the impact of the Excellence Award Model, primarily due to the fact that no randomized or controlled studies were found. The authors called for more knowledge on the relationships of organizational development and performance improvement.

Coleman et al conducted a review of articles published since 2000 that used key CCM papers as a reference, and concluded that organizations who had implemented most, if not all, of the 6 areas of the model demonstrated improvement in care. While more study of the cost-effectiveness of the model still remains, it was noted that the CCM serves as a positive framework for guiding practice redesign.

In the United States today, the majority of medical groups contain less than 50 physicians. There are approximately 59,500 medical groups with less than 50 physicians and only 678 with more than 50 physicians. Based on their available resources, the multiple aspects of the CCM may seem too demanding for these smaller medical groups to tackle. What quality improvement model might these groups use?

Solberg et al introduced a simpler conceptual framework that has evolved from literature and his many years of experience (see Figure 2). While it acknowledges the importance of organizational context and the need to attend to internal and external facilitators/barriers, it proposes 3 key components are needed for improvement in quality: priority, change process capability and care process contents. For success, priority for change begins with senior leaders and extends to all levels supported by appropriate resources and ongoing monitoring. Emphasized is the importance of change process capability, requiring attention to several components related to change management: skilled leaders at multiple levels, a common framework for managing the process, adequate data and other resources including time, trust and accountability of all involved. The care process content component identifies the need for systems

Figure 2

Conceptual framework for practice improvement

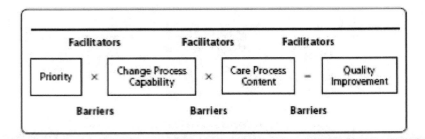

The Center for Medical Home Improvement, Crotched Mountain Foundation. Reprinted with permission.

and professes to support clinical care decisions and self-management support.

Another commonly used model for quality improvement is the Plan-Do-Study-Act cycle (PDSA). This model was developed by Associates in Process Improvement (API). (See Figure 3.) It is an action-oriented approach based on asking 3 main questions, followed by the Plan-Do-Study-Act cycle (PDSA). This model drives clarity to identify the aim, the measurement of success and the intervention (IHI website). See www.ihi.org/IHI for additional information. Institute for Health Care Improvement (IHI) is an independent, not-for-profit organization helping to lead the improvement of health care around the world. IHI organizes their information by topic, covering such categories as leading systems improvement to the how-to's surrounding specific conditions, such as diabetes. Under each topic, content is provided on how to assess your current state based on components of the Chronic Disease Model, followed by how to improve, measures to consider, evidence-based changes that have been implemented, improvement stories, links to pertinent resources and literature, frequently asked questions and emerging content.

Figure 3

PDSA model for improvement

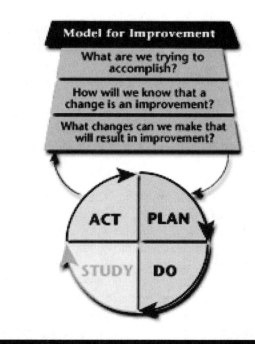

Figure 4

International Diabetes Center's model of patient centered team care

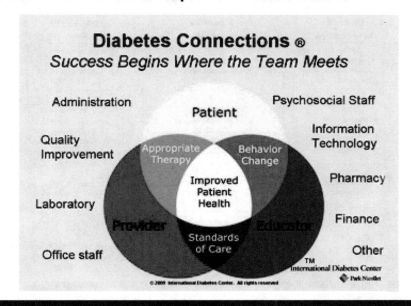

International Diabetes Center at Park Nicollet saw the need to translate the 6 key concepts of the CCM and those highlighted by Solberg and others into a comprehensive implementation model, designed to improve quality through a team-based approach. At its core is the belief that *success begins where the team meets* (see Figure 4). Improved health for the individual with diabetes is central, with recognition that relationships between key team members (patient, provider and educator/CDE) with support from multiple internal and external stakeholders equal improved outcomes.

With the Patient-centered Team Care model as the backdrop, IDC developed its Diabetes Connections Model, by blending organizational change and performance improvement components with its rich history of effectively translating research to practice training and dissemination tools. It was first tested in the *Partners in Advancing Care and Education Study* that was conducted between 2002-2004. In that study, sig-nificant improvements in diabetes care were demonstrated in 10 diverse health care settings.

Diabetes Connections Model is implemented in 3 phases (assessment, training and follow-up consulting) over ~2 year period of time (see Figure 5). Part team building, professional training and ongoing implementation consulting, it is intended to mobilize and guide health care organizations, in creating and maintaining a plan to improve the systems and process they need in order to deliver optimal diabetes care and education. Examples of how IDC translated the 6 key components of the CCM follow (see italicized areas below).

Phase I involves commitment from high-level leaders that program implementation is a key priority for the organization. Site champions and key stakeholders are identified and engaged through written assessments, interviews, observation, data review and participation in a design team session that includes: visioning, identification of strengths and challenges, and priority setting.

Figure 5

Diabetes Connections® model

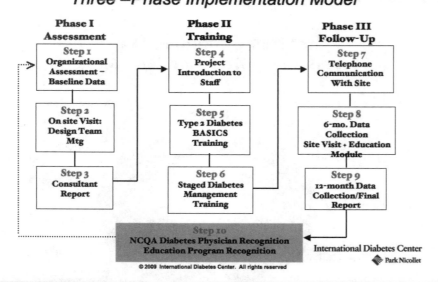

Diabetes Connections ®
Three –Phase Implementation Model

Recommendations and specific action items are made, based on the data provided, priorities of those involved and the gaps that were uncovered. *(CCM: During Phase I, multiple representatives from all 6 areas [community, health systems, self-management support, delivery system design, decision support and clinical information system] are engaged in the assessment activities, identifying strengths and gaps, and contributing to priority setting.)*

Phase II involves general staff introduction to the project, followed by all-staff training that builds knowledge and staff involvement, as they clearly identify the importance each team member can make in contributing to success. 2 of IDC's training programs are provided, Type 2 Diabetes BASICS training designed for educators and Staged Diabetes Management™ training designed for clinicians, office staff, diabetes educators and other team members identified by the organiza-

tion. *(CCM: The focus in Phase II is primarily on health system and delivery system design, decision support and self-management support for all care team members. At the close of each training program, the opportunity is provided to build on the original implementation plan. Often, specific needs in the areas of clinical information technology and community are also identified for ongoing follow-up.)*

Phase III involves continued program implementation as organizations act on identified strategies, monitor their impact (PDSA Cycle) and audit their care processes and outcomes at regular intervals. During this time, IDC provides monthly phone consultations for the next year and conducts a follow-up site visit at the 6-month mark to support the site champions in the change process needed to achieve national benchmarks for diabetes care and education. At that same time as the site visit, the organization selects 1 of 2 CME modules (Insulin or Hypertension Management) they feel

Figure 6

Diabetes Center Model

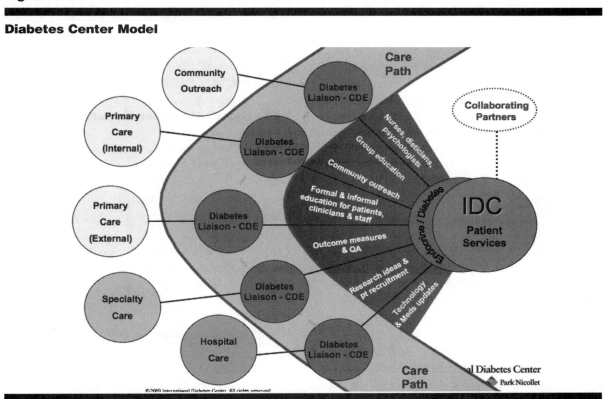

will be most helpful to the primary care clinicians in the organization. *(CCM: Phase III facilitates ongoing accountability and celebration of performance improvement strategies in all 6 of the key CCM components. Organization have stated that IDC's model provided the framework to improve their diabetes care and has positioned them to initiate other new opportunities.)*

Currently, IDC is identifying how to best replicate this model in community settings engaging multiple physician groups. In addition, IDC and its parent organization, Park Nicollet Health Services, have designed implementation models to support change at an organizational level, and at the point of care delivery. At the core is the Diabetes Guidance Council, a group that provides a forum for consensus building, communication, integration and coordination of care between all individuals, and programs providing diabetes care-related services across the system. With accountability comes the satisfaction that voices are heard, redundancies are minimized, and the latest research is being translated to promote best care delivery.

The Diabetes Center Model supports the patient and clinician and other community entities by utilizing Certified Diabetes Educators (CDEs) embedded within practices and across specialty lines to foster care through registry review, patient engagement, care education and a communication link to enhance clear transition of the patient across the care pathways. The intention is to have the care reside with the primary provider. An IDC medical director will be available as a resource to educators and providers when needed (see Figure 6).

With the spotlight on the current health care crisis, there is hope that key barriers previously identified, such as lacking or minimal reimbursement, inadequate technology, etc., may be addressed as efforts are made to provide workable solutions for the population as a whole. Just as models of care require priority setting from the leadership and at all levels, so will changing health care. Each professional and patient has a voice. Working together, change can happen.

National professional and quality improvement organizations play a key role in influencing health care improvement. It is imperative to have an understanding of the work and focus of these organizations to fully understand how they influence and impact the health care system. This section highlights only a few of the professional and quality improvement organizations that play a key role in shaping health care delivery, especially in the area of diabetes management. A more complete list of national organizations is listed in Section 9, APPENDIX 1.

American Diabetes Association (ADA)

Founded in 1940, the ADA is the nation's leading nonprofit health organization in diabetes research, consumer and health professional information, and patient advocacy. Their website (www.diabetes.org) contains extensive links and information for people with diabetes, health professionals and researchers. They are working to prevent and cure diabetes, and to improve not only the lives of people with diabetes but all those affect by diabetes. The ADA has programs in all 50 states as well as the District of Columbia. The following information highlights 3 major areas of ADA focus that serve to improve diabetes care and education.

Professional Education Opportunities

- Offers a variety of formats at the national, regional and local levels

- The Annual Scientific Sessions is the world's largest and most prestigious diabetes meeting

- Annual Advanced Postgraduate Courses offers cutting-edge clinical research in diabetes treatment and management

Diabetes Pro, Professional Resources Online

- Includes breaking news, clinical practice recommendations, clinical trials, webcasts, etc.

- Patient education materials

- Special interest information (eg, explanation of estimated average glucose [eAG] and eAG calculator)

My Food Advisor™

- A calorie and carbohydrate counting tool

- Features: recipes, ability to create a shopping list, add to your recipe box, etc.

- Assists the consumer with calorie and carbohydrate management and nutrition

Aligning Forces for Quality (AF4Q)

The Robert Wood Johnson Foundation (RWJF) launched the first phase of Aligning Forces for Quality in 2006 with a focus on ambulatory care (www.forcesforquality.org). Participants include 14 healthcare communities covering 11% of the US population. The goal in the first phase of the initiative includes public reporting of outcomes, quality care improvement and consumer engagement. Participants were provided grants and expert assistance to meet these goals. The rationale behind public reporting in each community is to:

- Use the same criteria to measure the quality of ambulatory care at health care organizations in their community

- Be reported in a fair, reliable and usable way that is understood by the consumer, who could be a health plan, employer or a patient

- Allow consumers to compare health care services and make an informed choice

- Cause health care organizations to improve their care, based on the outcomes and the fact that the consumer is going other places for care

In addition, The Robert Wood Johnson Foundation announced a $300 million grant to dramatically improve the quality of US health care. This second phase expanded the program to include inpatient care, as well as a focus on reducing racial and ethnic gaps in care and enhancing the central role that nursing plays in good health care.

The following is a brief overview of 2 communities and a sampling of their activities to date. The Diabetes Footprints Campaign in Cincinnati, Ohio focuses on type 2 diabetes. The major focus was on increasing patient awareness of how they should be engaging in the management of their disease through the use of a patient website. The website home page introduces the patient to 2 tools: a checklist for use at the doctor visit and a self-care checklist:

- ASK what your doctor should be doing for you

- LEARN what you should be doing for yourself

- ACT now to take care of your diabetes

Results of the Campaign will be available in 2010. In addition, local health plans are aligned and exploring new payment models to reward improved diabetes-related performance measures (see Section 4).

In Minnesota, Aligning Forces for Quality supported the launch of the Minnesota Diabetes Community Measures D5 Program. The focus was on creating a website for the patient to access information on how health care providers in the state perform on diabetes quality measures. Called the D5, it refers to five measures (HbA1c <7%, BP <130/80 mmHg, LDL <100 mg/dL, daily aspirin and tobacco-free). The D5 represents how well clinics are helping their patients manage their diabetes. It reports the percent of patients that have reached all 5 goals.

National Committee for Quality Assurance (NCQA)

The National Committee for Quality Assurance (NCQA) is dedicated to improving the quality of health care (www.ncqa.org). Founded in 1990, NCQA is dedicated to improving health care quality and committed to measurement, transparency and accountability at all levels of the health care system. They have the capability to bring together health plans, third party payers, physicians, policy makers and others who build consensus around health care quality issues. NCQA is known for its ability to develop technical specifications for measurement, and is looked to as the gold standard when evaluating health care quality and its measures are used in pay-for-performance programs.

NCQA accredits and certifies a wide range of health care organizations, including health plans and organizations that address disease management, credentials verification and other areas of care (www.ncqa.org). Examples of their measurement sets include:

• Healthcare Effectiveness Data and Information Set (HEDIS). A tool used for more than 90% of America's managed care health plans to measure performance on dimensions of care and service. PPOs participating in Medicare or the Federal Employees Health Benefit Program are also required to report HEDIS data. A comprehensive diabetes set is 1 of the areas addressed in the HEDIS measures

• Recognition Programs: NCQA developed a series of Recognition Programs that help identify doctors who provide quality care in a specific area. Health plans are using DPRP in a variety of ways, ie, adding Recognition seals to directories to help identify high-quality physicians, utilizing DPRP as means for P4P and, in some cases, supporting data entry to assist physicians in achieving this status

NCQA uses recognition status to incent physicians and medical groups to collect and submit data on clinical performance. Physicians achieving NCQA recognition lets patients and others in their community know they are publicly recognized for providing the highest-quality care. To date, nearly 10,000 physicians have been recognized for the following NCQA physician recognition programs:

• Diabetes Physician Recognition Program (DPRP)

• Back Pain Recognition Program (BPRP)

• Heart/Stroke Recognition Program (HSRP)

• Physician Practice Connections (PPC)

• PPC- Patient-Centered Medical Home (PPC-PCMH)

Diabetes Physician Recognition Program (DPRP) is a voluntary program that recognizes physicians who use evidence-based measures and provide excellent care to their patients with diabetes. Recognition is available for adult and/or pediatric populations. Health care organizations can apply as 1 entity or as individual physicians. If applying individually, 25 chart audits/eligible physician need to be submitted. If applying as an organization, 200 chart audits are submitted to NCQA.

DPRP Program has established 10 benchmark measures of quality in the following areas:

• HbA1c (<7%, <8% and >9%, considered out of control)

• Blood pressure (<130/80 mmHg)

• LDL control (<100 mg/dL and >130 mg/dL considered out of control)

• Dilated eye examinations

• Nephropathy assessment

• Foot exam

• Smoking status and cessation advice or treatment

While voluntary, DPRP measures are utilized by other organizations and pay-for-performance programs, such as Bridges to Excellence, to reward physicians for the quality care they provide (see Section 4). In addition to physician recognition programs, NCQA offers accreditations to health plans, wellness programs and others, and offers certification to physician organizations, credentials verification organizations and others.

American College of Physicians (ACP)

The American College of Physicians (www.acpoline.org) is the largest medical specialty organization of internal medicine physicians, with >126,000 members. Their mission is to bring quality and effectiveness to health care through high standards and professionalism.

ACP hosts an annual scientific meeting with over 260 sessions on a variety of topics. Their website includes information and opportunities for education and recertification, clinical information and guides on running a practice. To support their members in the area of diabetes management, ACP has created practical tools for the clinician and diabetes educational materials for patients.

American Academy of Family Practice (AAFP)

AAFP (www.aafp.org) is a national medical organization with a membership comprised of >94,000 family physicians, family medicine residents and medical students nationwide. Founded in 1947, their mission has been to promote the science and the skill of family medicine, and to ensure high-quality and cost-effective health care. A link on their website, www.familydoctor.org, offers a wide variety of information for the consumer and patient education handouts for physician use.

The Scientific Assembly is the AAFP's largest meeting for continuing education, typically drawing more than 17,000 physicians and visitors. Their website includes information and opportunities for education, clinical guidelines and resources for practice transformation.

Collaboration – ACP and AAFP

In 2005, IBM questioned the value of the health care it was purchasing for its employees and concluded that health care in the United States fails due to the way primary care is financed in comparison to other industrialized countries. IBM noted further that primary care is the only medical group charged with treating the whole patient. They were also interested in the models for patient-centered care that were being defined and trialed by primary care physician organizations.

The Patient Centered Primary Care Collaborative (PCPCC) (www.pcpcc.net) was created in late 2006 and included the American College of

Physicians, the American Academy of Family Physicians and other primary care physician organizations. Several large national employers approached PCPCC, asking them to develop a process to facilitate improvements in the patient-provider relations, and to develop a more efficient and effective mode of health care delivery. In February 2007, the ACP, AAFP, American Academy of Pediatrics (AAP) and American Osteopathic Association (AOA) collaborated and released the Principles of Patient-Centered Care (see Section 5 for details). These principles are used in state initiatives or they have developed their own using PCMH as a guideline. In achieving these goals, the PCPCC has become 1 of the major developers and advocates of the Patient-centered Medical Home (PCMH) model in America.

The PCPCC created an open forum for health care stakeholders to communicate and collaborate on improvements in the health care system. It also serves as an important link for continued education for federal and state government and individual physician practices on the medical home model as a viable form of health care delivery. PCPCC is now a coalition of over 200 members including major employers, consumer groups, patient quality organizations, third party payers, labor unions, health care centers, physicians and many others who have joined to develop and advance the patient-centered medical home.

American Association of Clinical Endocrinologists (AACE)

AACE (www.aace.com) was founded in 1991. Before this time, clinical endocrinology had no voice to the Health Care Financing Administration (HCFA) or representation in the health policy-making of influential physician societies. AACE efforts are directed to quality and cost-effective patient care. The association has more than 6000 members in the U.S. and in 91 foreign countries. AACE has created numerous evidence- and expert opinion-based guidelines and algorithms for treating diabetes and other endocrine disorders. They also establish and promulgate blood glucose and HbA1c targets that are used as standards by other quality improvement organizations.

Table 1

Overview of Diabetes-specific Measures Being Used to Assess the Quality of Diabetes

Organization	A1C test	A1C <7%	A1C <8%	A1C >9%	BP< 130/80	BP< 140/80	BP≥ 140/90	LDL screening
HEDIS	x	x[a]	x	x	x	x		x
NCQA		x		x	x		x	
DPRP (Adult)				x		x		
PQRI[b]								

continued

Table 1 (continued)

Overview of Diabetes-specific Measures Being Used to Assess the Quality of Diabetes

Organization	LDL <100	LDL ≥130	Monitoring nephropathy	Foot exam	Eye exam	Smoking Stats & cessation
HEDIS	x		x	x		
NCQA	x	x	x	x	x	x
DPRP (Adult)	x		x	x	x	
PQRI[b]						

[a]Diabetes measures for health plans only
[b]Diabetes specific measures only; PQRI requires additional information

3. Transparency of Data

The American College of Endocrinology (www.powerofprevention.com) was established in 1993, and is the scientific and educational component of AACE. They foster the science of endocrinology toward improvement in patient care and public health. To meet their mission, ACE develops educational prevention and disease awareness programs and activities. The programs have moved from focus on the members to include patient-based awareness campaigns. Their website also includes a link for patients and family.

American Medical Group Association (AMGA)

The American Medical Group Association (www.amga.org) evolved since its beginning in 1949, from the American Association of Medical Clinics to the American Group Practice Association in 1974 and, in mid-1996, to the American Medical Group Association (AMGA). Their mission is to improve health care by backing multispecialty practices so they will be the preferred model for care. The members of AMGA care for 95 million patients in 47 states. The average member medical group has 286 physicians and 20 satellite locations. Benefits of membership include political advocacy, education and networking programs, benchmarking services, publications and financial and operations assistance, group purchasing of life insurance and disability insurance.

Members of AMGA participated in the 3-year demonstration project from CMS, the Medicare Physician Group Practice (PG) Demonstration, which began in 2005. The project included 10 physician groups with the goal of improving its delivery of care for patients with congestive heart failure, coronary artery disease and diabetes. The results of this, and other projects aligning with AMGA, show that an organizational structure, resources and information are critical to success. The CMS demonstration resulted in $17.4 million in savings for the Medicare program and earned $16.7 million in incentive payments (see Section 4 for more detail).

Today, the need for transparency is widely recognized, for its importance in engaging multiple stakeholders in understanding and having a voice in contributing to positive change. In the health care arena, the words *transparency* and *public reporting* have been part of the vocabulary for over a decade. The growing prevalence of diabetes (23.7 million – diagnosed and undiagnosed) and the mounting costs of management of diabetes and its comorbidities ($174 billion) have gained the attention of both the public and private sector. Employer groups, government, clinicians, health plans and consumers recognize the need to improve quality and demonstrate value.

Transparency of data, public reporting and accountability is a key tactic in facilitating improvement. Doing so exposes the current state of diabetes care, provides opportunity for deserved recognition and engages communities in dialogue surrounding dissemination of information, learning from what is working and fostering performance improvement activities to address the gaps.

The charge before us is clear. It is not whether to have transparency in health care, it is how to do it well. In a recent paper, it was noted that identifying what performance measures are used and how they are determined demands more transparency in itself. Areas, such as insuring the accuracy of the data, respecting the privacy of the patient and determining effective methods for communicating the results, all need to be considered. Both at a national and state level, organizations are wrestling with these issues, with increasing attention being paid to the results.

The following is not intended to be an exhaustive review, but rather a summary of the development of transparency of diabetes-specific quality data over the last 15 years, with insights to the various types of measures being used today.

Transparency of Data in the Ambulatory Care Setting

As early as 1993, the Institute for Clinical Systems Improvement (originally called Institute for Clinical Systems Integration) was developed as a result of a challenge from the Business Health

Care Action Group (BHCAG), a coalition of large employer groups in Minnesota. Recognizing the rising costs of health care, BHCAG asked health care groups to demonstrate their ability to produce outcomes for the care they provided. 3 organizations and 1 health plan picked up the challenge. James Reinerson, CEO of Park Nicollet Medical Center, led its development, along with HealthPartners and Mayo Clinic, sponsored by HealthPartners. There was 1 central mission: to help its participating organizations improve the quality and value of the health care they provide. Today, ICSI has grown to include 56 medical groups, representing about 85% of Minnesota physicians, and 6 health plans are participating. Its early work served as a model for other US regional health care collaboratives. (www.icsi.org.)

As interest in outcome data grew, the need for a standard measurement soon became apparent. To address this issue, The Diabetes Quality Improvement Project (DQIP), funded by the Balanced Budget Act of 1997, was formed in 1997 to establish a set of diabetes-specific performance and outcomes measures that would allow for fair comparisons of health care plans and stimulate improvement in quality, while developing data that could be easily understood by the payers and consumers. It was a public/private coalition that rapidly expanded to include representatives from the ADA, the Foundation for Accountability (FACCT), the Health Care Financing Administration (HCFA), the National Committee for Quality Assurance (NCQA), the American Academy of Family Physicians, the American College of Physicians, and the Veteran's Administration (www.ncqa.org). The DQIP became known as the National Diabetes Quality Improvement Alliance (NDQA) from 2001-2006. It remains a collaboration of 13 public/private organizations dedicated to developing and maintaining a national performance measurement set for diabetes.

A result of the efforts of the DQIP was demonstrated in the publishing of *A Diabetes Report Card for the United States Quality of Care in the 1990s in the Annals of Internal Medicine* in 2002. This was the first report card to be published on the quality of diabetes care using set, standard measures to document diabetes care across the country.

The Physician Quality Reporting Initiative (PQRI) was developed by CMS in response to the 2006 Tax Relief and Health Care Act (TRHCA; P.L. 109-432) requiring the establishment of a physician quality reporting system, including an incentive payment for eligible professionals (EPs) who satisfactorily report data on quality measures for covered services furnished to Medicare beneficiaries during the second half of 2007 (the 2007 reporting period). While PQRI requires the report of multiple measures beyond diabetes, the NCQA's Diabetes Physician Recognition Program (DPRP) has been accepted as a diabetes registry for submission of PQRI data on behalf of eligible professionals seeking payment in 2008. For more details on the Diabetes Physician Recognition Programs, see www.ncqa.org.

National Quality Forum

The National Quality Forum (NQF), is a not-for-profit public/private organization, founded in 1999, that brings together representatives from all parts of the health care systems to develop a national strategy for health care quality measurement and reporting. They have established a process for establishing consensus on "best in class" standards and their measurements. NQF's endorsement has become the "gold standard" for health care performance measures. The diabetes measures endorsed by NQF are those measures listed by NCQA.

In August 2006, the Bush Administration issued an executive order, committing the federal government's health care programs to move forward in providing consumers with easy-to-use information about the quality and price of their health care (www.hhs.gov/valuedriven). In response to this order, the DHHS reached out in November 2007 to engage the private sector employer groups to help provide more "transparent" health care information to consumers, by supporting 4 "cornerstone" principles for health care:

1. Using interoperable health information technology (through which data can be communicated and exchanged among different information systems, software applications and networks)

2. Measuring and reporting health care quality

3. Collecting and reporting information on health care prices

4. Implementing programs, such as pay-for-performance reimbursement systems or high performance networks, which encourage consumers to use high-quality, cost-effective services

National Business Coalition on Health

The National Business Coalition on Health (NBCH) has urged its membership of over 60 employer-led coalitions across the United States, representing over 7000 employers and approximately 2 million employees and their dependents, to sign the DHHS "letter of support" for changing the principles of health care, and have listed resources on its website. For information on local business coalitions and their activities in improving quality care in their communities, visit www.nbch.org.

American Health Quality Association

The American Health Quality Association (AHQA) represents the national network of Quality Improvement Organizations (QIOs) and other professionals dedicated to promoting and facilitating fundamental change that improves the quality of health care. QIOs are located in nearly every major, urban community/state and work under contract to Medicare. They actively engage multiple stakeholders in the community to focus on supporting the implementation of best practice amongst physician groups, as well as facilitating public awareness of outcomes measures (www.ahqa.org).

Robert Wood Johnson Foundation

Robert Wood Johnson Foundation (RWJF) has been a leader in the quality movement through funding early development of quality measures and some of the first pay-for-performance experiments. In 2006-2007, RWJF initiated Aligning Forces for Quality (AF4Q), a multimillion dollar initiative involving 14 communities across the United States: Cincinnati, Cleveland, Detroit, Humboldt County (CA), Kansas City (MO), Maine, Memphis, Minnesota, Puget Sound, South Central Pennsylvania, West Michigan, Western New York, Willamette Valley (OR) and Wisconsin. In the area of public reporting, AF4Q is focused on improving the quality of information that is provided on physician performance, as well as making sure that consumers have access to the information. AF4Q sites are bringing various team members together—physicians, medical groups, health plans, patients and data experts—to determine what measures to use, establish consensus on a measurement data set and establish the methodology for data abstraction. Every effort is being made to aggregate data from a number of sources with the focus on producing reliable results. There is a belief in rewarding quality outcomes, as well as having the opportunity to identify areas that are needing attention. With the community approach, AF4Q sites provide a venue to determine effective ways of public reporting, encourage open dialogue and seek strategies to support performance improvement, through open dialogue and shared learning from other participating communities.

Transparency of Data in the Inpatient Setting

The Hospital Quality Alliance (HQA), formed in 2002, is a national public-private collaboration that is committed to making meaningful, relevant and easily understood information about hospital performance accessible to the public, and to informing and encouraging efforts to improve quality. The HQA advances measures endorsed by the NFQ. A website hosted by the DHHS, www.HospitalCompare.hhs.gov, compares performance measures on more than 4000 hospitals. Diabetes-specific measures include Diabetes in Adult, DRG 294: average Medicare payment paid to hospital and number of Medicare payments treated. www.HospitalCompare.hhs.gov Data is updated quarterly and is obtained from 4 data sources: claims data, medical record data, survey data and data from other organizations, such as The Joint Commission (TJC). One can access Quality Net (www.qualitynet.org) to view the Inpatient Quality Measures established for 2009. Currently, there isn't a specific category for diabetes. Yet, with the significant cost of inpatient diabetes care, one expects that this will be an area of focus in the future.

The Agency for Healthcare Research and Quality (AHRQ) has, as part of its mission, to translate research into practice and improve health quality, and develops products to assist state leaders who aim to improve diabetes care in their states. Their website provides access to a variety of measurements. Their 2004 National Health Care Quality Report includes 4 measures for hospital admission that, evidence suggests, could potentially have been avoided through high-quality outpatient care. Data was collected from 38 participating states on the following measures:

- Hospital admissions for uncontrolled diabetes per 100,000 population

- Hospital admissions for short-term complications of diabetes per 100,000 population

- Hospital admissions for long-term complications of diabetes per 100,000 population

- Hospital admissions for lower extremity amputations in patients with diabetes per 100,000 population

There has been great progress in the journey to bring transparency of diabetes quality data and public reporting from its infancy stage to one that is providing trusted results. Efforts to bring key stakeholders together, promoting open dialogue, are occurring nationally (www.thenationaldialogue.org/healthit) as well as locally (see Section 10). The need for transparency on establishment of measurement is being communicated in multiple venues. Genuine attempts to identify measures that reflect quality outcomes, as well as process and cost measures, are being addressed. Not an easy task, with the current demands of health care and the mix and challenges of data abstraction (paper and electronic medical records, claims data.) Yet, progress is definitely being made. Measures are improving which reflect engagement by many sources. Perhaps it requires pause to recognize and celebrate the progress to date.

4. Pay-for-Performance (P4P)

Numerous pay-for-performance (P4P) programs have sprung up throughout the United States in an attempt to improve health care, by incenting or rewarding physicians for delivering quality care. The concept gained traction after the 2001 Institute of Medicine report *Crossing the Quality Chasm: A New Health System for the 21st Century* was released that recommended incentives to physicians to drive much-needed change in the delivery of health care. The report clearly states that payments to physicians must "recognize quality, reward quality and support quality improvement." Currently, P4P programs cover a broad range of health care services including: preventative care (immunization and cancer screening), chronic care (diabetes and asthma), acute care (treatment of respiratory infections and back pain) and inpatient care. While P4P is not perfect, it has been called the "best worst choice" to balance individual physician autonomy and accountability with safety and quality standards. Centers for Medicare and Medicaid Services (CMS) has not overlooked P4P as a potential way to reward physicians delivering high-quality health care. CMS has several demonstration P4P projects underway that are designed to provide information needed, as they move into an era of value-based purchasing (VBP). CMS is moving from being a "payer" to a driver of quality improvement, with accountability for showing value for money spent.

Outpatient P4P Programs

The American Medical Association (AMA) has weighed in on P4P and created guidelines for the implementation of P4P programs. Table 2 summarizes the AMA guidelines for P4P. These guidelines were developed to provide some ground rules for third party payers, employer groups and CMS, when creating programs. They were required because of expressed concerns over P4P, including: the potential to undermine patient and physician autonomy, appropriate quality indicators, unfairness to physicians serving lower socioeconomic groups, potential to go from rewarding quality to financial penalties for lack of adherence and lack of adequate reward to compensate fairly for increased administrative burden. On the last point, early P4P programs did not offer adequate incentives to justify changing processes

of care to improve quality of care. While the range of incentives span from less than 2% to nearly 40% of annual physician compensation, the most common number quoted is ~10% bonus as incentive to change practice to improve quality.

The exact number of outpatient P4P programs is difficult to determine, because programs are continually being added, withdrawn and changed. It is clear that there are more than 100 P4P programs, covering more than 75 million lives. More than half of health maintenance organizations (HMOs) have 1 or more P4P programs. Table 3 summarizes some of the largest P4P programs that have published information on the program specifics and outcomes. Collectively, the improvements in health care attributed to P4P are modest. For example, early results of the PacifiCare Quality Incentive Program in a network of physician groups in California showed a very modest increase in A1C testing of 2.1 percentage points, that was similar to contemporaneous regional control organizations without P4P. Preliminary benchmarks have focused on improving screening, not metabolic or outcome measure. The mere existence of improved screening does not necessarily translate into improvement in the outcome measure. A study in a large network of federally qualified heath centers in Chicago showed P4P increased numbers of A1Cs collected (the P4P goal), yet did not show improvement in A1C value.

Inpatient Pay-for-Performance Programs

P4P has been heralded as a way to improve quality and safety in the hospital setting. The rationale is that the transparency afforded by comparing a consistent set of quality measures among different hospitals will drive quality and safety. The financial incentives are coupled with P4P programs, providing the much-needed resources for investing in infrastructure and process changes. The list of quality measures is quite exhaustive and depends on the particular P4P program. The most common clinical conditions with examples of quality measures are summarized in Table 4, and these are recommended by the National Quality Form, American Heart Association, CMS 7th Scope of work indicators and Joint Commission Core

Table 2

Summary of American Medical Association P4P Program Guidelines

Area	Recommendation
Quality Measures	1. Primary goal is to promote safe and efficient patient care, not monetary savings
	2. Performance measures must be evidence-based with input by practicing physicians and appropriate professional association(s)
	3. Performance measures must be able to be improved and scored in terms of relative and absolute improvement
	4. P4P program must be piloted and phased in over reasonable period time
Patient/Physician Relationship	1. Programs must support the patient/physician relationship
	2. Program cannot limit access to improved care and must not disadvantage patients on a basis of socioeconomic and geographical location
	3. Performance measures must be established considering some level of patient noncompliance
Physician Participation	1. Participation must be voluntary with ability for physicians to opt-in or -out without risk of punitive action (change to existing contract relationship or reduction in practice viability)
	2. Programs should encourage broad participation that is not dependent on size of practice or information technology resources (eg, EMR, patient registry)
	3. Physicians should be assessed as a group rather than individually
	4. High-performing physicians should be studied and processes shared with others
	5. Performance should not be used punitively for purposes of credentialing, licensure and certification
	6. Physicians have ability to respond to reported data with assurance data is secure from unauthorized access
Program Rewards	1. Use rewards, not penalties
	2. Rewards should cover additional expenses incurred in pursuit of quality improvement
	3. Physicians should not be disadvantaged because they provide care for underserved/uninsured patients

Measures (see Section 9). Currently, more than 40 hospital P4P programs have been established and reviewed extensively. Table 5 summarizes 3 major hospital P4P programs.

Summary of Inpatient P4P Programs

A dearth of controlled studies showing the impact of P4P on inpatient care process improvements is apparent. However, some preliminary learnings have been identified. Not all hospitals show improved care process improvements with the introduction of P4P programs, and others show only modest improvement over contemporaneous control hospitals. Another issue facing inpatient P4P programs is whether to provide incentives to the highest performers (eg, those organizations performing in the highest decile or quartile) vs. incentives based on meeting an absolute threshold. The concern with the former model is that it automatically excludes a high percentage of organizations, driving lower performers away from QI initiatives because, even with improved performance, they may never catch the leaders. Concern over the latter model is that it may not drive improvement measures as high as possible, because once the benchmark is achieved, there is less incentive to keep progressing.

Alternative models that provide P4P incentives based on change in performance from baseline to follow-up, coupled with meeting absolute thresholds, need to be considered. For example, Organization A and B have heart failure composite quality scores of 48% and 68%, respectively. After a 2-year quality improvement initiative, Organization A and B improve to 66% and 74%, respectively. If the threshold for payment is 70%, Organization A would not receive P4P incentive while Organization B would. In reality, Organization A demonstrated greater percentage point improvement in the heart failure composite score than Organization B, and should be rewarded for that improvement. Organization B should also be incented, because they have exceeded the established quality cut-point.

Similar to outpatient P4P programs, the payments are normally not going directly to enhance physician or diabetes care team salary, but rather to sup-port the actual QI program. This is important, because the underlying principle is that the incentive should not be for rewarding what are considered best practices, yet should be supporting the tremendous concerted efforts of QI departments to modify processes, ultimately leading to improved patient care and outcomes. A survey of hospitals participating in P4P programs revealed that the process changes and additional staff required to meet established incentive benchmarks may actually be significantly greater than the incentive itself. Moreover, a recent study of application of American College of Cardiology/American Heart Association acute MI guidelines in 54 hospitals participating in P4P revealed no significant incremental improvement in acute MI care or outcomes vs. 446 control hospitals. Overall, inpatient P4P programs appear to only be part of the solution to improving hospital performance.

Table 3

Outpatient Pay-for-Performance Program Summary Area Recommendation

Pay-for-Performance Performance Initiative	Players	Measures/Benchmarks	Dollars at stake	Result (Diabetes Specific)	References
CMS Physician Group Practice (PGP) Demonstration Project	10 Large Physician Groups (Billings Clinic, MT; Dartmouth-Hitchcock Clinic, NH; The Everett Clinic, WA; Forsyth Med. Group, NC; Geisinger Clinic, PA, Marshfield Clinic, WI, Middlesex Health System, CT; Park Nicollet Health Services, MN, St John's Health System, MO, University of Michigan MI)	27 quality measures in diabetes, CHF, and CAD; started in 2006 through 2009	Incentive if group achieves per capita savings compared to others in the community not assigned – awarded 80% of savings if quality measures are met	• Interim results showed improvement in all 27 quality measures • Medicare expenditures grew more slowly in PGP demonstration than contemporary controls • $16.7 million in incentive payments	http://www.cms.hhs.gov
California P4P Program	Integrated Healthcare Association (IHA) provides leadership; CA Health Plans (Aetna, Blue Cross, Blue Shield, CIGNA, Health Net, Kaiser, PacifiCare, Western Health Advantage); ~250 Physician Groups representing over 40,000 physicians	Preventive care, chronic disease care and acute care based on 9 NCQA and HEDIS Clinical Measures; 40% score on preventative care and management, 40% on patient satisfaction and 20% on IT solutions	$145 million in incentives paid out in 1st 5 years of program; $65 million in 2007; payments made based on percentile (<50th percentile no incentive, 50-74th percentile 1/2 incentive, >75th percentile full incentive)	• Overall, consistent small improvement in A1C and LDL testing and goal attainment • Increased screening for nephropathy • Chronic Disease Management increased likely hood of meeting goals	www.iha.org; Cutler et al 2007;
Bridges to Excellence – a site of Rewarding Results	Funded by Robert Wood Johnson Foundation and supported by Center of Medicare and Medicaid Services (CMS). Initiative of large employers (GE, Proctor and Gamble, Verizon, Raytheon, UPS, Humana, Ford), health plans (Aetna, Blue Cross and Blue Shield of Ohio, Kentucky, Illinois, Alabama, Massachusetts, Tufts Health Plan, United Healthcare, Harvard Pilgrim, and Humana) and Physician groups in Boston, Albany, Cincinnati and Louisville.	3 BTE Programs Diabetes Care Link[a]; Cardiac Care Link; Physician Office Link[a] The diabetes care benchmarks are adapted from NCQA/ADA Diabetes Physician Recognition Program	Diabetes: $80-100/patient for physicians who qualify for NCQA/ADA Diabetes Physician Recognition; up to 10% of physicians annual income will be paid to physicians who meet of exceed targets in the 3 areas.	• 2003 13 NCQA/ADA recognized physicians to 1,293 in 2006 with 2.4 million in rewards • In Massachusetts, average $1,403/physician/year • BTE recognized physicians have improved A1C and lipid testing along with more eye and kidney screening compared to non-recognized physicians • Electronic medical records critical to improved performance	Bridges to Excellence 2003-2008 Five Years On: Bridges Built, Bridges to Build; http://www.bridgestoexcellence.org); Rosenthal 2008

(Continued)

Table 3 (continued)

Outpatient Pay-for-Performance Program Summary Area Recommendation

Pay-for-Performance Performance Initiative	Players	Measures/Benchmarks	Dollars at stake	Result (Diabetes Specific)	References
PacifiCare Quality Incentive Program (QIP)	Pacific Care Health Systems, a very large health plan based in California; 300 large physician groups under contract with PacifiCare with average of 10,000 enrolled patients;	Ten IHA Domains: A1C, cervical cancer screening, mammography, childhood immunizations, LDL in CAD patients, satisfaction with PCP, medical group,, referral process, and specialist PCP communication	$0.23 per member per month for each of 10 domains meeting or exceeding 75th percentile based on 2002 performance; $276,000 for each 10,000 enrollees if all 10 domains met	• $3.4 million in first year of program • Improvement in cervical cancer screening versus control organization without P4P • A1C testing improvement similar to control org • Modest improvement • Increase in A1C testing	Rosenthal et al. 2005
ACCESS P4P Program	Community Health Network (ACCESS) largest group of federally qualified health centers (FQHCs) in Chicago.	50 Procedures listed on Health People 2010 Guidelines; diabetes related measures included completing diabetes flow sheet, A1C measurement, foot exam; other measures for immunizations, preventive screening, etc.	Physician base salary reduced ~15% with opportunity to earn $5 dollars per procedure included in P4P program capped at $5 times the number patients seen in the year.	• Increase in number of people with diabetes and no documented A1C receiving A1C test • No significant change in A1C level • Lowest performers improved the most	Coleman, 2007

5. Patient-centered Medical Home

Over the last decade, the definition of a medical home has evolved, from the intent of a depository for medical records for children to the upcoming Center for Medicaid and Medicare Service (CMS) medical home demonstration project that includes a model for reimbursement. The principles and examples of pilot medical homes are described below. Many national organizations have contributed to the development of the current principles of a patient-centered medical home, and description of their individual contribution to the patient-centered medical home is beyond the scope of this chapter. Thus, this section must be considered an overview highlighting several projects and initiatives.

Principles of a Patient-centered Medical Home

The principles of a patient-centered medical home, developed by the American College of Physicians, the American Academy of Family Physicians, the American Academy of Pediatrics and the American Osteopathic Association were also accepted by 13 other specialty healthcare organizations and the American Medical Association, and are described in Table 6.

The National Committee for Quality Assurance (NCQA) has released standards for the patient-centered medical home. Recognition is available on 3 levels, based on meeting required elements

Table 4

Common Inpatient P4P Clinical Conditions and Quality Measures

Clinical Condition	Quality Measure
Acute Myocardial Infarction (AMI)	• Aspirin upon arrival and prescribed at discharge
	• ACE inhibitor or ARB for left ventricular systolic function
	• Beta-blocker upon arrival and prescribed at discharge
	• Thrombolytic and percutaneous coronary intervention (PCI) within 30 minutes and 120 minutes of arrival, respectively
	• Inpatient mortality rate
Coronary Artery Bypass Graft (CABG)	• Prophylactic antibiotic recived within 1 hour prior to surgical incision
	• Prophylactic antibiotic selection for surgical patients
Heart Failure (HF)	• Assessment for left ventricular function
	• ACE inhibitor or ARB for left ventricular systolic function
	• Smoking cessation advice/counseling
Community-acquired Pneumonia (CAP)	• Oxygenation assessment within 24 hours of arrival
	• Blood culture collected prior to administration of antibiotic
	• Appropriate antibiotic based on current recommendations
	• Pneumococcal screening and vaccination
	• Smoking cessation advice/counseling
Hip and Knee Replacement	• Prophylactic antibiotic recived within 1 hour prior to surgical incision
	• Prophylactic antibiotic selection for surgical patients
	• Prophylactic antibiotic discontinued within 24 hours after surgery

Table 5

Inpatient Pay-for-Performance Program Summary

Pay-for-Performance Performance Initiative	Players	Measures/Benchmarks	Dollars at stake	Result (Diabetes Specific)	References
Premier Hospital Quality Incentive Demonstration (HQID)	CMS sponsored starting in 2003; 262 hospitals across 38 states	Acute myocardial infarction, coronary artery bypass graft, congestive heart failure, pneumonia, hip and knee (see Table XX-?)	2% or 1% diagnosis related group (DRG) bonus payment for 1st and 2nd deciles, respectively; financial penalty after 3rd year for bottom 2 deciles.	• $24.5 million bonus paid over first 3 years • Bonus from $2147 to $385,342 during 3rd year • Average 15.8 percentage point improvement in composite scores for all 5 conditions • Lowest performing hospitals showed greatest improvement • Financial incentive showed 4-5 percentage better improvement than public reporting hospital controls • CMS approved extension through 2009	Linenauer, 2007; Premier HQID Fact Sheet June 2008; Mehrotra 2009
Hawaii Medical Service Association (HMSA)	HMSA is independent licensee of Blue Cross Blue Shield of Hawaii; all 17 hospitals in Hawaii eligible	Points awarded for: 1. Participation in AHA's "Get with the Guidelines Coronary Artery Disease" 2. Length of Stay and complication rates in 18 common surgeries and obstetrics. 3. Patient and physician satisfaction 4. Successful implementation of QI program	$9 million in 2004	• $24.5 million bonus paid over first 3 years • Bonus from $2147 to $385,342 during 3rd year • Average 15.8 percentage point improvement in composite scores for all 5 conditions • Lowest performing hospitals showed greatest improvement • Financial incentive showed 4-5 percentage better improvement than public reporting hospital controls • CMS approved extension through 2009	Berthiaume 2004; Bethaume 2006; Mehrotra 2009
Blue Cross Blue Shield of Michigan	86 hospitals that have contracts with Blue Cross and Blue Shield of Michigan	Process measures for acute myocardial infarction, congestive heart failure, community acquired pneumonia and participation in other QI projects (eg, patient safety initiatives	Up to 4% DRG bonus payment for related conditions	• DRG bonus resulting in $30,000 to $4,000,000 per hospital • Overall cost-effective for health plan due to	Reiter 2006; Nahra 2006; Sautter 2007; Mehrotra 2009

and completing a data collection. Therefore, practices may have different capabilities of the patient-centered medical home principles.

The model shown in Figure 7 from the Center of Medical Home Improvement shows the coordination from the personal physician of medical home principles through acute illness management, preventative care management and chronic condition management.

The State of Primary Care in the United States

Reports on primary care in the United States show that medical students often reconsider internal medicine and family practice due to declining revenue, their high levels of indebtedness and the excessive workload which is partly attributed to primary care physicians in practice choosing to retire early. Further studies report that only 2% of students will pursue careers in internal medicine. This is alarming, as primary care has the potential to reduce costs while still maintaining quality. It is also known that individuals living in states with a higher ratio of primary care physicians to population are more likely to report good health than those living in states with a lower ratio.

The role of the primary care provider is essential to the redesigning of health care and PCMH. An editorial in the *Annals of Internal Medicine* titled Primary Care: Too Important to Fail closes with the following:

"We would be wrong to spend time debating which needs to come first: payment reform, attention to workforce, building an infrastructure for primary careor a focus on care coordination. Each of these activities is critical and contributes to success of the others. By the same token, we cannot build a reformed health care system on an endangered primary care enterprise. We must invest now. Primary care is too important to fail."

Figure 7

The medical home model (created by w. Carl Cooley, MD)

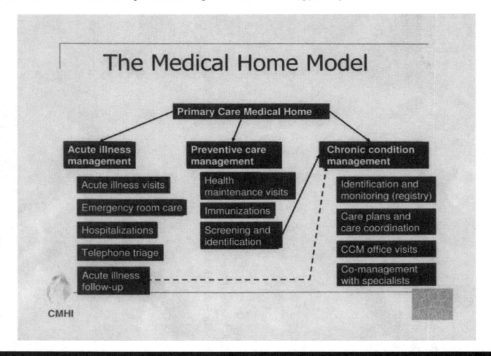

The Center for Medical Home Improvement, Crotched Mountain Foundation. Reprinted with permission.

Keystone III Conference and Future of Family Medicine Project

In January 2000, the Family Practice Working Party (WP) recognized the frustration of family physicians in trying to provide high-quality care with the current health care delivery system, which was not fostering their primary health care role. In October 2000, the Keystone III conference was called by the Working Party to "examine the soul of the discipline of family medicine, and to take stock of the present and grapple with the future of family practice." (www.AAFP.org.) The conference determined that a review was needed of the role of family medicine and plans for the future. The Future of Family Medicine (FFM) project was initiated by the leadership of 7 national family medicine organizations in 2002, to include consulting research followed by a task force.

Consulting Research

Through focus groups and interviews with family physicians, people whose care was or was not provided by a family physician, employers, payers, government and others, the goal was to identify strategies for the practice of family medicine to meet the need of patients. The recommendations were presented in August 2003, and in essence called for system-wide changes that included that every American have a medical home.

Task Force

In response to the work of the consulting research, the task force convened, and their final report was published as a supplement to the March/April 2004 issue of *Annals of Family Medicine*. Recommendations proposed included a system where the patient is the center of their care decisions, and that family practice operate on a *New Model* of delivering care. Features of the New Model include principles and capabilities of the patient-centered medical home:

• Open-access scheduling

• Online appointments

• Electronic health records

• Group visits

• E-visits

• Chronic disease management

• Web-based information

• Team approach, where clinical staffs are more involved in providing care

• Use of clinical practice guideline software

• Outcomes analyses

Implementation

The implementation phase of the project began in early 2004, when the AAFP took the lead role in creating a new initiative, **TransforMED,** to put the FFM recommendations into action (www.transformed.com/transformed.cfm).

Beginning in June 2006, TransforMED launched a 2-year National Demonstration Project to test their model of flexible, patient-centered care. 36 practices were selected to participate. 18 practices were engaged in facilitated implementation of the TransforMED Medical Home Model (see Figure 8). 18 practices were engaged in self-directed implementation. Results of this project will be reported in 2009. (www.transformed.com/ndp.cfm.)

Center for Medicaid and Medicare Service

In our fee-for-service payment system, an arrangement that rewards volume over value is a barrier to models such as PCMH (Commonwealth Fund). There are models that would enable the U.S. to provide quality, affordable care for every American. The Commonwealth Fund report to the Senate Committee on Health, Education, Labor and Pensions notes that we spend twice what other nations spend on health care, yet there is overwhelming evidence of inappropriate care, missed opportunities and waste within the US health care system.

Figure 8

TransforMed patient-centered medical home model

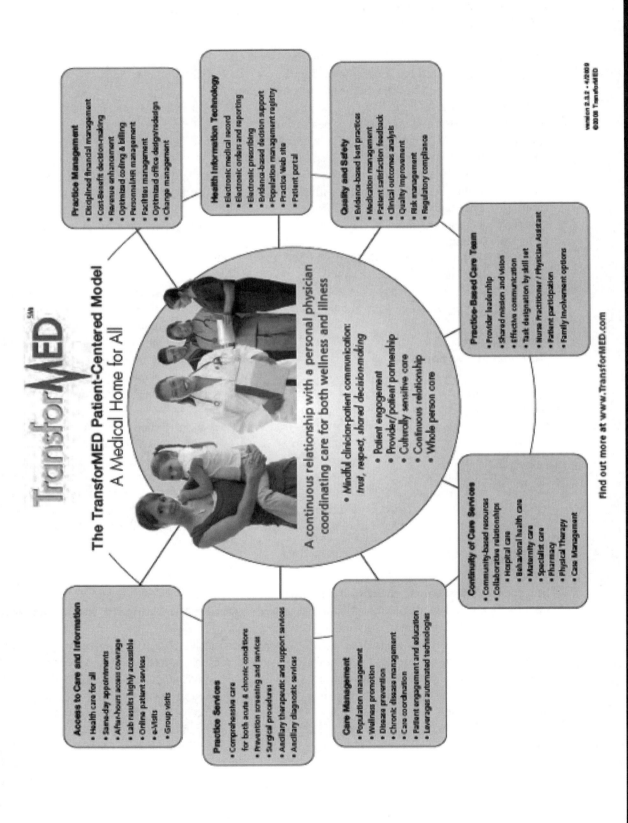

Table 6

Principles of a Patient-centered Medical Home

Personal physician	The patient will have a physician who will coordinate their care, whether acute, chronic or preventative
Physician-directed medical practice	The physician leads the team of health care professionals in their practice. The team members are responsible for the care of the patient
Whole person orientation	The physician provides for the patient's care throughout their life or refers to an appropriate professional for care
Enhanced access	Elements: same-day appointments, email between physician/staff and patient, scheduling online, triage by phone
Payment	Elements: reflect value vs. volume, recognize care other than traditional face-to-face, adjustment for patient severity and burden, adopt health information technology, rewards for achieving quality measures
Care is coordinated and/or integrated	Patient's care is coordinated across all health care entities (nursing home, specialist, etc.) and the patient's community (family, Meals On Wheels, etc.). Through information technology, assure that the patient receives the prescribed care when and where it is needed
Quality and safety	Elements: care plan is created by physician, patient and, possibly, their family, use evidence-based medicine. Clinical outcomes are gathered and action taken of deficits, practices are recognized by a non-governmental agency to assure that their capabilities meet patient-centered care, patients are engaged in care decisions and assured that their needs are being met

Table 7

Medical Home Demonstration per Patient per Month Payment Rates

Medical Home Tier	Patients with HCC Score <1.6/month	Patients with HCC ≥1.6 /month
Tier 1	$27.12	$80.25
Tier 2	$35.48	$100.35

Available at ww.cms.hhs.gov Accessed on May 8, 2009

Rewarding Value

As part of the Tax Relief and Health Care Act of 2006, the legislators created a 3-year Center for Medicaid and Medicare Service (CMS) Patient-centered Medical Home (PCMH) demonstration project. This project will commence in 2010 and will be conducted in 8 states, involving 400 practices, 2000 physicians and 400,000 Medicare beneficiaries. The purpose is to determine if medical homes reduce costs and improve the quality of health care. The demonstration project will be completed in 2012. This project involves care management reimbursement and incentive payments to physicians. CPT codes have been identified, and fees will be adjusted using the Hierarchal Condition Code (HCC) scores to reflect severity and burden to the physician.

Payment will be based on the practices' capabilities as outlined by the CMS version of NCQA PCMH recognition (www.ncqa.org). A Tier 1 medical home must meet 17 basic capabilities, such as tracking referrals, using a health assessment plan, reviewing all medications, using an integrated care plan, etc. Tier 2 must meet the requirements for

Table 8

National Organizations Sponsoring Medical Home Models

American Academy of Pediatrics (1967)	• First introduced medical home, with the intent to have a central location for archiving medical records of children with special needs
	• 2002 model expanded to include accessibility, continuous, comprehensive, family-centered, coordinated, compassionate and culturally sensitive care
	• 2005 focusing to include all children and youth
Community Care of North Carolina (2000)	• States Medicaid program
	• Implemented components of the medical home: disease management, evidence-based clinical practice and an emphasis on a physician-led team approach
	• Savings to the state was $195-$215 million in 2003 and between $230 and $260 million in 2004
Health Care Quality Survey The Commonwealth Fund (2006)	• Survey of more than 2830 adults nationwide • Outcome: when minorities have a medical home, racial and ethnic differences in terms of access to medical care disappear
The Patient Centered Primary Care Collaborative (2007) tals,	• Members: major employers, consumer groups, patient quality organizations, health plans, labor unions, hospi-physicians and others >400 members • Members agree it is essential to support a better model of compensating physicians
	• Purpose: develop and advance the patient-centered medical home
	• Several pilots are being developed in both public and private sectors

Tier 1, plus 4 other capabilities (eg, electronic medical record, coordination of care including follow-up of inpatient and outpatient care, performance measures and reporting to physicians [see Table 7]).

Summary

Table 8 highlights 4 additional national organizations that have played a part/been involved in the evolution of patient-centered medical homes. This list is not meant to be inclusive. In 2009, results from the TransforMED National Demonstration Project will be released. In the following years, there will be outcomes from the Center for Medicaid and Medicare Service (CMS) Patient-centered Medical Home (PCMH) demonstration project and The Patient-centered Primary Care Collaborative. Results from these projects have the potential to affect our health care delivery system to move towards patient-centered medical homes, with payment for value and not volume.

Introduction

Delivering patient care in a group medical visit (GMV) was first described in the 1970s for well-child appointments, and has expanded since to include primary care and specialty practice. GMVs have not been widely accepted by many physicians, due to numerous concerns including: quality of care, patient confidentiality, visit structure/logistics, resistance to change and reimbursement. Originally, the concept of GMVs , also known as shared medical visits or simply group visits, was to increase access to care and practice efficiency. As the number of providers using GMVs increased in the past decade many more benefits have been demonstrated (see Table 9). GMVs are well suited for the management of chronic diseases, such as type 2 diabetes, because the same self-management skills and education is required by all patients, and the presence of the chronic disease provides a common bond. GMVs are differentiated from drop-in group medical appointments (DIGMAs) that are not disease-specific and function more to ease access to care by having open slots for any patient to fill. The impact of GMVs is far-reaching and consumer trends for cost-effective care and education may drive an increase in their utilization, as patients look for value for their health care dollar (see Section 7).

GMV Planning and Structure

Preparation and planning are key elements of successful GMVs. Participation in a GMV is by invitation only, because not all patients are good candidates due to psychological, emotional, language or learning barriers. Pre-visit planning includes review of the patient chart or electronic medical record prior to the visit to determine what laboratory tests, immunizations and referrals are needed. Pre-visit labs or point-of-care testing for A1C, lipids, albumin/creatinine ratio, and serum creatinine (eGFR) has been shown to make the visit more meaningful. The literature describes several different agendas that are often modeled after early work by Beck et al, who developed cooperative health care clinics (CHCCs) for geriatric HMO patients. Most visits are 2 hours in length and follow an agenda similar to the one described

Table 9

Overview of Group Medical Visits

Area/Topic	Benefit
Patient outcome	• Improved diabetes related standards of care • Reduced number of headaches • Reduced weight • Improved glycemic control
Healthcare utilization	• Reduced visit to Emergency Center • Decreased urgent care visits • Decreased inpatient admissions • Lower outpatient visit charges
Satisfaction	• Improved patient satisfaction • Improved physician satisfaction • Improved communication with physician • Better access to care
Patient adherence	• Increased visit to nutrition specialist • Increased self-monitored blood glucose (SMBG) • Increased healthy eating behaviors

in Table 10. The typical number of patients varies from 8-12 or more.

Patients are asked to come 30 minutes prior to the start of the GMV, to allow for collection of insurance information, copayments, vital signs and any missing laboratory data that may be obtained using point-of-care testing. The visit is started with time allocated for socializing that allows interaction and support between patients with a common medical condition. The provider kicks off the visit with an introduction of all staff and participants. The Health Insurance Portability and Accountability Act (HIPAA) requires that patients sign a confidentiality form, because protected health information (PHI) will be shared as part of the GMV. Patients must be made aware that they must not share other's PHI outside of the GMV.

A significant amount of time is committed for a single educational topic related to diabetes. The physician starts the education session off, and may turn many of the topics over to others on the diabetes team. The diabetes educator can discuss self-management skills, pharmacists can focus on diabetes medications, registered dietitians can discuss medical nutrition therapy, psychologists can reinforce health behaviors and emotional health, and exercise physiologists can show patients how to increase activity level. Some physicians call on local medical specialists (endocrinologists, ophthalmologists, podiatrists, nephrologists, etc.) to provide education on specific topics. The group is asked what topics they want to cover in future visits, highlighting the patient-centered care aspect of the process. Ample time is allotted for a question and answer session. Group facilitation skills are required, to prevent overly talkative patients from dominating the visit

Table 10

Sample Group Medical Visit Agenda

Time	Activity
15 minutes	Welcome and socializing
15 minutes	Introductions of staff and patients, confidentially forms
30-40 minutes	Education topic
15 minutes	Question and answer
30 minutes	Individual one-on-one

and to make sure more tentative participants have a safe environment to ask questions.

The final part of the GMV includes some time for one-on-one medical assessment by the physician. This is a critical aspect of the GMV, allowing individual assessment of metabolic control and surveillance for complications. Patients can ask questions in a private setting and bring up other medical concerns that require separate, individual visit(s). Prescriptions and referrals are completed as needed. Since the other members of the diabetes team are present at this time to ask/answer questions, this is the best time to gather additional medical information.

Coding for GMVs

A very common question regarding GMVs is how to code appropriately in order to be reimbursed for services rendered. Currently, the Centers for Medicare and Medicaid Services (CMS) have not created Procedural Terminology (CPT) codes specifically for GMVs. This does not mean that services rendered during the group visit cannot be coded and billed to CMS and third party payers. A survey of the literature regarding coding for GMV points to a similar theme, as coding of the GMV is done similarly as for individual visits. Table 11 contains a list of codes that may be considered for GMVs.

Table 11

CPT Codes for Group Medical Visits

Code	Comment
99213	Sometimes used, low complexity, low-to-moderate severity
99214	Most commonly used, moderate complexity, moderate-to-high severity
99078	Physician education in group (unclear on whether will be paid)
G0109	Group diabetes self management education; for ADA-recognized education programs
97804	Group Medical Nutrition Therapy; used by RD
96153	Group Health and Behavior Intervention; used by psychologist
99499	Unlisted E/M service

The question of increased productivity is often asked. Assume a typical GMV has 8-12 patients, and that it will require a minimum of 3 hours of the physicians' time to prepare, conduct and document the event. This approximates the number of patients with diabetes that can be seen individually during the same time period. Thus, GMVs are conducted more for patient and physician satisfaction and improved outcomes, rather than for increased productivity.

7. Consumer Trends

Consumer trends in accessing and purchasing healthcare have been undergoing a rapid evolution in the past few years. Major changes in how (and who) pays for health care have occurred, that are dramatically changing attitudes towards the price of health care vs. value. The value equation is:

$$\text{Value} = \frac{\text{(Clinical Outcomes + Patient Satisfaction)}}{\text{(Cost + Time)}}$$

The major shift being recognized by the consumer is that, as they increasingly bear the burden to pay for services, they are seeking the best outcome for the money spent. Patient satisfaction and time enter into the equation, because health care is being considered a service that should be readily obtained when needed. The section below describes consumer trends surrounding who is paying for health care, where health care is being delivered and what employers are doing to improve the health of their employees.

Who is Paying for Health Care?

10-20 years ago, employers and federal government were the primary funders of health care. Today, there is a dramatic rise in the number of uninsured/underinsured people, due to the shift in burden of paying from the employer to the employee. For example, from 1995-2005 there has been a 40% increase in out-of-pocket health care expenses. That percentage is even greater in those with chronic disease. Much of this increase is due to a shift of cost of health care from the employer to the employee, through the use of high deductible consumer-directed health plans (CDHPs) and health savings account (HSAs). CDHPs are often referred to as "catastrophic" plans, because a very serious injury, event or disease would need to occur in order to exceed the $10,000 (or higher) deductible required to be paid by the policy holder prior to the plan distributing funds. Even more traditional health care plans often contain hefty deductibles of $1000 or more, that must be paid by the policy holder before the plan pays. Increasing out-of-pocket expenses leads to a decrease in people accessing health care. This is especially serious for people with diabetes that should take part in regular, ongoing follow-up.

The natural reaction for someone paying for health care out-of pocket is to apply skills and knowledge in other areas, such as purchasing an automobile, to health care. The perceived value of health care becomes critical. Consumers seeking value compare prices for medical procures, medications and technologies against the quality or outcomes of the product or services. A prime example of this is Carol.com, a website designed to offer consumers the ability to compare and contrast the cost of medical services offered by numerous health care organizations in Minnesota. The range of services cover acute conditions and chronic disease. Patient satisfaction is listed, so patients can learn from others what experience they can expect. The intent is that consumers will take more interest and responsibility in their care, and that health care providers will then develop offerings to better meet consumers' needs at more competitive prices.

Where is Health Care Being Delivered?

1 unmistakable trend in health care is the desire of consumers to access health care where and when they find it convenient. The health care industry has responded by opening small clinics in major retailers and pharmacies throughout the United States. Feeding the need for quick and affordable health care, these small clinics are creating competition with more traditional clinics, group practices and integrated health care systems. Originally designed for more minor acute medical needs, they are expanding into management of chronic diseases, like diabetes.

Consumers are increasingly going online to access information on health care and care itself. For example, the Hawaii Medical Service Association (HMSA) offers 24/7 online physician appointments for anyone living in Hawaii. Cost is $10 and $45 for members and nonmembers, respectively. This overcomes many barriers to accessing care, including constraints of time, distance and cost. For patients with diabetes, this will comple-

ment routine office visits, by communicating glucose data to a physician for suggested adjustment in diabetes regimen.

What are Employers Doing to Improve Employee Health?

Employers are increasingly taking a more active role in health care, by encouraging their employees to participate in wellness and employee assistance programs (EAPs) to reduce cost while increasing productivity. A survey of companies offering wellness and health coaching to employers revealed that for every $1 spent on the wellness program, the employer saves $3-6 in reduced absenteeism and presenteeism (coming to work, but not able to function at full potential due to chronic conditions, such as diabetes, depression, back pain, etc.).

8. References

Models of Care

Bergenstal R. Treatment models from the International Diabetes Center: advancing from oral agents to insulin therapy in type 2 diabetes. *Endocrine Practice*. 2006;12(1):96-104.

Bodenheimer T, Wang MC, Rundall TG, et al. What are the facilitators and barriers in physician organizations' use of care management processes? *Jt Comm J Qual Saf*. 2004;30(9):505-514.

Coleman K, Austin B, Brach C, Wagner EH. Evidence on the Chronic Care model in the new millennium. *Health Aff*. 2009;28(1):75-85.

Etzwiler D. Diabetes translation: a blueprint for the future. *Diabetes Care*. 1994;17:1-4.

Institute of Medicine. *Crossing the Quality Chasm: A New Health System for the 21st Century*. Washington, DC: National Academy Press; 2001.

Mazze RS, Strock E, Simonson GD, Bergenstal R. *Staged Diabetes Management-A Systematic Approach*. 2nd ed. Minneapolis, MN: Wiley Publishing; 2004.

Mazze RS, Powers MA, Wetzler HP, Ofstead CL. Partners in advancing care and education solutions study: impact on processes and outcomes of diabetes care. *Population Health Management*. 2008;11:297-305.

Medical Marketing Lists, Medical Market. Available at www.mmslists.com. Accessed May 8, 2009.

Minkman M, Ahaus K, Huijsman R. Performance improvement based on integrated quality management models: what evidence do we have? A systematic literature review. *Int J Qual Health Care*. 2007;19:90-104.

NIDDK. National Diabetes Statistics: 2007 fact sheet. Bethesda, MD: U.S. Department of Health and Human Services, National Institutes of Health; 2008.

Rickheim P, Weaver T, Flader J, Kendall DM. Assessment of group versus individual diabetes education. *Diabetes Care*. 2002;25:269-274.

The Plan-Do-Study-Act (PDSA) cycle was originally developed by Walter A. Shewhart as the Plan-Do-Check-Act (PDCA) cycle. W. Edwards Deming modified Shewhart's cycle to PDSA, replacing "Check" with "Study."

Wagner EH, Austin BT, Davis C, Hindmarsh M, Schaefer J, Bonomi A. Improving chronic illness care: translating evidence into action. *Health Aff (Millwood)*. 2001;20:64-78.

National Organization Websites

www.diabetes.org

www.forcesforquality.org

www.rwjf.org/qualityequality/af4q/about.jsp

www.ncqa.org

www.acponline.org

www.aafp.org

www.pcpcc.net

www.aace.com

www.amga.org

Transparency of Data

Aron D, Pogach L. Transparency Standards for Diabetes Performance Measures. *JAMA*. 2009;301(2):210-212.

HEDIS. 2009 Technical Update Comprehensive Diabetes Care. Volume 2. October 1, 2008.

NIDDK. National Diabetes Statistics: 2007 fact sheet. Bethesda, MD: U.S. Department of Health and Human Services, National Institutes of Health; 2008.

National Quality Forum Compendium, 2000-2005. Available at www.qualityforum.org. Accessed on May 8, 2009.

National Health Care Quality Report. AHRQ Publication No. 08-0040. Available at www.AHRQ.gov. Accessed on May 8, 2009.

President Bush's Executive Order. August 22, 2006. Available at http://www.hhs.gov/valuedriven/fourcornerstones. Accessed May 8, 2009.

Saaddine J, Engelgau M, Beckles G, Gregg E, Thompson T, Venkat Narayan KM. A diabetes report card for the United States: summary of care in the 1990's. *Ann Int Med*. 2002:136(8):565.

2006 Tax Relief and Health Care Act (TRHCA) (P.L. 109-432). See 2008 PFS Final Rule. November 27, 2007, 72 Fed. Reg. 66222, at 66336-66359.

National Business Coalition on Health. Available at www.nbch.org. Accessed May 8, 2009.

American Health Association on Quality. Available at www.ahqa.org. Accessed May 8, 2009.

Aligning Forces for Quality. Available at www.af4q.org. Accessed May 8, 2009.

Hospital Quality Alliance Available at www.hqa.org. Accessed May 8, 2009.

Hospital Compare. Available at www.HospitalCompare.hhs.gov. Accessed May 8, 2009.

Institute for Clinical Systems Integration/About ICSI/ICSI History. Available at www.icsi.org. Accessed May 8, 2009.

National Committee for Quality Assurance. Available at: www.ncqa.org. Accessed May 8, 2009.

Pay-for-Performance (P4P)

AMA. Guidelines for Pay-for Performance Programs. June 21, 2005.

Berthiaume JT, Tyler PA, Ng-Osoria J, LaBresh KA. Aligning financial incentives with "Get With the Guidelines" to improve cardiovascular care. *Am J Manag Care*. 2004;10:501-504.

Berthiaume JT, Chung RS, Ryskina KL, et al. Aligning financial incentives with quality care in the hospital setting. *J Healthc Qual*. 2006;28:36-44.

Coleman K, Reiter KL, Fulwiler D. The Impact of Pay-for-Performance on Diabetes Care in a Large Network of Community Health Centers. *J Health Care Poor Underserved*. 2007;18:966-983.

Committee on Quality of Health Care in America, Institute of Medicine. Crossing the quality chasm: a new health system for the 21st century. 2001.

Cutler TW, Palmieri J, Khalsa M, Stebbins M. Evaluation of the relationship between a chronic disease care management program and California pay-for-performance diabetes care cholesterol measures in one medical group. *J Manag Care Pharm* 2007;13:578-588.

Damberg CL, Sorbero ME, Mehrotra A, et al. An environmental scan of pay for performance in the hospital setting: final report. US DHHS Assistant Secretary for Planning and Evaluation Report. November 2007.

Endsley S, Baker G, Kershner BA, Curtin K. What family physicians need to know about pay for performance. *Fam Pract Manag*. 2006;13(7):69-74.

Glickman SW, Ou FS, DeLong ER, et al. Pay for performance: quality of care and outcomes in acute myocardial infarction. *JAMA*. 2007;297:2373-2380.

Lindenauer PK, Remus D, Roman S, et al. Public reporting and pay for performance in hospital quality improvement. *N Engl J Med* 2007;356:486-496.

Mehrotra A, Damberg C, Sorbero MES, Teleki SS. Pay for performance in the hospital setting: what is the state of the evidence? *Am J Med Qual.* 2009;24:19-28.

Millenson ML. Pay for performance: the best worst choice. *Qual Saf Health Care.* 2004;13:323-324.

Nahra TA, Reiter KL, Hirth RA, et al. Cost-effectiveness of hospital pay-for-performance incentives. *Med Care Res Rev.* 2006;63(suppl):49S-72S.

Premier Hospital Quality Incentive Demonstration Rewarding Superior Quality Care Fact Sheet. June 2008. Available at www.cms.hhs.gov/HospitalQualityInits/. Accessed May 8, 2009.

Reiter KL, Nahra TA, Alexander JA, Wheeler JR. Hospital responses to pay-for-performance incentives. *Health Serv Manage Res.* 2006;19:123-134.

Rosentahl MB, Frank RG, Zhonghe L, Epstein AM. Early experience with pay-for-performance: from concept to practice. *JAMA* 2005;294:1788-1793.

Rosentahl MB, Landon BE, Normand SL, et al. Pay for performance in commercial HMOs. *N Engl J Med.* 2006;355:1895-1902.

Rosenthal MB, de Brantes FS, Sinaiko AD, et al. Bridges to excellence recognizing high quality care: analysis of physician quality and resource use. *Am J Mang Care.* 2008;14:670-677.

Sautter KM, Bokhour BG, White B, et al. The early experience of a hospital-based pay-for-performance program. *J Healthc Manag.* 2007;52:95-108.

Patient-centered Medical Home

AAFP, AAP, ACP, AOA. Joint principles of the patient-centered medical home. February 2007. Available at www.pcpcc.net. Accessed May 8, 2009.

Cooley WC, Center for Medical Home Improvement. The medical home: building a new brand name for quality care. April 25, 2008. Park Nicollet Learning Day

Medical home demonstration per patient per month payment rates, overall and by patient HCC score. Available at www.cms.hhs.gov. Accessed on May 8, 2009.

Zerehi M. How is a shortage of primary care physicians affecting the quality and cost of medical care?: a comprehensive evidence review. American College of Physicians. White Paper. 2008.

Meyers DS, Clancy CM.. Primary care: too important to fail. *Ann Intern Med.* 2009;150(4):272.

Future of Family Medicine Project. Available at www.aafp.org. Accessed on May 8, 2009.

Spann SJ. Report on financing the New Model of family medicine. Ann Fam Med. 2004;2:S1-S21.

The Future of Family Medicine. Available at www.transformed.com/ffm.cfm. Accessed on May 8, 2009.

National Demonstration Project. Available at www.transformed.com/ndp.cfm. Accessed on May 8, 2009.

Davis K. The Commonwealth fund, Invited Testimony Hearing on "Crossing the Quality Chasm in Health Care Reform" to the Senate Committee on Health, Education, Labor, and Pensions. January 29, 2009.

CMS Medical Home Demonstration. Fact Sheet. January 9, 2009. Available at www.cms.hhs.gov. Accessed on May 8, 2009.

National Committee for Quality Assurance. Available at www.ncqa.org. Accessed on May 8, 2009.

Group Visits

Beck A, Scott J, Williams P, et al. A randomized trail of group outpatient visits for chronically ill older HMO members: the Cooperative Health Care Clinic. *J Am Geriatr Soc*. 1997;45:543-549.

Jaber R, Braksmajer A, Trilling JS. Group visits: a qualitative review of current research. *J Am Board Fam Med*. 2006;19:276-290.

Noffsinger E, Sawyer DR, Scott JC. Group medical visits: a glimpse into the future? (enhancing your practice). *Patient Care*. 2003;37:18-27.

Consumer Trends

Halverson D, Glowac W. Healthcare tsunami: the wave of consumerism that will change U.S. business. Madison, WI. Wave Strategy, LLC; 2008.

9. APPENDIX 1: National Organizations

Note: The appendix is not meant to be all inclusive.

AAFP American Academy of Family Practice
www.aafp.org

• One of the largest national medical organizations

• >94,000 family physicians, family medicine residents and medical students nationwide

• Founded - 1947

• Mission has been to preserve and promote the science and art of family medicine and to ensure high-quality, cost-effective health care for patients of all ages

• Entrenched in patient-pentered medical home

ACP American College of Physicians
www.acponline.org

• Largest medical specialty organization

• >125,000 physicians - internists, internal medicine subspecialists, medical students, residents and fellows

• Founded - 1915

• Mission is to enhance the quality and effectiveness of health care by fostering excellence and professionalism in the practice of medicine

• Entrenched in patient-centered medical home

ADA American Diabetes Association
www.diabetes.org

• Nation's leading nonprofit health organization providing diabetes research, information and advocacy

• Founded - 1940

• Conducts programs in all 50 states and the District of Columbia

ADA American Dietetic Association
www.eatright.org

- Nation's largest organization of food and nutrition professionals

- Founded - 1917

- > 68,000 members

- Mission: *Empower members to be the nation's food and nutrition leaders*

AMA American Medical Association
www.ama-assn.org

- Nation's largest physician group

- Founded - 1847

- Advocates on issues vital to the nations health

- Mission is to promote the art and science of medicine and the betterment of public health

AF4Q Aligning Forces for Quality
www.forcesforquality.org

- National program of the Robert Wood Johnson Foundation (RWJF)

- Designed to help communities across the country improve the quality of health care for patients with chronic conditions such as diabetes, asthma, depression and heart disease

AHRQ Agency for Healthcare Research and Quality
www.ahrq.gov

- 1 of 12 agencies within the Department of Health and Human Services (DHHS)

- Committed to helping the nation improve our health care system

- Mission is to improve the quality, safety, efficiency and effectiveness of health care for all Americans

CHI Center for Health Improvement
www.centerforhealthimprovement.org

- An independent, nonprofit, prevention-focused health policy center

- Dedicated to improving population health and encouraging healthy behaviors

- Provides technical assistance for the RWJF AF4Q in 14 community collaboratives

CMS Centers for Medicaid and Medicare Services
www.cms.hhs.gov

- Comprehensive website

- Information on CMS programs (Medicare, Medicaid, SCHIP) as well as information (regulations and guidance, research, statistics, data and systems, outreach and education, resources and tools)

HEDIS Health Plan Employer and Data Information Set
www.ncqa.org

- Initiated in 1989 by a small group of HMO, corporate and benefits executives dedicated to find a way to compare health plans objectively

- Today, 90% of America's health plans use the tool to measure performance on important dimensions of care and service

- Consists of 71 measures across 8 domains of care

- HEDIS makes it possible to compare the performance of health plans on an "apples-to-apples" basis

ICSI Institute for Clinical Systems Improvement www.icsi.org

- An independent, non-profit organization

- Facilitates collaboration on health care quality improvement by medical groups, hospitals and health plans

- Operates in the state of Minnesota and in adjacent areas of surrounding states

IHI Institute for Healthcare Improvement

- Independent not-for-profit organization

- Helping to lead the improvement of health care throughout the world

- Founded – 1991

- Programs by topic: leadership, patient safety, hospital operations, outpatient care, improvement methods

- Works to accelerate improvement by building the will for change, cultivating promising concepts for improving patient care and helping health care systems put those ideas into action.

TJC The Joint Commission
www.jointcommission.org

- An independent, not-for-profit organization

- Accredits and certifies more than 15,000 health care organizations and programs in the United States.

- Accreditation and certification is recognized nationwide as a symbol of quality that reflects an organization's commitment to meeting certain performance standards

Leapfrog
www.leapfroggroup.org

- Founded - 1998

- A group of large employers working together to use the way they purchased health care to have an influence on its quality and affordability. They recognized that there was a dysfunction in the health care market place with no way of assessing its quality or comparing health care providers

- A 1999 report by the Institute of Medicine gave the Leapfrog founders an initial focus – reducing preventable medical mistakes. The report found that up to 98,000 Americans die every year from preventable medical errors made in hospitals alone. In fact, there are more deaths in hospitals each year from preventable medical mistakes than there are from vehicle accidents, breast cancer and AIDS. The report actually recommended that large employers provide more market reinforcement for the quality and safety of health care. The founders realized that they could take 'leaps' forward with their employees, retirees and families by rewarding hospitals that implement significant improvements in quality and safety. Funding to set up Leapfrog came from the Business Roundtable (BRT) and The Leapfrog Group was officially launched in November 2000. Leapfrog is supported by the BRT, The Robert Wood Johnson Foundation, Leapfrog members and others

NBCH National Business Coalition on Health
www.nbch.org

- Non-profit, membership organization

- Represents 60 business and health coalitions, over 7000 employers and 25 million employees and their dependents across the United States

- Dedicated to value-based purchasing of health care services through the collective action of public and private purchasers

- eValue8™ is the nation's leading evidence-based request for information (RFI) tool, used by coalitions and major employers to assess and manage the quality of their health care vendors

NQF National Quality Forum

- The NQF is a not-for-profit membership organization created to develop and implement a national strategy for health care quality measurement and reporting. A shared sense of urgency about the impact of health care quality on patient outcomes, workforce productivity, and health care costs prompted leaders in the public and private sectors to create the NQF as a mechanism to bring about national change

• Established as a public-private partnership, the NQF has broad participation from all parts of the health care system, including national, state, regional and local groups representing consumers, public and private purchasers, employers, health care professionals, provider organizations, health plans, accrediting bodies, labor unions, supporting industries and organizations involved in health care research or quality improvement. Together, the organizational members of the NQF will work to promote a common approach to measuring health care quality and fostering system-wide capacity for quality improvement

CMS PGP Centers for Medicare and Medicaid Services Physician Group Practice

• Currently, Medicare reimburses physicians and other health care providers on the number and complexity of the services provided to patients. There is good evidence that by anticipating patient needs, especially for patients with chronic diseases, health care teams that partner with patients can intervene before expensive procedures and hospitalizations are required. The Physician Group Practice demonstration is designed to encourage this and other preventive efforts

Patient Centered Primary Care Collaborative
www.pcpcc.net

• Founded - 2007

• Members: major employers, consumer groups, patient quality organizations, health plans, labor unions, hospitals, physicians and others; >400 members

• Members agree it is essential to support a better model of compensating physicians

• Purpose: develop and advance the patient-centered medical home

• Several pilots are being developed in both public and private sectors

RWJF Robert Wood Johnson Foundation
www.rwjf.org

• Founded - 1936

• Mission is to improve the health and health care of all Americans

• Goal: to help society transform itself for the better

10. APPENDIX 2: Websites that Provide Information on Data Transparency and Public Reporting

- American Health Association on Quality www.ahqa.org

- AHRQ at http://www.innovations.ahrq.gov/qualitytools

- Aligning Forces for Quality www. af4q.org.

- California Office of the Patient Advocate www.opa.ca.gov

- Health & Human Services Hospital Compare www.hospitalcompare.hhs.gov

- Health Partners Quality Measurement www.healthpartners.com/portal/143.html

- Health Scope (CA Health Care Quality Ratings) www.healthscope.org

- Hospital Compare www.HospitalCompare.hhs.gov

- Hospital Quality Alliance www.hqa.org

- Institute for Clinical Systems Integrations www.icsi.org

- JCAHO Quality Check www.qualitycheck.org

- Leapfrog Group www.leapfroggroup.org/cp

- Massachusetts Health Quality Partners www.mhqp.org

- Minnesota Community Measurement www.mnhealthcare.org

- National Committee for Quality Assurance www.ncqa.org

- National Association of Health Data Organizations www.nahdo.org

- National Business Coalition on Health www.nbch.org

- NY Health Accountability Foundation www.nyshaf.org/index/hmo_report_card

- OR Assn of Hospitals & Health Systems Price Point www.orpricepoint.org

- The Dartmouth Atlas of Health Care www.dartmouthatlas.org

- A National Dialogue on Health Information Technology and Privacy http://www.thenationaldialogue.org

Chapter 15: Diabetes Technology: Insulin Pumps and the Artificial Pancreas

Judy L. Shih, MD PhD
Howard Wolpert, MD

Contents

1. Insulin Replacement Therapy

2. Continuous Subcutaneous Insulin Infusion Pumps

3. Artificial Pancreas

4. References

CHAPTER 15: DIABETES TECHNOLOGY: INSULIN PUMPS AND THE ARTIFICIAL PANCREAS **383**

Overview

Patients with type 1 diabetes are insulin-deficient, due to autoimmune destruction of the insulin-producing beta cells and, thus, must be treated with insulin replacement therapy. In contrast, type 2 diabetes is characterized by hyperglycemia, insulin resistance and relative impairment of insulin secretion, as a consequence of progressive loss of beta cell function. Over time, insulin replacement therapy may also be necessary in patients with type 2 diabetes, in order to maintain glucose levels in the target ranges.

The Diabetes Control and Complications Trial (DCCT) demonstrated that improved glycemic control with intensive therapy compared to conventional therapy effectively delays the onset and slows the progression of diabetic retinopathy, nephropathy and neuropat-hy in patients with type 1 diabetes.[1] In the DCCT, the *intensive therapy* cohort received a regimen consisting of multiple daily injections (MDI) of long-acting and rapid-acting insulin, or continuous subcutaneous infusion of rapid-acting insulin via an insulin pump to mimic normal physiologic insulin secretory patterns. Based on the findings of the DCCT, *intensive therapy* is now considered the standard of therapy for management of type 1 diabetes.

The clinician must have an understanding of normal physiologic insulin secretion, in order to develop a rational insulin replacement regimen customized to the individual patient, and to better understand the utility of newer technologies in diabetes. Normal physiologic insulin secretion consists of 2 components: 1.) basal insulin, which controls blood glucose levels in between meals and during periods of fasting by regulating hepatic glucose production; and 2.) meal time (bolus) insulin (Figure 1).

Basal insulin requirements are not constant, and vary throughout the day and overnight. In adolescents and adults, basal insulin requirements tend to decline during the early nocturnal period, from approximately 11PM to 2AM, and then increase, from approximately 3AM to 7AM. This latter increase in insulin requirements is known as the *dawn* phenomenon and is related to nocturnal growth hormone spikes.

Meal-related endogenous insulin secretion into the portal circulation is extremely rapid and consists of an initial secretory burst, known as the "first phase" insulin secretion, and is followed by a more prolonged "second phase" of insulin secretion, which is sustained until euglycemia is restored. These complex secretory dynamics keep peak postprandial glucose levels usually below 140 mg/dL, and return glucose levels to the preprandial range within 90-120 minutes.

Basal/Bolus Insulin Replacement Regimens

A basal/bolus insulin replacement regimen is the optimal approach in the treatment of type 1 diabetes, and is designed to mimic normal physiologic patterns to the greatest degree possible (Figure 1). These regimens consist of a long-acting insulin injection (glargine or detemir), which represents the basal insulin requirement for a patient, and multiple rapid-acting insulin injections (aspart, lispro or glulisine) given at meal times to cover postprandial glycemic excursions (Figure 2). During the early phases of type 2 diabetes, when there is still residual beta cell function, a relatively simple insulin replacement program, consisting of either long-acting or fixed-dose premixed insulins

Figure 1

Normal physiologic insulin levels: basal-and meal-stimulated insulin secretion

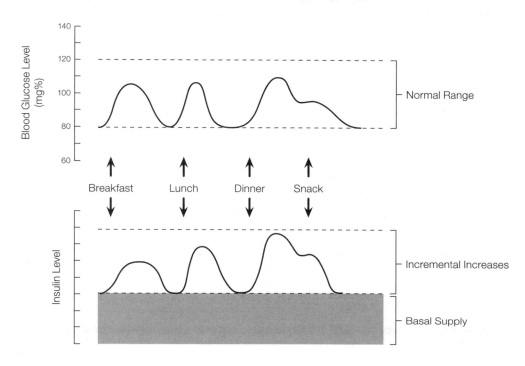

Figure 2

Schematic showing twice-daily injection of short-acting (regular) and intermediate NPH insulin

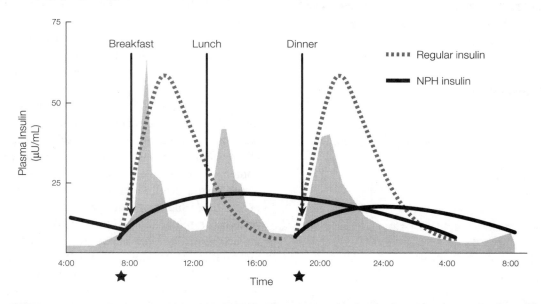

Figure 3

Schematic showing basal insulin (glargine or detemir) and mealtime rapid-acting insulin, such as aspart, lispro or glulisine

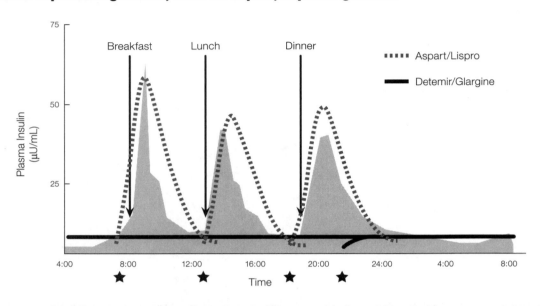

Table 1

Practical Means of Providing Basal Insulin in a Physiologic Insulin

Replacement Program

Insulin glargine given daily
(at bedtime or before breakfast, or twice daily)

Insulin detemir given twice daily
(at breakfast and supper or bedtime)

NPH given before breakfast, before supper, and at bedtime

NPH given in small doses before each meal, and a larger dose of NPH at bedtime

(such as 75/25 or 70/30), will provide satisfactory control of glucose levels (Figure 3). However, as insulin deficiency progresses with type 2 diabetes, a multi-component, basal/bolus-like insulin replacement regimen, similar to that required of patients with type 1 diabetes, will become necessary.

Although basal/bolus insulin injection regimens more closely mimic normal physiology, some patients may find that added daytime (particularly lunch time) injections may not be practical or convenient. Thus, an alternative regimen that utilizes a split/mixed-insulin approach might be more appropriate. Such a regimen would consist of pre-breakfast rapid-acting insulin and NPH (intermediate-acting insulin), pre-supper rapid-acting insulin and bedtime NPH. However, this type of program has several limitations: if lunch and snacks are not eaten at consistent times during the day, there is a risk for hypoglycemia from the morning NPH.